KT-430-443

Total Health

Total Health

The essential family guide to conventional and complementary medicine

**Diana Austin Hilary Bower Jackie Creswell Tor Davies
Tessa Thomas Juliet Walker Belinda Whitworth
Consultant editor Dr David Peters MB ChB DRCOG MFHom MRO**

MARSHALL PUBLISHING • LONDON

A MARSHALL EDITION
CONCEIVED, EDITED AND DESIGNED BY
MARSHALL EDITIONS LTD
THE ORANGERY
161 NEW BOND STREET
LONDON W1Y 9PA

First published in the UK in 1998 by Marshall Publishing Ltd

Copyright © 1998 Marshall Editions Developments Ltd

All rights reserved including the right of reproduction in whole or in part in any form.

Hardback ISBN 1-84028-177-4
Paperback ISBN 1-84028-090-5

PROJECT EDITOR THERESA LANE
PROJECT ART EDITOR HELEN SPENCER
EDITORS ANNA FISCHEL, ANNE JOHNSON
DESIGNERS PHIL GAMBLE, SARA MATHEWS
EDITORIAL ASSISTANT JAMES RANKIN
DESIGN ASSISTANT PHILLIP LETSU
INDEXER CAROLINE SHEARD
MANAGING EDITORS CLAIRE CURRIE, ANNE YELLAND
EDITORIAL DIRECTOR SOPHIE COLLINS
ART DIRECTOR SEAN KEOGH
PICTURE EDITOR ZILDA TANDY
DTP EDITOR LESLEY GILBERT
EDITORIAL COORDINATOR BECCA CLUNES
PRODUCTION NIKKI INGRAM

Originated in Singapore by HBM Print
Printed and bound in Portugal by Printer Portuguesa

Note: Every effort has been taken to ensure that all information
in this book is correct and compatible with national standards
generally accepted at the time of publication. This book is
not intended to replace consultation with your doctor,
complementary therapy practitioner or other healthcare
professional or to replace professional first aid training. The
authors and publisher disclaim any liability for loss, injury
or damage incurred as a consequence, directly or indirectly, of
the use and application of the contents of this book.

Note: The terms "he" and "she", used in alternate articles,
refer to people of both sexes, unless a topic or sequence of
photographs applies only to a male or female.

Foreword

Advances in scientific research and technology mean that doctors know more about disease than ever before. New medicines are constantly being developed, life-support and intensive care improve all the time and patients can recover more quickly after modern microsurgery. However, doctors still do not have all the answers, and many disorders cannot be cured. The best way to prevent such illnesses is through a healthy lifestyle.

Taking care of both mind and body is essential for overall wellbeing. It is an approach that has long been recommended by complementary practitioners. Increasingly, doctors recognize the importance of promoting good health, and many of them find complementary therapies valuable, too. In fact, many of their patients use both approaches simultaneously.

Diet plays an important part in maintaining good health. A well-balanced diet contributes essential vitamins, minerals and other nutrients that help the body to function properly and fight off diseases. By maintaining a good diet, taking regular exercise and learning how to relax – without tobacco or excessive alcohol – you will be well on your way to improving your health.

Contents

INTRODUCTION

Chapter 1
COMMON HEALTH PROBLEMS

Chapter 2
COMPLEMENTARY THERAPIES

Chapter 3
HEALTHY EATING

Chapter 4
ESSENTIAL FIRST AID

SEE ALSO
Stress   76–77

How healthy are you?

Being healthy is not just a matter of not being ill. It is about actively getting the most out of your life. To do this your body has to work efficiently, with plenty of energy. You should also be prepared to cope with life's ups and downs, which requires effective techniques, loving relationships, enough time to work and play and a positive outlook.

Your health is determined partly by genetic inheritance – the body you were born with – and partly by external factors. But even a sound and healthy constitution can be harmed through neglect or abuse. Although there is much still to be discovered, research has been able to identify certain factors that speed up the decline of vital organs, including smoking and the overuse of alcohol. There are others that definitely slow down the aging process – for example, regular exercise and a healthy weight.

So how can you tell how healthy you are now? There are various tests that signal if your body is functioning well. Your doctor can measure your blood pressure, blood sugar or cholesterol level; at home, you can check your pulse rate (see box, facing page) and calculate your body mass index (see p.258). Complementary therapists say they can detect signs of physical malfunction in the irises of your eyes or on your tongue.

CHECK YOUR LIFESTYLE

The more you can answer yes to the questions below, the healthier you are. If you have a no answer, you should try to correct the situation.

- Do you eat mainly fresh unprocessed food (pp.262–69)?
- Is your weight right for your height (p.258)?
- Are you a nonsmoker or have you given up (pp.20–21)?
- Are you a moderate drinker (pp.20–21 and p.255)?
- Can you put your worries aside and relax (pp.14–15)?
- Do you spend time with friends and relatives?
- Can you climb three flights of stairs without gasping and becoming breathless?
- Do you go for a walk, play with children, work in the garden, dance, visit a gym, vacuum the house or do other energetic activities at least twice a day, five days a week (pp.10–11)?
- Do you fall asleep quickly at night and sleep well (pp.16–17 and pp.80–81)?
- Do you wake up most mornings feeling lively and looking forward to the day?

PHYSICAL HEALTH

Having a body that functions effectively denotes good physical health. This means having a heart and lungs that pump efficiently, vital organs that work without strain, a healthy immune system and supple muscles and strong bones. One way to achieve this is with exercise. Although most of us will never be super athletes, we do wish to be able to do what we want without struggle and strain, whether it is playing football with the children, carrying the washing, running for the bus, or staying the pace at a disco.

It is never too late to start exercising. For example, researchers in Great Britain have found that people between 75 and

93 years of age who exercised gently for 12 weeks increased the strength of their thigh muscles by about 25 percent. This is a rejuvenation of strength of 16–20 years.

You can contribute to your physical health by following preventive methods for looking after your body. These include taking advantage of medical checks such as cervical screening or blood pressure tests, regularly having your eyes tested and seeing a dentist, protecting your skin from sunburn and practising safe sex (see p.169). Following ergonomic procedures at work, such as sitting with the correct posture at a computer, and operating machinery safely, including wearing a seat belt in your car, are also important.

If you do have an illness, it is still important for you to take care of yourself. Proper attention to a temporary illness such as a cold can help you recover more quickly. Chronic conditions such as diabetes or heart disease require following your doctor's instructions diligently to alleviate symptoms and complications.

MENTAL HEALTH

There is a common belief that happy, positive people are healthier. Numerous research studies have established clear links between a positive state of mind and good physical health. There are many other studies that suggest deliberately cultivating a positive state of mind can help fight off ill health.

Much of this has to do with stress, the word now used to denote all kinds of pressures. But stress itself is not the ultimate culprit – it is how you cope with it that matters. A certain amount of creative tension is a stimulus that can motivate and empower a person. However, too much pressure can create constant anger or worry, which, in turn, can lower your resistance to illness.

CHECK YOUR PULSE

Your "resting" pulse gives an idea of how efficiently your heart is working. Find your pulse in either your wrist or neck when you first wake up and count the beats for 15 seconds. Multiply this figure by four to get a heart rate per minute and see how you fare on this chart.

Age	20–29	30–39	40–49	50+
Men				
Excellent	< 60	< 64	< 66	< 68
Good	60–69	64–71	66–73	68–75
Fair	70–85	72–87	74–89	76–91
Poor	> 85	> 87	> 89	> 91
Women				
Excellent	< 70	< 72	< 74	< 76
Good	70–77	72–79	74–81	76–83
Fair	78–94	80–96	82–98	84–100
Poor	> 94	> 96	> 98	> 100

You should see your doctor if your rating is poor. How soon your pulse returns to normal after exercise is another indicator of how fit your heart is. Ideally, it should return to normal after 4 to 5 minutes.
< = less than > = more than

WAYS TO KEEP HEALTHY

If you know that you have an unhealthy lifestyle, try to set yourself realistic targets, tackling one area of weakness at a time, with a determination to improve.

■ Eat a more balanced diet, choosing appetizing and varied foods, and try to maintain a healthy and stable weight.
■ Keep your alcohol intake within government-prescribed safe limits.
■ If you smoke, look at ways to stop.
■ Take more exercise – any increase is beneficial.
■ Visit the doctor if you have a persistent health problem (see pp.24–25).
■ Consider how you might cultivate better ways to cope with stress. ■

SEE ALSO
Eating for high energy
256–257

An active life

Regular exercise has a vital part to play in the quality of your life. It keeps muscles and bones in good health, improves the efficiency of the heart and lungs, flushes the vital organs with nutrients and enhances flexibility and strength. It also tunes up the immune system and sparks off brain chemicals that produce feelings of wellbeing.

It used to be thought that exercise must be vigorous to achieve any meaningful benefits, but recent research shows that even as little as 15 minutes of moderate physical activity twice a day, five times a week can actively improve your health. Studies also show that people who take less than 30 minutes of physical activity a week have almost double the danger of dying prematurely from coronary heart disease and greatly increased risks of many other illnesses, ranging from diabetes to colon cancer.

PHYSICAL AND MENTAL BOOSTS

Leading an active life has an impact on all the systems of the body. During exercise the heart beats faster and stronger, speeding up the flow of blood throughout the body. This increases the supply of nutrients and removes waste products more rapidly, preventing the build up of fatty deposits that set the scene for heart disease and stroke. Over time, the heart muscle becomes stronger, which improves its efficiency and allows it to work harder with less effort. At the same time, blood pressure decreases.

The lungs and respiratory system also become more effective, bringing in more oxygen with less work. Muscles throughout the body become larger and consume more energy; in turn, fat stored in the body is broken down and metabolized, helping to reduce excess fat. These benefits help increase energy levels and stamina. Bone density also increases, which reduces the risk of osteoporosis.

Exercise benefits both your ability to concentrate and your mental health. It increases your alertness, reduces tension

Joining a gym gives you the advantage of using a variety of equipment under professional supervision, and enlisting with a friend can be an incentive for keeping up with regular visits. However, walking faster and farther than usual, playing outdoor games with children or going for an enjoyable swim are also excellent ways to exercise – without having to make radical or time-consuming changes.

and triggers brain chemicals known as endorphins, which contribute to feelings of wellbeing.

TYPES OF EXERCISE

There are all sorts of ways to achieve moderate activity. The aim should be to incorporate into your routine some aerobic exercises, muscle toning exercises and exercises to improve flexibility.

Aerobic exercise increases the efficiency of your lungs and heart. It enables your heart to pump blood around the body efficiently and without strain and helps your body use oxygen more effectively. Good activities are brisk walking, jogging, swimming, dancing, cycling and squash. Any exercise that you can do for at least 12 minutes without a break and that makes you breathe heavily is good.

Improving the condition of your muscles helps protect them and the surrounding bones against injury and makes everyday tasks easier. Swimming, running, or weight-training are good activities, but household tasks such as vacuuming, window cleaning, vigorously cleaning the car and lifting shopping and children count, too.

Stiff, unused muscles and ligaments are easily injured. Regular gentle exercise increases the blood flow and helps joints and muscles stay supple and mobile. Because most types of exercise include elements of stretching, you should always warm up with gentle stretching before you begin your routine, thus avoiding muscle injuries.

MAKING A START

There are many everyday opportunities to improve your level of fitness. Make it a rule to use stairs rather than lifts, walk up escalators, walk or cycle on short trips instead of taking the car, attack housework with vigour and play energetic games with your children.

Set realistic goals if you want to make your life more active. Your body needs time to limber up and, if you set too hard a pace, you may become discouraged or even hurt yourself. If you are a little out of shape, start slowly, gradually building up the time and effort you put in as you gain strength and confidence. Set short-term targets – a commitment to walk every morning for two weeks, a certain time for a length of the swimming pool or 20 sit-ups without pain.

Remember, there is no such notion as being too old to start. Research shows that those who start regular moderate exercise in their 70s can add a year to their life expectancy; starting in your late 30s adds an average of two and a half years. ■

CAUTION

If you are out of shape or have a major health problem, always see your doctor before embarking on a new exercise routine.

EXERCISE TIPS

Regular exercise provides a number of health benefits, improves your physical appearance, boosts self-esteem, reduces stress and enhances your mood. Here are a few suggestions to help you get started:

- Make 30 minutes (or two 15-minute sessions) of moderate exercise five days a week your goal.

- Moderate exercise includes whatever raises your heartbeat, makes you feel warm and makes you breathe more heavily than usual. Examples are brisk walking, football, tennis, aerobics, cycling, table tennis, dancing, do-it-yourself activities, gardening, housework and playing with children.

- Start slowly and build up as you gain confidence. In a matter of weeks there will be a noticeable increase in your stamina.

- If you are older or have certain medical disorders such as heart disease see your doctor before starting a regime.

- Remember to do a few stretches before and after exercising.

- Join a gym or exercise class with friends, family, children or workmates for motivation and enjoyment.

CAUTION

You should seek professional help if you think that you have problems with hostility, anxiety or depression.

Your emotional life

There is nothing unhealthy about strong emotions. In some situations, anger, fear or sadness may be appropriate responses. But if one of these is colouring your whole life, it can undermine your wellbeing.

The body and mind have a mode for emergencies – the stress response. This response helps us cope with short-term dangers, but if it keeps going or is continually triggered without time for adequate relaxation between bursts of effort, health problems arise. Major life changes or daily hassles can undermine health, depending on your style of coping and your skills at managing stress.

One study found that the employees most likely to have a heart attack were those with the least control over their work. The most damaging part of their emotional strife was not the work but the feeling of not being in control.

An ability to cope with stress and other emotions will help you handle difficult situations such as the death of a close friend or relative, getting married or the breakup of your marriage, having a baby, changing house or jobs, financial or legal problems and retirement. Inappropriately strong emotions or lack of emotional expression may be a sign that you are not coping well. Try to seek advice or support.

EXPECTING THE IMPOSSIBLE

Many people set themselves up for a stressful life by unwittingly cultivating unrealistic expectations of both themselves and others. Most people harbour some

Relatively minor upheavals such as redecorating can be highly stressful. Plan ahead and talk problems through with your partner so that you both assert your own view. Communication and appropriate anticipation will go a long way toward making change exciting rather than tense.

myths that put them under strain, especially fear of being found wanting physically, intellectually or emotionally.

If you feel you must always win the approval of those around you, much of your time will be spent doing what others want, or what you think they want, which can create feelings of anxiety. Conversely, if you believe making mistakes or failing is unacceptable, you create unreasonable pressure for yourself and others. This can lead to intolerance, confrontation and anger. Another trait that can cause stress is to feel there must always be a perfect solution to any problem. Such thought patterns destine you to disappointment at least some of the time, particularly if other people are involved.

These unrealistic expectations may stem from the attitudes of parents and teachers, from your peers or from society. Regardless of how they develop, they put strain on your emotional life and stop you developing healthy methods of avoiding or dealing with difficult situations.

KNOW YOUR TEMPERAMENT

People who bottle up negative emotions and sorrow may be able to express themselves only in aggressive, hostile outbursts and mistrust. People blessed with an optimistic, tolerant, humorous attitude to life generally have higher self esteem and handle stress more easily.

It is not a simple matter to change patterns of behaviour. Psychotherapy can help to moderate habitual pessimism and depression and instil self respect and a positive outlook. Try to improve your relationships with others: listen to their opinions, learn to be tolerant and forgiving and avoid outbursts, which only lead to conflicts. Once aware of your own susceptibility to stress, it is much easier to do something about it (see box, right). ∎

ARE YOU STRESS PRONE?

Are your attitudes setting you up for an excess of stress? Answer the following questions, giving only one "yes" answer to each number. Look for the appropriate result below, based on the type of question (A, B or C) you responded yes to the most.

1 a. Are you competitive and aggressive in work and in sports and games?
   b. If you lose a few points in a game do you give up?
   c. Do you avoid confrontation?

2 a. Are you ambitious and anxious to achieve a lot?
   b. Do you wait for things to happen to you?
   c. Do you find excuses to put things off?

3 a Do you do things quickly and often become impatient?
   b. Do you rely on other people to spur you into action?
   c. Do you often rerun events of the day, worrying about them?

4 a. Do you talk fast, loudly and emphatically and interrupt a lot?
   b. Can you take no for an answer with equanimity?
   c. Do you find it difficult to express your feelings and anxieties to others?

5 a. Do you get bored easily?
   b. Do you like having nothing to do?
   c. Do you accommodate other people's wishes, not your own?

6 a. Do you walk, talk and eat quickly?
   b. If you forget to do something, do you not bother?
   c. Do you bottle things up?

Results

Mostly As
You live at a high-stress pace and might be prone to coronary heart disease and other stress-related illnesses. Slow down and take time to relax. Look at your philosophy of life and perhaps take up a noncompetitive hobby in your leisure time.

Mostly Bs
You have a relaxed attitude toward life. However, a certain amount of stress is healthy and a spur to positive achievement. If you want to achieve more, consider being less laid back.

Mostly Cs
You create stress by inaction. Start a campaign to build up your confidence, self esteem and assertiveness. Make a list of your good points and concentrate on them.

Learning how to relax

Relaxing should be one of the easiest acts, but by the time we are adults many of us need to learn – or rather relearn – how to achieve it. Children can switch off and become immersed in play, yet for adults in today's fast-paced life, finding time to unwind can seem like just another demand, another "must do" in a busy schedule.

Relaxation is an essential ingredient for maintaining an active life. It is not a luxury – you should not wait until you collapse because your body and mind cannot take any more. Stretch a rubber band repeatedly without a break and in time it will lose its suppleness and may even snap. The same goes for your mind and body. All work and no play makes a person increasingly ineffective in all areas of life. Tiredness saps performance, tasks take longer and mistakes are more likely.

Constant tension also affects the physical flow of the body, transmitting strain to muscles, causing aches and pains, disrupting digestion and raising blood pressure. Appetite can be affected with missed or rushed meals adding to the energy loss. Many people hyperventilate, taking shallow, rapid breaths into only the top section of their lungs. This not only increases feelings of tension but can cause a variety of other worrying symptoms.

All these effects can be countered with relaxation. There are innumerable ways to relax mind and body. Some are "quick fixes" that help you cope with immediate moments of stress, pressure or anger. The old remedy of counting to 10 and breathing deeply, right down into the abdomen, is based on solid science – it slows the heart rate, tempers the "flight or fight" reaction and gives the mind a few seconds to think. Taking a short break at intervals throughout the day – going for a brief walk, reading a chapter in a book or stretching for a few minutes – also helps to lower your pressure threshold.

TIME FOR YOURSELF

One key to keeping your exposure to stress in the beneficial zone is to ensure that you do not neglect your friends in favour of work or family commitments and that you have interests outside your daily routine. Allow yourself time every day to do what you enjoy – whether it is sewing, painting, reading or watching your favourite television programme – and make sure you regularly do things purely for fun. Meeting friends, a movie or meal out, a walk in the park or around

A PRESCRIPTION FOR RELAXATION

- Spend 10 to 15 minutes daily on a body-mind relaxation technique such as meditation.
- Take a 5- or 10-minute break outside at least once every day.
- Do something completely unconnected with your work life two or three times a week.
- Do not neglect your friends and family. Turn to them for support, and be there to return the favour.
- Relax in a candlelit bath before going to bed.
- Laugh as much as possible.

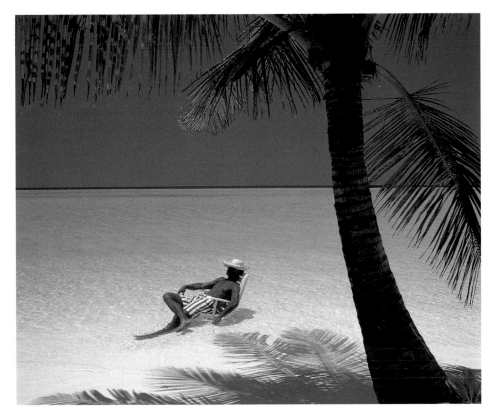

If you do not have the luxury of escaping to a peaceful desert island, you can learn a visualizing technique that takes you there in your imagination. With peace of mind restored and your body relaxed, you will be able to concentrate better and complete tasks with energy, efficiency and enthusiasm.

town are other antidotes to pressure, while talking over problems with those close to you can help you unwind and put challenges into perspective. Research suggests that a good laugh not only relieves pressure, but also has beneficial effects on your general health.

LONG-TERM MEASURES

Practising regular relaxation techniques can help build a calm, stable platform from which you can leap into life. Research has demonstrated that routine relaxation sessions – 10 to 15 minutes a day – can lower blood pressure, improve sleep, increase energy levels and enhance concentration and memory.

Which approach you follow depends on what you enjoy. Yoga and tai chi ch'uan are ancient disciplines that combine coordinated movement and postures with controlled breathing to reduce physical tension and clear the mind. Progressive muscle relaxation and visualization (see p.65), meditation and prayer focus on quietening the body and mind. Practices such as aromatherapy, massage, shiatsu massage and reflexology can foster an environment where tension ebbs away and the body's natural restorative process starts to work. Other studies suggest that stroking a pet, such as a cat or dog, listening to music or looking at beautiful objects can produce similar effects, even to the extent of reducing blood pressure.

Daily relaxation has great benefits, but it is also important to plan longer periods of relaxation. Take regular holidays – if possible, away from your home – even if you go away for only a day or weekend to the beach or the countryside, where you can properly unwind. You may be surprised at just how different life can look when you return. ∎

SEE ALSO
Sleeping disorders **80–81**

Your biological clock

In response to the natural world, our brains and bodies follow the cycles of light and dark by waking and sleeping. Sleep takes up about one-third of our lives and is the time when the body restores and repairs itself. The brain receives uninterrupted time to organize and store the constant stream of information it takes in every day.

Good sleep is an essential ingredient for promoting physical and mental health. Your sleeping pattern is regulated by the "biological clock". This natural timer is synchronized by the 24-hour, or circadian, cycle of light and dark, as well as by other daily clues. It ensures that the body's "housekeeping" functions, such as waking, sleeping, eating, waste disposal and repair, occur at regular, appropriate times. The biological clock triggers changes in hundreds of substances and processes, from hormones and brain chemicals to body temperature, heart and breathing rates and urine production.

Research suggests that this internal clock may be positioned in two particular areas of the midbrain, sited just above the optic nerves. The electrical and chemical output of these clumps of brain cells are thought to prompt other brain areas to make the hormones that stimulate or suppress our various body systems, according to the circadian cycle.

One of these hormones, melatonin, regulates sleepiness. Secreted by the pineal gland in the brain, melatonin is released as daylight fades, inducing sleepiness. It is switched off again at dawn, signalling to the body that it is time to wake up. Melatonin levels are highest in the winter when days are short and lowest in the summer months when days are long.

JET LAG

Just how important sleep is to regulating the body's processes can be seen from the problems that occur when our regular

From conception to birth, a foetus spends nearly all its time asleep and seemingly dreaming. A baby sleeps about 16 hours a day, and this progressively lessens – an adult needs about eight hours sleep a night. As a person grows older, he spends less time dreaming when asleep.

Sleep patterns

Hours

Time awake

REM (dreaming sleep)

NREM (dreamless sleep)

Age in years   Conception   0   5   10   20

patterns are disrupted by long-distance plane flights. When changing time zones quickly, the internal body rhythms fall out of kilter with the local time. While your body and brain are saying sleep, your new location's light-dark cycle, temperature changes, mealtimes and human activities are saying stay awake. The result is "jet lag", and the characteristic symptoms include fatigue, irritability, hunger, headache, lightheadedness and vagueness, as the body tries to forget its old schedule and adapt to the new one. People who work during night shifts can have similar problems.

One of the most effective ways to adjust your body clock is to seek exposure to bright light at hours of the day appropriate for your new time zone and schedule. This helps your body reset its clock. Some research also suggests that taking supplements of melatonin in the evening to encourage sleep may help shorten this adaptation time.

FLUCTUATING SYMPTOMS

Circadian rhythms can also influence the way our body deals with ill health. For example, it is thought that the reason many asthmatics often feel worse in the morning is due to the cyclic release of hormones at that time. This has implications for the management of asthma and when drugs are best taken.

Without sleep, the body cannot rest and repair itself at all – most people know instinctively that the best way to recuperate from a bout of flu or sickness is to "sleep it off". Blood pressure drops while you are sleeping, and breathing and heart rate slow down. At the same time, the body releases more growth and sex hormones. Sleep could also be a survival mechanism – a way of conserving energy at times of inactivity.

When you are asleep, two distinct patterns of slumber alternate throughout the night: deep, dreamless, nonrapid eye movement sleep, known as NREM, and rapid eye movement sleep, or REM, when you dream. NREM predominates and is itself divided into four levels, ranging from light to deep sleep.

WHAT HAPPENS DURING SLEEP?

When you fall asleep, you drift first into NREM, spending about 90 minutes sinking down through the four levels and back up again. This is broken by a 10 to 15 minute burst of REM, during which your body is almost completely immobile, except for the rapid flickering of the eyeballs. However, your brain is almost as electrically active as it is in waking hours and dreams occur. It is thought that dreams are the brain's way of sorting information gathered during waking hours for memory storage or disposal.

This pattern repeats itself throughout the night, although time spent in NREM becomes gradually shorter and REM time lengthens. The last REM period before waking often lasts up to an hour. ∎

KEEPING YOUR SLEEP RHYTHMS IN ORDER

- Allow enough time for sleep and make sure you go to bed and wake up at about the same time each day.
- Do not go to bed feeling hungry or straight after a heavy meal.
- Do not spend too much time in a brightly lit bathroom before going to bed.
- Sleep in total darkness.
- Pull the curtains back as soon as you wake.
- If flying across time zones, spend several hours in bright light during the morning of arrival, do not sleep until it is dark and let the dawn light wake you.

SEE ALSO
The medicine cupboard
313

CAUTION

■ During pregnancy, discuss with your doctor any drugs you take. Drugs taken by the mother can enter the foetus's bloodstream. Some drugs are safe, but others are known to be harmful to a foetus and for most drugs there is no firm evidence either way.
■ Never give aspirin to a child 12 years of age or younger: it has been linked to a dangerous condition known as Reye's syndrome. Use paracetamol instead.

Ask the pharmacist's advice before buying over-the-counter medicine, but let him know if you are taking any prescription drugs. You should ask him or your doctor for advice whenever you take prescription drugs.

Using medicines safely

The more information the better is a good philosophy when it comes to using medicines safely. Knowing what you are taking, and why, will help ensure you gain the maximum possible benefit with the minimum risk of harm. If you can, have a list of potential questions ready to ask the doctor or pharmacist.

Always closely follow the instructions you are given, whether by the doctor, pharmacist or on the packet, especially if the medicine is for your use at home. (Some medicines, such as anticancer drugs, are administered only by doctors or nurses.) For example, there are good reasons for being told to take a drug with food: certain medicines can irritate an empty stomach lining. If the label dictates that you take the medicine first thing in the morning, this may be because it is when your body chemistry needs the help.

Some drugs may need to be taken a certain number of times a day if they have a specific efficacy period; if you take these doses unevenly throughout the day, you could be unprotected part of the time. Remember, too, to check whether "four times a day" means during waking hours or whether you need to wake up in the night to take it over a 24-hour period.

NAMING ITS CONTENTS

Make sure that you know the generic, or nonproprietary, name of your medicine, not just the brand title. The generic name describes the active ingredient, and several different brands can contain the same active ingredient.

Once the patent of a proprietary drug runs out (usually after 20 years), generic versions can also be made. Doctors are often encouraged to prescribe these because they are usually just as effective but often cheaper. Knowing the generic name prevents confusion and duplication: some people, unknowingly, end up taking a double dose of the same medicine because it has different names.

TAKING THE MEDICINE

Find out how long you will be taking the drug. Some, such as antibiotics, are not fully effective unless you take the whole course. Others have harmful effects if you stop taking them suddenly, so you should remember to visit your doctor in advance if you need a repeat prescription.

Some drugs work spectacularly fast. Glyceryl trinitrate, for example, provides

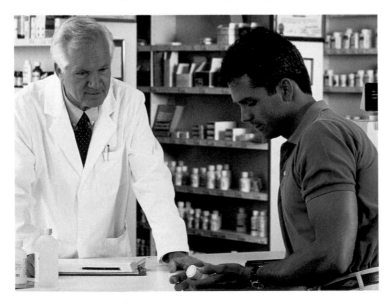

almost immediate relief from the chest pain of angina. Others work more slowly and there may be no real benefit for several weeks. Ask what to expect so that you do not give up taking a drug just when it starts to take effect.

Many drugs have side effects. They may appear immediately but subside after a few days, or they can appear much later as the dose builds up in your body. It is important to report any persistent side effects to your doctor. Remember, too, that one drug can interact with another. Always inform your doctor or pharmacist of other medicines you are taking at the same time. While some side effects can be serious, most are an inconvenience that may have to be put up with until the condition is treated.

WHAT TO ASK

Whether your doctor has prescribed a medication or you are buying it from a pharmacist, it is worth asking the following questions about it:

■ What are the trade and generic names of the medicine?

■ What kind of medicine is it? For example, it might be an antihypertensive, a cholesterol-lowering drug or a painkiller.

■ How does it work in the body?

■ Does it have any side effects?

■ How often should it be taken and for about how long ?

■ When is the best time of day to take it?

■ Are there any foods or drinks that should be avoided when taking the drug?

■ What should be done if a dose is accidentally missed?

■ What are the signs that it is working?

Finally, remember that drugs are not appropriate for all illnesses. Do not expect to get a medicine every time you visit the doctor. Good medical care often means knowing when not to prescribe. ■

ANTIBIOTIC ABUSE

The use of antibiotics is soaring, but many prescriptions are inappropriate. Antibiotics kill bacteria. They are useless against coughs and colds, which are mostly caused by viruses. Even when antibiotics are called for, many people fail to finish the course prescribed because they feel better. The bacteria that haven't been killed off become more resilient to attack and become resistant to antibiotics, and these are left to multiply.

When you need antibiotics...

■ Bacterial meningitis

■ Pneumonia

■ Tuberculosis

■ Severe acne

■ Bacterial cystitis

■ Sexually transmitted infections

■ Before or after major surgery

...and when you don't

■ Colds, sore throats, chicken pox, shingles, mumps, measles, herpes — all caused by viruses

■ Most cases of diarrhoea and vomiting.

OVER-THE-COUNTER MEDICINES

Drugs for minor ailments can increasingly be bought "over-the-counter" without a prescription. They are often lower strengths than those prescribed by a doctor, but remember that they are still medicines. Even everyday drugs can be dangerous in overdose – taking too many paracetamol, for example, can cause serious liver damage. Always take notice of the maximum dosages recommended, and be careful combining medicines.

SEE ALSO

Heart disease	35–39
Acupuncture	212–213
Alcohol	255

Smoking and drinking

For those who decide to stop smoking tobacco or drinking alcohol, the main ingredient of success is self motivation. Nevertheless, there are all sorts of strategies and techniques that may help boost your resolve.

Tobacco and alcohol, as well as certain drugs, are hard to give up because the body depends on the chemicals that those substances provide, and it becomes physically and emotionally addicted to them. When the body is deprived of these chemicals, it usually goes through "withdrawal" symptoms.

For example, every puff on a cigarette rapidly delivers a burst of nicotine to the body and brain. When this wears off, the body reacts first with restlessness, then with increasing anxiety and irritability, at which point the smoker lights up. Many people believe tobacco calms them down, when in fact it is the nicotine in the tobacco that is stimulating them in the first place. Smoking tobacco has numerous negative effects on your body such as an increased risk of cancer.

GIVING UP TOBACCO

The most important strategy is to pick a specific "quit day" and stick to it. It may help if it is a day when something out of the ordinary is happening – perhaps starting a new job or going on holiday. You should stop completely: research shows that trying to cut down slowly is less effective in the long term.

Before you stop, keep a smoking diary for several days. Write down for each

In the long term, abuse of alcohol and smoking can have devastating effects on the brain, heart, liver, lungs and other organs in your body. Although alcohol in moderation is acceptable, it is better for your health to never smoke tobacco.

EFFECTS OF ALCOHOL

Slurred speech and blurred vision; reduction of memory, concentration, judgment and coordination; inappropriate emotional responses

Skin becomes flushed as blood vessels at surface widen; can cause excessive heat loss

Abnormal heartbeat; the force of heart muscle contraction decreases

Cirrhosis of the liver

Inflammation of the stomach lining

Water loss from kidneys, causing dehydration

EFFECTS OF SMOKING

Headaches; lack of oxygen and narrow blood vessels lead to stroke

Tar in smoke can trigger cancer in the oesophagus; tobacco also causes cancer of mouth and throat

More mucus is secreted, causing chronic cough; increased susceptibility to infection; risk of lung cancer and emphysema

Faster heartbeat; build up of atheroma blocks arteries; blood pressure rises; carbon monoxide enters blood

Increased acid causes stomach ulcer

cigarette smoked what you were doing at the time, who you were with, how you were feeling and how much you enjoyed or needed it. Then ask yourself: what or who stimulates me to have a cigarette; which ones could I easily have not had; and which could I not have done without and why? Use your answers to devise strategies that will help you deal with these moments when you stop. Feelings of craving last about three minutes, so plan distractions that take that long such as making a phone call, brushing your teeth or filing a nail.

It helps to change your routine so that you avoid situations in which you would have had a cigarette. Replace the morning cup of coffee that went with the first puff of a cigarette with orange juice, bypass the shop where you bought your cigarettes and avoid lunch with your smoking friends until the cravings pass. Taking up a new and absorbing hobby can help, as can enjoying little treats as the days pass or counting up the money you are saving.

HELPFUL AIDS

Various devices to cope with withdrawal symptoms are available. Nicotine replacement therapies in the shape of chewing gum, skin patches or nasal sprays,can help heavy smokers. The aim is to gradually reduce the patch size or the strength of the gum or spray. Use them as part of a well-defined stop-smoking plan. Studies show the best boost to success is joining a stop-smoking support group.

Other gadgets include filters to remove some of the tar and nicotine, herbal cigarettes, which contain no nicotine but still produce tar and carbon monoxide, and gums that make cigarette smoke taste foul. All may provide brief support but do not stop the nicotine craving, nor do they break the physical activity of smoking.

ALCOHOL DEPENDENCE

Drinking alcohol in moderation has its benefits. However, compulsive, long-term heavy drinking can lead to alcoholism and cirrhosis of the liver, a potentially fatal condition. Heavy drinkers find it difficult to wean themselves off alcohol and cope with the withdrawal symptoms. Professional psychological, social or physical treatment tends to be more successful than self help if the drinker is to be cured in the long term. Living with an alcoholic can take its toll on the family members: they may benefit by seeking help from local support groups.

Beating an addiction to drugs also requires professional help to wean the body off its dependency. ■

CAUTION

When you stop smoking be prepared for withdrawal symptoms, which include restlessness, coughing, an upset stomach, dizziness and insomnia. All the symptoms will decrease over two or three weeks, leaving you feeling fitter and with greater self respect.

WHEN YOU STOP SMOKING

After...	Effect on the body
20 minutes	Blood pressure and pulse rate return to normal; circulation improves in the hands and feet.
8 hours	Oxygen levels in the blood return to normal; chances of heart attack start to fall.
24 hours	Carbon monoxide is eliminated from the body; lungs start to clear out mucus and other debris.
48 hours	Nicotine is no longer detectable in the body; the ability to taste and smell improves.
72 hours	Bronchial tubes relax and breathing becomes easier; energy levels increase.
2 to 12 weeks	Circulation improves throughout the body, making physical activity easier.
3 to 9 months	Breathing problems such as coughing, shortness of breath and wheezing decrease; overall lung function increases by 10–15 percent.
5 years	Risk of heart attack falls to half that of a smoker.
10 years	Risk of lung cancer falls to half that of a smoker; risk of heart attack falls to the same as a nonsmoker's.

Chapter 1

COMMON HEALTH PROBLEMS

WHETHER YOU SUFFER FROM A TEMPORARY illness or a chronic disorder, the more information you have about the problem, the better equipped you will be to handle it. You will be more prepared to decide what warrants a visit to the doctor and what doesn't: should you contact the surgery to treat conjunctivitis, painful periods, a strained muscle or fatigue?

Knowledge often makes it easier to cope with caring for a family member with a chronic condition such as a child with asthma or a parent with Alzheimer's disease. It will also help you take preventive measures, which are usually easier to follow than treating an illness. For example, there are many steps you can take to reduce the risk of diseases that are prevalent today such as heart attacks, diabetes and cancer.∎

SEE ALSO
How healthy are you? 8–9
Using medicines safely
18–19
Essential first aid 292–313

CAUTION

■ *Do not attempt self-diagnosis. See your doctor.*
■ *Do not stop taking prescribed medicine without first talking to your doctor.*
■ *Tell your doctor and complementary practitioner about treatments prescribed by the other.*

When to see your doctor

A visit to the doctor's surgery used to be prompted only by feeling ill. Nowadays, you and your family might visit for 101 reasons, as much to do with staying healthy as being sick.

You might go to the doctor for a regular test such as a cervical smear, for help to lose weight or stop smoking, for guidance on family planning or for children's immunizations. And, of course, you'll visit when you are feeling ill.

Sometimes it is difficult to know what symptoms warrant a visit. Every winter, for example, doctors are deluged with patients suffering from coughs and colds, although most cannot be treated. The best thing to do is to curl up in bed with lots of fluids and let your immune system go to work (see pp.26–27).

There are particular symptoms that you should always report to a doctor (see box, left). It is also important to inform your doctor's surgery if a symptom worsens or persists for more than a few days.

Contact your doctor during office hours if possible rather than late at night. Illness always seems more frightening at night and it is easy to think your symptoms are a sign of serious illness. They probably are not but if you are unsure, seek advice. Most doctors operate a telephone advice line staffed by doctors or nurses.

VISITING YOUR DOCTOR

To save time, write down what you want to say to the doctor or ask him before your visit. You will need to explain when you first started feeling ill or noticed something unusual and whether you have had it before. Describe precisely what the pain or problem feels like, even if it seems embarrassing or silly – doctors are used to it. Think of what makes your condition better or worse, such as heat or the time of day. You should also inform your doctor about what medicines you are taking, including complementary remedies and those from the chemist.

Doctors are trained to interpret the symptoms and warning signs of disease.

WARNING SIGNS OF SERIOUS ILLNESS

The following should always be reported to a doctor:

■ Weight loss of 3 kg (7 lbs) or more without a known reason.

■ Any change of shape, size or skin texture in a breast, a lump or thickening in a breast or a discharge or bleeding from a nipple.

■ Any change, swelling or lump in a testicle or persistent, complete failure to have an erection.

■ Feeling thirsty without an obvious reason.

■ Any unexplained dizziness.

■ Any change in a skin spot, wart or mole, such as changing colour, growing bigger or thicker, itching or bleeding.

■ Coughing up blood; loss of blood when urinating or from the bowels; or unexpected vaginal bleeding after intercourse, between cycles or in menopause.

■ Black stools or any persistent change in bowel habits.

■ Frequent indigestion or acid belching.

■ Difficulty in swallowing, or huskiness or hoarseness in your voice that continues for more than three weeks.

■ Any first, severe or unusual headache.

■ Any unexplained leg pain or frequent, persistent back pain.

■ Any sore that does not heal or unexplained swellings.

In most cases they can treat you there and then on the basis of your medical history and your description of your symptoms – physical examination is often not necessary. Occasionally, your doctor may refer you to a consultant in one area of medicine for specialist treatment.

You can ask the doctor questions, too, if you feel unclear about what is causing the problem, how it is normally treated or what you can do to help. You may also want to know if there are any long-term effects and if there is anything you can do to prevent it from happening again. ∎

CAUTION

Never give aspirin to a child 12 years of age or younger: it has been linked to a dangerous condition known as Reye's syndrome. Treat a fever with paracetamol.

WHEN IT'S AN EMERGENCY

The following can be signs of serious illness in either adults or children. Dial 999 for an ambulance or go straight to the Accident and Emergency department of a hospital.

Problem	Warning signs
Severe chest pain	Pain accompanied by paleness, feeling sick or cold, sweating or having breathing difficulties that last for more than 10 minutes.
Breathing difficulties	If the person has shortness of breath, is gasping, gulping or wheezing, is choking or is unable to speak or drink.
High temperature or fever	If the temperature in an adult rises over 40°C (104°F), perhaps with a stiff neck, cramps or vomiting.
Severe wounds	Such as deep cuts or wounds where the bleeding will not stop, as well as injuries where the edges of the wound cannot be pulled together, are difficult to clean or are red and inflamed.
Head injuries	Are serious if the person has passed out; developed double vision; seems confused, drowsy or dizzy; or cannot remember what has happened to him.
Broken bones	A bone may be broken if the person can put no weight on it, a limb is twisted awkwardly or the person is in great pain and feels nauseous.
Sudden severe pain	Is serious if it lasts more than 10 minutes and there is no apparent reason.
Loss of consciousness	When the person cannot be woken up.
Bad burns or scalds	Heavy blistering or broken skin, a burn that covers a large area or is on the face, or skin that has turned white or black may require medical attention. For a sunburn, consult a doctor if the person has large burned and blistered areas, is shivery, queasy, vomiting, feverish or suffering from palpitations.
Vomiting and diarrhoea	May be serious if accompanied by worsening stomach pains or blood.

DANGER SIGNS IN CHILDREN

Seek help right away if a child:

∎ Has any violet-coloured spots that don't fade when pressed.

∎ Has breathing difficulties.

∎ Is in pain when breathing in.

∎ Is vomiting violently.

∎ Is weak, drowsy or confused and doesn't react to you.

∎ Cannot sit up properly or bend his head forward.

∎ Less than six months with an armpit (axillary) temperature over 38.3°C (101°F) or a rectal temperature over 39.7°C (103.5°F).

SEE ALSO

Vaccinations   120–121

Your immune system

The immune system consists of an extraordinary set of specialized cells and substances that work together to protect the body from invading foreign substances such as bacteria, viruses, chemicals, dust and pollen. When it is healthy and fully functioning, it can banish infections and pollutants with barely an outward sign.

Some natural immunity is passed on from a mother to her child not only in the womb, but also after childbirth in the mother's milk – as long as the child breast-feeds. The immune system, however, mostly develops as you grow up and are continually exposed to the numerous, potentially dangerous organisms inside and outside the body.

The system depends on two closely connected key players: lymphocytes (white blood cells) and antibodies, which neutralize invading germs. Lymphocytes are manufactured in bone marrow and transported throughout the body by a colourless fluid called lymph via the lymphatic system, a network of vessels.

Antibodies are produced by certain types of lymphocyte in response to contact with a foreign attacker. They are specific to that attacker and, once made, the manufacturing cell "remembers" the attacker's shape and trigger and instantly starts producing the correct antibodies if it appears at some other time. It is because of this ability to remember that you can be artificially immunized against certain diseases with vaccinations.

THE ROLE OF ANTIBODIES

Antibodies cling on to foreign cells. They either neutralize the poisonous substance that the attackers pump into the bloodstream or mobilize groups of blood protein, which break down the invader cell walls, dissipating their contents. Antibodies can also act as "flags" to alert the large white cells called macrophages, which engulf attackers. Other white cells, called cytotoxic T-cells, act similarly to antibodies, locking on to particular infecting organisms and destroying them, while T-cells – known as natural killers – can recognize and destroy foreign substances even if they have never come across them before.

The actions of the immune system explain some of the physical symptoms that we sometimes feel. For instance,

Scavenger white cells known as macrophages travel throughout the body to devour dead cells and debris, as well as any unwelcome invaders. The colour-enhanced yellow macrophage below has been magnified 6000 times.

TIPS FOR A HEALTHY IMMUNE SYSTEM

- Stop, or at least cut down, smoking – it decreases the levels of some immune cells (pp.20–21).

- Eat a balanced diet with plenty of fresh vegetables and fruit and unprocessed foods (pp.238–91).

- Learn how to reduce stress (pp.76–77). While hormones released during moderate, short-term stressful situations can quicken healing, prolonged stress depletes immune processes. A good self-image and a healthy attitude to life can help you cope with stress.

- If you're neglecting your diet or are stressed, take vitamin and mineral pills (p.249).

- Spend 15 minutes walking, cycling, swimming, gardening or doing housework twice a day, five days a week. Exercise increases the efficiency of the lymph network.

- Research shows that one or two alcoholic drinks a day are not harmful. Binging is. Drink alcohol only in moderation.

- Allow yourself six to eight hours' sleep – this is important to give the body's cells a chance to replenish.

THE WHITE BLOOD CELLS

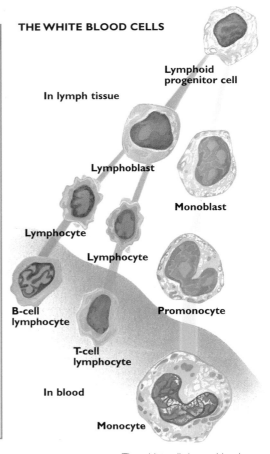

Lymphoid progenitor cell

In lymph tissue

Lymphoblast

Monoblast

Lymphocyte

Lymphocyte

B-cell lymphocyte

Promonocyte

T-cell lymphocyte

In blood

Monocyte

The white cells in our blood are made in the lymph system tissue. They stem from lymphoid progenitor cells and develop via lymphoblasts and monoblasts into lymphocytes or promonocytes. Lymphocytes become either B-cells or T-cells and promonocytes mature into monocytes, which enter the blood. The B-cells are the origin of cells that secrete antibodies. Monocytes can transform into the large white cells called macrophages.

lymph nodes swell in the neck, armpits and groin as lymphocytes multiply and antibodies are produced. When blood vessels dilate and leak to let immune cells rush to a spot under attack, that area becomes inflamed. And pus is largely made up of dead macrophages, which have finished their job in devouring foreign cells.

Unfortunately, not all immune reactions are beneficial. The immune system can overreact or react abnormally and cause allergic disorders such as asthma and hayfever. It can also be tricked by abnormal genes and viruses into seeing some of the body's own cells as foreign. As a result it attacks and destroys those cells, causing autoimmune diseases such as diabetes, rheumatoid arthritis and multiple sclerosis.

MIND OVER MATTER

The immune system is not just physical. Doctors have long known that the mind and a patient's attitude can make a difference in overcoming disease. When cancer patients are asked to use positive images – for example, to imagine their white cells conquering their tumour – levels of lymphocytes, antibodies and natural killer cells increase.

When you are tired or stressed or when you indulge in an unhealthy lifestyle – such as smoking, drinking too much, staying up late, eating poorly or not exercising – the immune system becomes depleted, slower to react and less effective. This makes you vulnerable to attack by infection and illness. You can boost your system and return it to peak condition by following the tips in the box above. ∎

CAUTION

Only stop taking asthma medication on your doctor's advice, not just because you have been symptom free for a while. Preventive medicine may get rid of your symptoms, but it does not mean that you no longer have asthma.

Asthma

One of the most common chronic diseases in the industrialized world, asthma affects roughly six percent of the population of western Europe and the United States. It is indiscriminate in its targets, extending across social boundaries and affecting both men and women, old and young, city residents and country dwellers.

The typical signs of asthma are feeling short of breath, tightness in the chest, wheezing while breathing out and a persistent cough. The symptoms occur when the thousands of tiny airways in the lungs constrict and their linings swell, hindering the flow of air into the chest.

In normal lungs this type of inflammation occurs in tiny areas thousands of times a day. It is an essential part of healthy functioning because it gets rid of hostile factors such as germs, dust and pollutants that are breathed in with the air. In asthmatics, however, the airways are in a constant state of low-level inflammation. When asthma sufferers encounter certain irritants, their airways overreact, becoming dangerously narrow and potentially reducing the crucial supply of oxygen to the body.

WHAT CAUSES ASTHMA?

It is believed that 30 percent of people inherit a genetic potential to develop asthma, although they do not necessarily go on to have the condition. The genes involved create what is known as an atopic tendency and are the same ones that make people susceptible to eczema, and allergies (see pp.125–29). For most

HOW ASTHMA AFFECTS THE LUNGS

The tiny branching airways of the lungs are called bronchioles. In an asthma sufferer, the bronchioles constrict and mucus builds up in them. The narrowed airways make it difficult to breathe and can cause an asthmatic to wheeze. Coughing can also occur, which dislodges mucus from the inflamed bronchioles. Inhaling a reliever drug widens the bronchioles so that the sufferer can breathe properly.

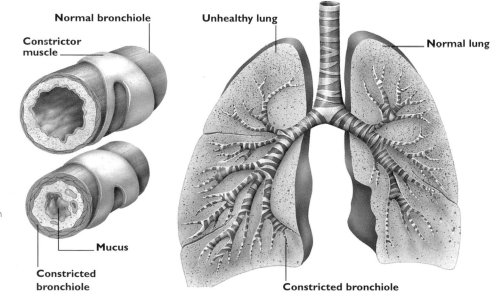

Normal bronchiole

Constrictor muscle

Mucus

Constricted bronchiole

Unhealthy lung

Normal lung

Constricted bronchiole

people, however, the initial trigger is a widespread virus called rhinovirus, which is responsible for many coughs and colds.

It seems the first attack of asthma sets off the inflammatory process and from then on the lungs are primed to overreact to a variety of other trigger factors (see box, below). Some of these – such as exercise, smoke and pollution – are known as irritants and often cause a mild reaction in normal lungs. Others, such as house dust mites (which live on shed flakes of dead skin), pollen and pet hair, are normally harmless, but cause an

ASTHMA TRIGGERS AND HOW TO AVOID THEM

Causes	Preventive measures
Common cold viruses	Avoid close contact with people with colds.
Exercise	Properly treated asthma should not interfere with exercise. Use reliever medication before beginning an activity.
Tobacco smoke	Do not smoke and avoid smoky environments, especially when pregnant or with a young child. Ban smoking at home if your child has asthma.
Air pollution	Watch pollution levels, particularly in summer and, if possible, avoid going outside on high-risk days.
House dust mites	Vacuum frequently, including your mattresses. Use synthetic mattress covers, pillows and duvets. Wash bedding every week at 60°C (140°F). Keep wardrobe doors closed so that dust does not settle on clothes. Wash soft toys regularly or put them in the freezer to kill mites.
Cold air	On cold days, particularly if it is windy, place a scarf around your face to prevent a sudden intake of cold air.
Pollen and grass	Avoid long grass and taking walks in the evening when pollen levels are higher than in the daytime. Keep car and house windows closed. Choose low-pollen plants for your garden.
Mould spores	These grow in almost any warm moist area and are released mostly in autumn and summer or on damp days. Remove mould and avoid damp houses. Open windows and let fresh air in if it's not the pollen season.
Furry or feathery animals	Don't acquire any new pets. Keep those already part of the family out of the bedrooms and always groom them outdoors.
Stress	Explore ways to lower your stress levels and to avert panic if asthma symptoms begin. Learn to breathe with your diaphragm.
Occupational triggers (including chemicals, glues, acids, dyes, fumes, animals, grains, wood, coffee bean and tea dust)	Use protective equipment such as masks and protective clothing. Talk to the health and safety officer at your workplace about how to reduce exposure, for example, by using extractor fans or sealing off equipment that produces hazardous substances.
Medicines, particularly aspirin-based	Always ask a pharmacist's advice before buying over-the-counter medicines.

CAUTION

Look for the colour coding on asthma medication to avoid confusion. Relievers are always in a blue inhaler. Preventer inhalers may be light or dark brown, maroon or orange, but never blue.

To use an inhaler correctly, exhale, then breathe in slowly and deeply as you trigger the aerosol.

inflammatory reaction in susceptible individuals. Airborne substances at work can make asthma worse and can even cause the condition in someone who did not have it before. People working with chemicals, laboratory animals or in dusty environments are particularly at risk and it is important to report any signs of wheezing or chest tightening to both a doctor and the health and safety officer.

MAKING A DIAGNOSIS

Asthma can be tricky to diagnose. The first step is to try to build up a picture of the illness. A doctor might ask you whether anyone else in the family has asthma, if your chest hurts or if you have had a recurrent cough, how you feel at different times of the day (asthma is often worse at morning and night) and whether you have been exposed to trigger factors.

The doctor may also listen to your chest with a stethoscope to see if you wheeze

when you breathe out, and he may ask you to blow into a simple apparatus called a peak flow metre; it measures the speed at which the air comes out of the lungs. The faster the air comes out, the less narrowing of the airways there is. If it is still unclear whether you have asthma, you may be asked to do a simple exercise test, such as quickly stepping on and off a box for a few minutes, after which your peak flow will be measured. Exercise provokes wheezing in 90 percent of uncontrolled asthma cases.

CHILDREN AND ASTHMA

Detecting asthma in young children can be difficult because at least 30 percent wheeze at some time during their first five years. Also, peak flow metres used to assess older children and adults cannot be used with those under six years of age.

Typical symptoms of asthma in young children are wheezing and sometimes a troublesome cough, particularly at night, with colds or with exercise. Tiredness and listlessness during the day can also be a clue as undiagnosed asthmatic children often have trouble sleeping.

It's almost impossible to protect your child from all triggers. Banning smoking at home and trying to reduce the allergens that an infant is exposed to in the first three months of life can help. The latest research shows that children with a family history of asthma may be protected from its worst effects if they are breast-fed for the first four or five months of life. Many children grow out of asthma, but those who have it at the age of 14 are likely to carry the tendency into adult life.

TREATMENT

Asthma requires regular treatment to keep it under control. There are two key types of drugs: preventers, which are used to

HOW SAFE ARE STEROID DRUGS?

There is often concern about the side effects of the cortico-steroids that are present in asthma preventer drugs. In particular, parents worry that they can inhibit their child's growth. There is no evidence to show that this happens with the steroid dosages normally used for asthma. Because asthmatics usually inhale steroids, they are delivered straight to the lungs in low doses and little is absorbed into the rest of the body.

In rare cases children with severe or uncontrolled asthma may need to take high doses of steroids in tablet form, which can cause bones to thin and increase blood pressure and weight gain. In these cases it is important to weigh up the side effects of the drug with the child's quality of life – and even his chances of survival. Severe or untreated asthma can itself inhibit growth and may also be life threatening. You should bear in mind, too, that the corticosteroids used for treating asthma are quite different from the anabolic steroids that have earned such a bad reputation in body building.

curb the underlying inflammation in the airways, and relievers, which are used to treat asthma symptoms at the time they occur. Preventers work by reducing the sensitivity of the airways. The drugs prevent blood vessels from dilating and leaking, thereby stopping the immune system's inflammatory processes from narrowing the airways.

Corticosteroids and cromoglycates are the two main types of preventer drug. Both are usually taken two to four times a day with an inhaler (see below, right). Patients should start to feel better after a few days. Preventers must be taken regularly to maintain their effect.

RELIEVING SYMPTOMS

Unlike preventers, which work long term, reliever medication eases asthmatic symptoms instantly. Relievers are used as soon as symptoms of asthma appear or, if recommended, before exercise. They should give almost complete relief for four to six hours. The medicines used are often referred to as bronchodilators because they relax the muscles surrounding the airways. This allows the airways to open up and the person to breathe.

Relievers are short-term aids and have no effect on the underlying inflammation. Making little use of reliever medication is a sign that your asthma is well controlled. If you have to use it more often than prescribed, or wheezing wakes you at night, tell your doctor. Your preventer medicine may need to be increased.

Sudden asthma attacks can be frightening but your doctor should give you a strategy for coping. This may include sitting down and trying to relax your breathing, using your reliever inhaler again and contacting your doctor or going to the hospital casualty department if things do not improve. ∎

After an acute attack, an asthmatic may spend time in hospital on a nebulizer. The machine enables staff to give high doses of a reliever drug in the form of a fine mist and to monitor progress. In severe cases, nebulizers may be used at home.

A spacer is easier for children to use because it allows the child to breathe normally while inhaling the drug. The blue one here is for adults who may have trouble with coordination.

TAKING MEDICATION FOR ASTHMA	
Equipment	**How it works**
Inhaler	This device turns medication into a fine mist that can enter the airways of the lungs. Metered dose inhalers deliver a precise "puff" of drug carried on high-pressure gas. Dry powder inhalers use a capsule that shatters when you suck on the device and releases a fine powder of medicine. It demands less coordination.
Spacer	A valved mouthpiece is attached to one end of a large-volume plastic container, which has a hole to hold an inhaler. The medicine is puffed into the container and then breathed in normally instead of in one breath. Spacers help babies and children and those who have difficulty coordinating their inhaler technique.
Nebulizer	A machine that turns liquid medication into a fine mist, a nebulizer enables a much higher dose of medication to be given. It is used in hospitals for acute attacks and sometimes to help babies and young children.

CAUTION

Because influenza can develop into pneumonia, an annual flu vaccination is recommended for the elderly and people with chronic diseases. A vaccine that protects against the pneumococcus bacterium – the most common cause of pneumonia – is available.

Chest infections

Lower respiratory tract infections – often called chest infections – are common. While the body can fight off many of these with the help of a few days in bed, some can become more serious or chronic.

Bronchitis, pneumonia and pleurisy are all infections affecting different parts of the lung. Bronchitis – an inflammation of the large branches, or bronchi, of the lung – develops when a bacterial or viral infection prompts an overproduction of the mucus normally produced in the airways to keep them moist. Excessive mucus can make you cough, while inflammation can cause the airways to narrow and make you feel breathless and unwell.

Pneumonia develops when an infection travels into the bronchioles (smaller tubes) and alveoli, the tiny air sacs at the end of each bronchiole through which oxygen moves into the bloodstream. The infection inflames the alveoli and fills them with fluid. This impairs the lungs' ability to pump oxygen into the bloodstream and around the whole body.

People with pneumonia usually lose their appetite and feel ill and feverish. They also suffer from a phlegmy cough, breathlessness and a feeling of tightness in the chest. If a sharp pain in the side develops, this can mean that the infection has spread to the lining of the lung, a condition known as pleurisy.

WHAT CAUSES INFECTION?

Most chest infections are caused by bacteria, a few by viruses. Some are simply breathed in and others live harmlessly in the throat unless you are fatigued. If your resistance is weakened by long-term illnesses, such as asthma (see pp.28–31), chronic bronchitis, heart disease, diabetes or cancer, or you are elderly and cannot move around normally, you will be more susceptible to chest infections. Smokers are also particularly vulnerable because cigarette smoke damages the lining of the bronchi and their resistance to germs.

More rare types of pneumonia are Legionnaire's disease, caused by germs in faulty air-conditioning or hot-water systems, and psittacosis, which is spread by some birds, including pet parrots.

Many adults have a bout of bronchitis at some time in their lives. It usually lasts a week or two, and most people overcome it without recourse to medical treatment. But if the condition does not improve after 10 days or so, you should go to your doctor. Acute infections like bronchitis and pneumonia put a great strain on the lungs and need to be controlled.

THE SPECTRE OF TUBERCULOSIS

Tuberculosis (TB) was a main cause of death in the first half of the 20th century. Improved social conditions curbed it in the developed world and antibiotic treatments were developed in the 1950s. But in recent years the number of cases has risen because of poor health among the homeless, the susceptibility of immuno-compromised patients and increasing antibiotic resistance among TB bacteria caused by failure to finish the course of treatment. In healthy people, the immune system fends off TB, and those who have not built up a natural immunity can be vaccinated. In the infected, a cocktail of antibiotics over nine months or a year is necessary to eradicate the disease.

DISEASES OF THE LUNGS

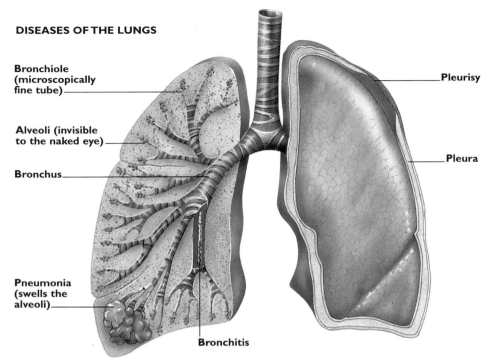

Bronchiole (microscopically fine tube)

Alveoli (invisible to the naked eye)

Bronchus

Pneumonia (swells the alveoli)

Bronchitis

Pleurisy

Pleura

Bronchitis, a common complaint of smokers, infects the bronchi (the large branches of the lungs) and the bronchioles (smaller tubes). Pneumonia is more serious: infection spreads to the bronchioles and alveoli (air sacs). Most dangerous – and painful – of all is pleurisy in which infection reaches the pleura, the membrane that surrounds the lungs.

Antibiotics are the main way of treating bronchitis and pneumonia because both are normally caused by bacteria. Viral infections, however, do not respond to antibiotics and the body's own natural defences are the only way to fight these. Pneumonia and pleurisy are deeply painful and require painkillers, and in severe infections oxygen can be lifesaving.

CHRONIC LUNG DISEASES

In emphysema, a fatal disease, the walls of the alveoli are gradually destroyed, making it difficult for the body to absorb oxygen. As a result the person becomes increasingly crippled by breathlessness, is often unable to walk more than a few metres and is prone to lung infections.

Chronic obstructive airways disease (COAD) is a combination of emphysema and chronic bronchitis. The latter disease is caused in the same way as acute (short-term) bronchitis, but instead of going away after a few weeks, symptoms such as cough, sputum and breathlessness

continue because of reduced resistance in the lungs and a gradual scarring and stiffening of the lung tissue.

A small number of emphysema cases are genetic, but the most common cause of emphysema and COAD is smoking. Even after long-term use of tobacco, stopping smoking dramatically reduces the risk of developing either condition. If one does develop, quitting can reduce symptoms.

There are no cures for COAD, but it is possible to ease symptoms. Cough mixtures are not much help, but broncho-dilator drugs similar to those used in asthma can help relax the airways and improve wheezing. Exercise is important. Pure oxygen, supplied with a mask or nose tubes, helps some patients. Those who have an advanced condition may need to be hooked up to oxygen most of the day. Physiotherapy exercises can help drain excess mucus and phlegm. Breathing retraining can help sufferers use their chest more efficiently, relieving breathlessness and panic. ∎

CAUTION

Most people who have pneumonia are treated at home, but about one in six becomes ill enough to need admission to hospital. Tell the doctor if any symptoms worsen – pneumonia becomes serious when infection spreads to other parts of the body. Most pneumonia sufferers make a complete recovery, but it can take some time to feel 100 percent fit again.

SEE ALSO

Losing weight	260–261
Hydrotherapy	236–237

CAUTION

Avoid clothes that can impair the free flow of blood up the veins, such as tight knicker elastic and garters. Anything that restricts the legs can cause the valve damage that leads to varicose veins.

Efficient valves prevent gravity pulling blood downward. When the valve no longer closes properly, blood forms pools in the vein, which cause swelling.

Varicose veins

Bulging, twisted purplish vessels called varicose veins are caused when the valves that keep the blood flowing toward the heart fail. Damaged valves allow blood to flow downward, collect and pool. This stretches and distorts the delicate structure of the vein, particularly where it is close to the surface of the skin and less supported by muscle.

The legs are more susceptible to varicose veins because it is there that pressure is greatest as blood is pumped against gravity back to the heart. The most common symptoms are aching, tired legs and swollen ankles. In some people the skin on their legs turns a brownish-blue: this is because toxins usually washed away by briskly flowing blood accumulate and the legs are poorly supplied with oxygen. There is also a higher risk of ulcers developing from even minor knocks because the legs are generally unhealthy.

Faulty valves often run in families, but they also occur in people who stand for long periods of time. Pregnancy and being overweight are other factors. Regular walking and a healthy weight can stop them forming. Wearing elastic support stockings, the simplest way of treating the problem, can also help prevent varicose veins. Support stockings are tightest at the ankle and loosen as they rise up the leg. The pressure they exert prevents blood from pooling by diverting it into the veins deeper in the legs, where the muscles are a more efficient pump to the heart.

SURGICAL TREATMENT

While stockings can greatly ease milder symptoms, they do little for the unsightly appearance of the veins or for severe pain. Many people ask for surgical treatment. The procedure, known as "stripping" the vein, involves inserting a long cable into the vein through a cut at the ankle. The cable is pulled out, with the offending vessel, through another cut in the groin.

Before operating, the surgeon uses X-rays or ultrasound examination to work out exactly which part of the vein system is causing the problem and to ensure that the deep veins are working reliably. The results of this small operation, often done as day surgery with a local anaesthetic, are usually excellent and a complete cure.

A third treatment involves injecting a special solution inside the vein, which scars it and makes it collapse. This is a reasonable treatment for mild cases, but there is a risk that the problem will recur. ∎

NORMAL VALVE

Open	**Closed**

ABNORMAL VALVE

Open	**Closed**

Heart disease

The heart is a muscle that pumps blood and its essential cargo of oxygen and nutrients around the body. Like all muscles, it needs oxygen to work properly. Its supply comes in via the two powerful coronary arteries that network deep into the heart muscle. When something goes wrong with this supply, the condition is life threatening.

The heart beats regularly and strongly thanks to the two coronary arteries that supply it with blood. When the artery walls fur up with atheroma (fatty sludge), blood cannot easily pass through. If the blood clots in one of these arteries, the result is a heart attack. Part of the heart muscle dies, and the dead area is replaced by scar tissue.

The term heart disease covers many conditions, including abnormal heart structure, valve defects and defects with the "pacemaker", which triggers a regular heartbeat. However, the biggest killer of the Western world is atherosclerosis – the build up of fatty sludge in the coronary arteries. This sludge, called atheroma, consists of cholesterol, proteins and tissue debris. It gradually narrows the arteries and restricts the vital supply of oxygen-rich blood to the heart. It also reduces the flexibility of the arteries, which can increase blood pressure and crack the normally smooth surface of the artery wall. Cracks create dangerous blood clots, which can block the artery completely.

A variety of risk factors bring about atherosclerosis. The mixture of narrowed vessels, high blood pressure and blood clots is known as coronary artery disease. It sets the scene for pain and heart attack.

ANGINA PECTORIS

Meaning pain in the chest, angina pectoris is the early warning system for coronary artery disease. It is caused when an artery is so furred up that blood has difficulty flowing to the heart. Most angina sufferers experience pain when something makes their heart beat faster, which increases its need for oxygen. The trigger could be climbing stairs or running for a bus, emotional upsets, excitement, cold weather, a heavy meal or sex.

Symptoms start as a tightness or heaviness on the chest and develop into pain, which can spread into the neck or left arm. It usually passes after a few minutes' rest or the use of medication. However, sometimes symptoms occur even when sitting down or resting. This is known as unstable angina and suggests the blockage is getting worse. Angina can alert you and your doctor to the state of your arteries and prompt lifestyle changes and the use of medication if necessary.

HEART ATTACK

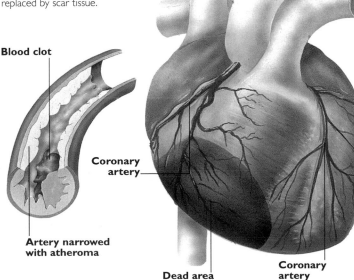

Blood clot

Coronary artery

Artery narrowed with atheroma

Dead area

Coronary artery

CAUTION

A heart attack starts with pains similar to angina, but instead of going away the pain builds up. The pain is accompanied by other symptoms such as sweating, nausea, breathlessness and weakness. If this happens, stop any activity and lie down. In case you lose consciousness, call for help. If the pain lasts for more than 10 minutes, call your doctor or for an ambulance.

HEART ATTACK

Myocardial infarction, or heart attack, is caused when a coronary artery is blocked by a blood clot or atheroma and a part of the heart muscle is starved of oxygen, killing it. This can be further complicated if muscle damage disturbs the heart's electrical pulse and triggers an arrhythmia (irregular beat). The most serious type is ventricular fibrillation – the vibration of the pumping chambers (ventricles) in the heart becomes uncoordinated and stops the heart pumping adequately.

Cardiopulmonary resuscitation and a shock treatment called defibrillation are vital to save the person's life. Heart attack victims are also prescribed drugs called thrombolytics, which dissolve the clot and limit muscle damage. After a heart attack, the dead area of the heart muscle is replaced by scar tissue. Fortunately, losing a small portion of muscle need not interfere with a return to normal activities, but reducing risk factors is crucial to avoid another attack.

HEART FAILURE

The term heart failure covers conditions where the heart becomes too weak to pump blood adequately. Heart attack damage, diseases such as cardiomyopathy, viral infection and high blood pressure weaken the heart muscle. Four one-way valves in the heart ensure blood flows in only one direction. However, if one of them fails to open or close fully, this valvular disorder can cause heart failure.

Heart failure weakens blood circulation and causes fluid to accumulate in parts of the body, particularly the legs and lungs. This causes symptoms such as fatigue, breathlessness and swollen ankles. There is no real cure for heart failure – other than heart transplantation – but drugs and lifestyle changes can ease symptoms.

The heart's beat can also be disturbed by faults in the pacemaking cells that trigger the coordinated contraction of the billions of cardiac muscle cells. Surgically implanting a tiny electrical "pacemaker" to stimulate the correct beat artificially often allows patients to lead a normal life.

RISK FACTORS

The risk of developing heart disease depends on a number of factors. The more you have, the greater your chance of a heart attack. The most important are a family history of heart disease, a high-fat diet, smoking and high blood pressure.

RECOGNIZING THE PROBLEM

Heart attacks, strokes and seizures are often confused. You should learn how to tell the symptoms of these conditions apart so that you will know what to do in an emergency:

Heart attack
Symptoms Sudden, persistent, crushing central chest pain that may spread to the left arm and to the jaw, neck, other arm, abdomen or back. The person may feel faint and have pale skin and rapid shallow breathing. The patient may suddenly collapse without warning. The heart can stop working altogether.
WARNING Do not give fluids. Place the person in the recovery position (p.301). If help is not near, be prepared for resuscitation if the heart fails (pp.296–97).

Stroke
Symptoms The person may appear drunk and disorientated, with slurred speech, a sudden severe headache, loss of balance, weakness or paralysis. Saliva may dribble from the mouth, bowel control may be lost and pupils may be of unequal size.
WARNING Do not give the person anything to eat or drink. Help her into the recovery position (p.301).

Seizure
Symptoms A child has violent, twitching muscles and fever. An adult will go rigid, have convulsions and lose consciousness.
WARNING Do not use force to restrain the person. After the seizure ends, place her in the recovery position (p.300).

LOWERING YOUR RISK OF HEART DISEASE

What to do	Why?	How?
Take exercise	Regular exercise increases beneficial high density lipoprotein (HDL) cholesterol, which protects against atherosclerosis. It also increases heart efficiency, lowers blood pressure, helps control body weight, balances blood clotting factors and reduces stress.	Take 15 minutes of moderate exercise (gardening, housework, brisk walking, dancing or swimming) twice a day five days a week. Moderate exercise should make you sweat slightly and breathe more heavily than usual.
Improve your diet	Low-fat diets promote a good balance of blood fats and help maintain a healthy weight.	Replace saturated fat such as butter with low or unsaturated fats. Eat plenty of fruit and vegetables. Reduce salt.
Maintain a healthy weight	Guard against developing diabetes, high blood pressure and high-risk, centrally-located fat. Weight around the abdomen strains the heart the most.	Combine a healthy diet with regular exercise. Involve the whole family if possible and seek support from groups such as Weightwatchers if you need to lose weight.
Stop smoking	This is the most important modifiable risk factor. Smokers under 50 years of age are twice as likely to die of a heart attack as nonsmokers. Smoking increases adrenalin and heart rate, raises blood pressure, reduces the blood's oxygen-carrying capacity and encourages thrombosis (blood clotting).	Use nicotine patches, gum, acupuncture, meditation and psychological approaches or willpower to quit. Ask your doctor for help and seek advice from friends or relatives who are former smokers. The more you smoke and the more years you smoke, the greater the likelihood of dying from a heart attack.
Lower your blood pressure	Up to 20 percent of adults have high blood pressure. It strains the heart and encourages hardening of the arteries, which raises pressure further. It runs in families but is also a product of lifestyle habits.	Reduce your weight, cut back on fatty foods and salt, stop smoking, drink alcohol moderately and lower your stress levels. If lifestyle changes are not successful, long-term drug treatment may be necessary.
Drink alcohol sensibly	Research suggests moderate drinkers have less risk of heart disease than teetotallers or excessive drinkers.	Moderate drinking is defined as four units of alcohol a day for men and three for women (p.255). A unit equals half a pint of beer, a glass of wine or one measure of spirits.
Reduce stress	A little stress keeps you alert and motivated but prolonged high levels raise adrenalin levels, heart rate and blood pressure. Stress does not cause heart disease but can be a trigger if arteries are already narrowed.	Learn to lower stress levels using techniques such as relaxation and meditation. Prevent too much stress by planning work, setting realistic goals and sharing burdens such as childcare and housework.
Control diabetes	Diabetes doubles the risk of heart attack and stroke, possibly because it is linked with weight gain, high cholesterol, high blood pressure and poor circulation.	Adhering to a pattern of regular healthy eating and a positive lifestyle strategy can significantly reduce the risk of heart disease and other conditions if you have diabetes.
Enjoy sex	A combination of exertion and excitement can bring on angina, but sex also releases stress and is good exercise.	If you can walk up and down 13 steps without chest pain, sex is unlikely to be harmful, but first take any drug prescribed.

ANGIOPLASTY

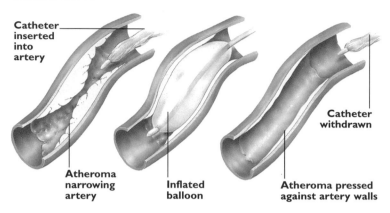

Catheter inserted into artery

Catheter withdrawn

Atheroma narrowing artery

Inflated balloon

Atheroma pressed against artery walls

Angioplasty widens the coronary artery so that the blood can flow more freely. It involves threading a catheter (a flexible tube) with a deflated balloon attached to its tip into the narrowed stretch of artery. The balloon is inflated and squashes fatty deposits against the artery walls.

These are also intertwined with other factors such as diabetes, being overweight, lack of exercise and stress.

You are at greater risk of having a heart attack if you have a close relative, such as a parent or sibling, who has had one, particularly if he was under 55 years of age. Members of a family tend to share bad habits, for example, eating the same fatty diet. They may also have inherited disorders such as familial hypercholesterolaemia. In this disease, the processes that remove cholesterol from the bloodstream are half as effective as normal.

High levels of cholesterol build up which, if uncorrected, can cause angina, heart attack and death in apparently healthy young adults or children. Familial hypercholesterolaemia affects 1 in 500 people. If one person in a family has it, all others must be tested so preventive action can be taken. If the disease is detected early and managed with a rigorously low-fat diet and cholesterol-lowering medication, the person can live into old age.

In Western societies the main dietary reason for developing high cholesterol is not high-cholesterol foods but eating too much saturated fat. There is now scientific evidence that a combination of a low-fat diet, exercise and relaxation training can reverse established coronary artery disease.

DIAGNOSIS

The doctor will take a look at your family history and your lifestyle to help her make a diagnosis. She will measure your blood pressure and may take blood samples to analyze cholesterol levels. She may also investigate the workings and structures of your heart using modern technology.

Electrocardiograms (ECGs) record the electrical activity of the heart. The test may be combined with riding a static bicycle or running on a treadmill to see what happens when you physically exert yourself. Echocardiograms use ultrasound (high frequency sound) to transmit detailed images of the entire moving heart. They are used to investigate patients with valve disease or structural defects. Today's techniques can even detect heart defects before a child is born.

Angiograms are X-rays taken of the heart after you are injected with a dye to reveal exactly where and by how much your heart vessels have narrowed. This investigation is essential before coronary surgery or angioplasty.

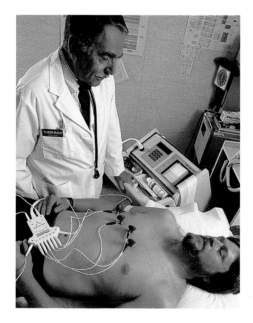

An electrocardiogram (ECG) picks out rhythm abnormalities, detects old or recent heart attacks and provides information on whether the heart is working under strain or enlarged. ECGs may be combined with an exercise stress test to mimic normal exertion and are sometimes taken over 24 hours using a portable machine.

TREATMENT

A range of medications is available to treat heart disease (see below). Other treatments involve surgery. In angioplasty the coronary arteries are widened to let blood flow freely again. Sometimes doctors also place a wire cage, or stent, into the section of artery to hold back the sludge. Angioplasty is simple and often requires only a day in hospital. It can be highly effective, but the widened artery may renarrow and need a second go.

If the arteries are severely blocked and drugs or angioplasty do not relieve pain, coronary artery bypass grafting may be needed. Surgeons sew in replacement stretches of artery or vein, usually taken from the leg, to bypass the blockage. A bypass operation generally takes five hours under general anaesthesia. The heart has to be stopped and its functions taken over by a heart-lung machine. Afterward, the patient is monitored for two to four days in intensive care. The patient often goes home a week later and can return to work and normal life after about six weeks.

Diseases of heart rhythm are often treated by fitting a pacemaker, a tiny electrical generator that stimulates the heart to beat, under a local anaesthetic. Complete recovery is normal. Faulty heart valves can also be replaced or repaired. ∎

MEDICATION FOR HEART DISORDERS		
Condition	**Type of drug**	**What it does**
Heart attack	Thrombolytics ("clot-busters") and anticoagulants such as aspirin, streptokinase, heparin and warfarin.	Dissolve blood clots and prevent more forming by reducing the stickiness of small blood cells. Used initially to break down blockage, as well as long term.
Angina	Nitrate	Rapidly relieves attacks by relaxing artery walls and increasing blood flow to the heart.
	Beta-blocker	Slows beat and force of the heart, decreasing its need for oxygen. Used long term to prevent attacks.
	Calcium antagonist	Relaxes artery walls and increases blood flow to heart. Some slow heartbeat and lower blood pressure.
	Potassium channel opener	Increases blood flow to heart and reduces workload.
Heart failure	ACE (angiotensin converting enzyme) inhibitor	Relaxes blood vessels by inhibiting angiotensin, a chemical with a powerful constricting effect.
	Digoxin	Derived from foxgloves (digitalis), it slows the heart.
	Diuretic	Reduces water and salt by increasing urine output.
Heart disease	Statin	Slows the production of cholesterol in the liver.
	Resin	Lowers lipid levels by stopping re-absorption of bile salts – cholesterol is used in replacing them.
	Fibrate	Reduces production of triglycerides and low density lipoproteins (LDL) in liver.
Hypertension	Beta-blocker, calcium antagonist, ACE inhibitor and diuretic.	Preventive drugs that reduce high blood pressure.

Sprains

Ligaments are tough pieces of fibrous, elastic tissue that attach one bone to another, holding a joint together and limiting its range of movement. There are a number of ligaments supporting each joint. If a ligament becomes overstretched or ruptures, the injury is known as a sprain (which should not be confused with a strain).

A sprain can be either an "acute" or "chronic" injury. An acute sprain occurs when there is a single injury, but if a ligament is persistently stressed by certain repeated activities or movement, it can develop into a chronic sprain.

Sprains occur when a joint is stretched beyond its normal range. When this happens fibres in the ligament rupture, along with small blood vessels, and the joint becomes swollen and looks bruised. When soft tissue such as ligaments, muscles and tendons are damaged, the injury sets off an inflammatory process characterized by four main symptoms: redness, pain, heat and swelling. Each of these represents an important part of the healing process.

THE SYMPTOMS

The severity of the symptoms varies with the degree of the injury. The pain in a sprain is caused by damage to nerve fibres at the injury site, irritation of the nerve endings by toxic substances released from the injured tissue and pressure on nerve endings because of the increased flow of blood in the injured area.

The redness of the skin is partly caused by the rupture of small blood vessels. The area flares up because blood vessels around the damaged tissue widen to increase the supply of nutrients and healing substances. The increased blood flow also helps to take away poisonous waste substances created by the injury, but at the same time it causes swelling.

THE ANKLE JOINT

Tibia

Fibia

Ligament (one of several – for clarity, others are not shown)

Sprains can occur in any joint, including the ankle, wrist, knee and elbow. The ankle is especially vulnerable because it has a wide range of movement, yet it still has to support the full weight of the body. Sprains account for approximately 80 percent of injuries to the ankle.

In a severe sprain, the joint may need splinting in a hospital. Or the ligament may require arthroscopy to reattach it. In this surgical procedure, an endoscope – a rigid tube with an attached lens – is inserted into the joint through a small incision. Instruments are inserted into another incision to repair the damage.

TREATING THE SPRAIN

With less severe sprains, treatment can relieve pain, minimize the bleeding and restore function to the joint. A process called RICE (rest, ice, compression and elevation) usually works best. The first step is to apply ice to the area. This causes blood vessels to contract and slows the rush of blood to the injury. To avoid ice-burn, wrap the ice in a thin wet cloth and apply it for 15–20 minutes at a time.

The area can then be strapped – or compressed – with an elastic bandage to reduce the collection of fluid around the damaged tissue. This will also relieve pain caused by the pressure of excess fluid on nerve endings. Bandaging should be tight enough to create some pressure against the skin but not so constricting that it causes further pain or restricts blood circulation.

The limb should be elevated to a horizontal position to prevent blood accumulating around the injury from the pull of gravity and to ease the passage of blood. It is crucial to rest the injured area to allow the damaged fibres time to repair. An ankle sprain can take 6–12 weeks to heal, and physiotherapy may be needed if it is slow to do so.

EASING THE PAIN

You can take nonsteroidal anti-inflammatory drugs (NSAIDs), such as ibuprofen, which also act as painkillers; they are available from a pharmacy. However, remember that although the pain will be numbed by the drugs, you should not be too energetic because the injury feels better – you may do more damage to the injury.

Depending on the severity of the sprain, pain can last for five to seven days, although it should lessen daily. Listen to your body; if the sprain is still painful continue to rest. If it feels stiff rather than painful, some gentle movement will be beneficial. The swelling may remain for longer. It is important to consult your doctor if the pain does not appear to be diminishing at all, in which case hobbling around could increase the damage to the joint. Sometimes it can be difficult to distinguish a sprain from a small fracture unless an X-ray is taken. ∎

OPTIONS FOR MUSCULOSKELETAL PROBLEMS

It is important to follow the RICE procedure (see text) for treating a sprain. However, there are complementary treatments for sprains – and other musculoskeletal problems – that can help alleviate the symptoms or reduce the recovery time.

- Gentle massage (pp.206–09) a few days after a sprain can improve circulation to the damaged tissues, which will increase warmth in the area and help speed healing.

- Studies have indicated that acupuncture (pp.212–13) can reduce pain and swelling, and it may help speed up the healing process. Practitioners use it to treat muscle and joint pain.

- Osteopaths (pp.230–32) and chiropractors (pp.234–35) use manipulation to release stiffness from muscles and joints. Depending on your posture or occupational activities, which may contribute to the problem, they may suggest exercises.

- A homeopath (pp.196–201) may use *Arnica* or *Ruta* to help an injury heal, *Rhus toxicodendron* for joints that are stiff on first movement and *Bryonia* for pain made worse by movement.

- Many complementary practitioners attribute long-term inflammatory problems in joints to diet, and research does suggest this link for some people with rheumatoid arthritis.

Strains

Fibres in a muscle or a tendon, which attaches muscle to a bone, may be overstretched or even torn. This type of injury is called a strain. Pain, tenderness and swelling may occur in the affected area.

Muscles and tendons are most at risk of strain when they are cold and tense, particularly as we age. Injuries normally occur when a vigorous movement is made too quickly. People who exercise too energetically without first warming up are particularly vulnerable to strains. Exercising with the wrong technique or poor equipment, especially footwear, or on uneven or hard surfaces, also makes limbs liable to strain. Some people have a mechanical imbalance, such as unequal leg lengths, which can cause the body to compensate in a way that makes them prone to injury.

If a muscle is overstretched, it can become tense and sore and go into spasm. Because muscle spasm restricts circulation, a vicious circle of pain and spasm can build up. Most joints are surrounded and protected by muscles. Because joints are easily injured, tendons and muscles are also prone to injury.

Because muscles need blood to provide oxygen for them to contract, they contain a large number of blood vessels. These bleed if muscle tissue is actually torn, but there is usually no bruising to be seen unless the skin has been damaged too.

FROM ACUTE TO CHRONIC

Strains are either the result of a sudden, violent force to a muscle and are called "acute" or develop over a long period of time and are known as "chronic". The least damaging of acute sprains are caused by a minor injury such as catching your thigh on a desk edge. A few muscle fibres are torn and there may be a small amount of bruising. A harder blow or stretch of the muscle or tendon results in more fibres being torn. You may be able to feel a bump, which is made up of liquid and blood, around the injury.

A more severe strain may require a visit to the hospital to check for fractures. You will probably be in considerable pain and the area will swell and look extremely bruised within a few hours. If the injury is to a leg or ankle, crutches may be useful.

A complete rupture is the most severe type of acute strain. A popping sound is often heard if a tendon has ruptured. If it is a muscle, the two ends will separate and you will see two bulges with a gap in the middle. The injury is likely to be excruciatingly painful with considerable

WHAT IS TENDONITIS?

Tendonitis is an inflammation that is often caused by simple overuse. The Achilles tendon at the back of the ankle and the tendons at the wrist are commonly affected by this injury, which may or may not cause swelling. You may be able to hear the inflamed tendon squeaking in its groove when you move it.

Achilles tendon damage is often caused by running downhill or uphill excessively. It may also occur in people who have recently changed their gym shoes if the heel of the shoe rubs the tendon during exercise.

Treatment involves applying ice for 15–20 minutes several times a day. Rest is essential. After the pain disappears, exercises that gently stretch the tendon are beneficial.

bruising and swelling, as well as muscle spasm around the area. You will need hospital attention followed by physiotherapy treatment.

Poor posture, mechanical imbalances and occupational overuse can all put muscle groups under long-term, or chronic, strain. If muscles become strained and tense in this way, they may be tender most of the time, and they can sometimes cause pain. Most neck and shoulder pain and tension headaches are caused in this way.

Generally, muscles repair more quickly than tendons. This is because of the large blood supply which constantly feeds muscles with nutrients and healing agents. Tendons may form knots of tough tissue called adhesions during healing, which can reduce their stretchability and cause problems later on. Physiotherapists can offer advice and rehabilitation exercises to help prevent this from occurring.

OTHER CONDITIONS

A stress fracture is simply a hairline fracture, commonly in a lower leg bone, and is usually caused by repeated stress such as training on hard surfaces or running long distances. You will probably have one or more tender spots along the shin bone. Most stress fractures mend after three to six weeks' rest, but severe ones may need to be immobilized in plaster. Diagnosis can only be confirmed from an X-ray.

Another form of strain is called a shin splint. The term covers many conditions, but often refers to soreness along the front of the lower leg. The pain may indicate a stress fracture. Shin splints can be caused by inflamed tendons in the leg, or by swelling of the periosteum, the thin tissue that covers the bone and provides a soft surface to which the tendons are attached.

TREATMENT

Whatever the cause, treatment for acute strains is the same: resting the injured area, applying ice wrapped in a thin wet cloth for 15–20 minutes at a time and applying moist heat such as steam all help to alleviate pain. If the condition continues, you may need to take an anti-inflammatory drug.

Chronic strains should be treated by a physiotherapist, sports massage therapist, osteopath (see pp.230–32) or chiropractor (see pp.234–35). Exercises may be recommended to improve posture or other mechanical problems. ∎

PROVOKING A STRAIN

When a muscle contracts it pulls on a bone – and also on the tendon that joins the two – which moves the limb. A strain is most likely to occur when a sudden force stretches the muscles or tendon. For example, playing tennis can cause "tennis elbow" because straining the forearm muscles inflames the tendon that attaches them to the humerus, the upper arm bone. (Tennis elbow does not always arise from playing tennis.)

Humerus

Tendon

Ulna

Muscle

Forearm

CAUTION

Repetitive strain injury should be treated as soon as possible. Some researchers believe that, if left untreated, the condition may lead to permanent tissue damage.

Wearing a supportive wrist brace relieves the symptoms of repetitive strain injury. If you operate a computer, try to limit your use of the mouse by becoming familiar with short-cut keystrokes, and make sure you take a brief rest from the keyboard every 20 minutes. During these rest breaks, you can also help your back by standing up and stretching.

Repetitive strain injury

The subject of several court cases by employees against employers, repetitive strain injury (RSI) affects many manually skilled workers who perform – as the name of the condition suggests – rapid repetitive tasks.

The term repetitive strain injury is loosely applied to a range of work-related disorders affecting the forearm, wrist and hand, and occasionally the shoulders and neck. It often involves chronic strain of the forearm muscles, which move the wrist and fingers.

Symptoms vary. Some people have an aching at work that clears up overnight or at weekends. Others experience an ache that develops during the day and does not resolve fully without several weeks' rest. Still others suffer persistent pain that takes months or years to improve.

People who work on production lines or use keyboards continuously may develop this condition if their muscles become tense, their working posture is poor or they cannot control their own work rate. Excess work load, poor time management, inappropriate work station setup and uncomfortable repetitive tasks may all be involved. Problems are often triggered by a change in the work situation such as a different keyboard.

A common form of the condition is tenosynovitis, in which the covering of the tendon in the wrist becomes inflamed. This makes it difficult for the tendon to move in the small channels in the wrist.

CHANGE AND REST

Repetitive strain injury can be cured, but treatment of the immediate problem must be accompanied by changes in the way you work to prevent a recurrence.

Complete rest is the priority if the problem is caused by acute tenosynovitis. Applying ice for 15–20 minutes several times a day and anti-inflammatory drugs may help. The wrists may have to be splinted for two to three days to prevent movement. Once the inflammation is curbed, start exercising the area with advice from a physiotherapist.

When you return to work, correct your seated posture. Your arms and wrists should be in line with the desk or work surface, at 90 degrees to the floor, so adjust your chair height accordingly. Use a wrist rest to ensure your wrists are level with your hands. Feet should be flat on the floor – use a footstool if necessary – with knees making a right angle with the floor. Your chair should support your lower back, with your shoulders relaxed. ∎

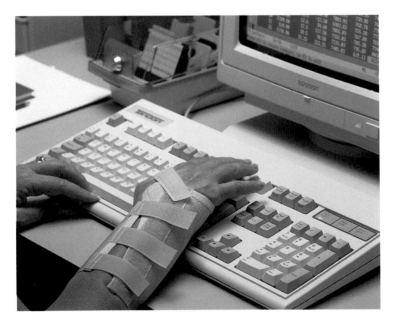

Muscle cramps

Cramps occur when a single muscle or a group of them suddenly goes into contraction. This causes sharp pain, which wears off only as the contraction eases.

Cramps are caused by various factors. The most common one occurs during exercise, which can lead to the muscle having insufficient chemicals for it to work properly. When you work a muscle, the cells burn blood sugar at a faster rate. The sugar combines with oxygen from the blood, and through complex chemical processes that take place in the muscle cells, the energy is used as the muscle contracts. The more vigorously or the longer you exercise, the faster this process must become to cope with the increasing demands of the muscles. If the muscle cannot deal with this process quickly enough to keep up with its energy requirements, lactic acid starts to be produced.

Lactic acid can produce energy, but it is inefficient. If you continue exercising, the acid builds up faster than it can be broken down. This causes normal muscle contractions to stop and triggers the characteristic burning sensation, seizure and pain of a cramp. A cramped, tense muscle will not allow proper blood flow through it, so the lactic acid can build up even more.

A cramp can also be triggered by losing salt and fluids, which alter the electrical balance involved in triggering muscle action. This loss can be caused by a high fever, excessive sweating in hot weather or prolonged exercise.

TREATING A CRAMP

To alleviate a cramp, you should stop exercising if you are doing so and try to gently stretch the affected muscles. This may make the cramp feel worse at first, but it will gradually improve.

You can massage the area to increase the supply of blood to the muscles. Applying heat or taking a warm bath will also encourage blood to flow. Be careful not to make the bath too hot or expose yourself to high temperatures too quickly; sudden change can put pressure on circulatory and temperature control systems.

Drink plenty of water to keep your body hydrated, especially when exercising in hot weather. Prolonged sweating may require replacing salt along with fluids.

You can try to prevent cramps by eating healthily to provide your body with the nutrients that improve the chemical efficiency of muscles. In addition, the fitter you are, the more oxygen your body can supply to your muscles and the less likely you are to suffer from cramp. ∎

RESTLESS LEG SYNDROME

About 15 percent of the population suffers from restless leg syndrome, which causes tickling, burning, prickling and aching sensations in the leg muscles. It is usually worse at night, and stress and large intakes of caffeine increase symptoms.

There is no single cure, but you can experiment with cooling or heating the legs, as well as gentle calf stretches and massaging the calves. Avoid stimulants, such as coffee, exercise and heavy meals, before going to bed. Try a relaxation routine (p.65) or yoga. As a last resort, your doctor can prescribe drugs.

CAUTION

If you think you have sprained your knee, follow the standard treatment – rest, ice, compression and elevation. However, if the joint feels unstable, if you cannot straighten the knee or if it is noticeably swollen, go to the doctor – you may have ruptured a ligament or torn a cartilage.

The ligaments in the knee and the discs of cartilage inside the joint and at the ends of the bones are the tissues often damaged during an awkward fall. You can manage without one of the cruciate ligaments, but if the knee keeps giving way, your doctor may suggest reconstruction surgery.

Knee injuries

The knee is a complex structure with many moving parts. It can be damaged in a number of ways, particularly in sports such as football, running and skiing, where the knee may be subject to sudden twisting.

One common knee injury is tearing of the cartilage. It can be caused by arthritis or by a twisting fall. In this type of injury, pain is usually on the inside front of the knee and the leg is hard to straighten and walk on and swells up.

Treatment involves 10 to 14 days' rest with the knee bandaged. If the cartilage has been dislodged, the knee may suddenly lock and unlock. In such cases, the cartilage may need to be removed under a general anaesthetic. Either way, gradual exercise helps mobilize the knee.

LIGAMENT DAMAGE

One of many ligaments in the knee, the tibial collateral ligament runs down the inside of your knee close to the skin. It is usually damaged or torn by an impact that forces the leg outward such as in a football tackle. In older patients, the injury can be the result of an old strain or bone degeneration. Initially, you will probably be able to walk comfortably, but within an hour the pain will become more severe and increase with time and the joint will swell. Treat it by following the standard RICE procedure (see pp.40–41).

Anterior and posterior cruciate ligaments form a cross within the knee joint. The posterior cruciate is commonly damaged in road traffic accidents where the knee hits the dashboard, thrusting the lower bone backward into the thigh.

Severe injury needs hospital attention. Diagnosis is usually made by inserting an arthroscope – a tiny camera on the end of a needle – into the knee. Whether surgical reconstruction is needed depends on how far the stability of the knee is affected.

"RUNNER'S KNEE"

The key symptom of runner's knee (patellofemoral stress syndrome) is an aching around the knee cap, especially when going up and down stairs. It results when the knee cap does not follow its usual smooth route between the upper and lower leg but swerves off course. The cause is an unequal pull on the knee cap because of a relative weakness of the muscles on the inside front of the thigh. The cure involves exercises to strengthen this muscle group, and these can be recommended by a physiotherapist. ∎

THE KNEE JOINT

Femur

Posterior cruciate ligament

Anterior cruciate ligament

Medial meniscus cartilage

Tibia

Fibular collateral ligament

Tibial collateral ligament

Fibula

CAUTION

In most cases, bursitis will settle without medication as long as the area is rested. However, it is important to treat infected bursae quickly to prevent the infection from spreading into the bloodstream, causing the serious condition of septicaemia (blood poisoning).

Bursitis

Bursae are small fluid-filled sacs that act as cushions between bones and muscles or tendons. The sacs prevent the tendons or muscles becoming worn as they rub over bony surfaces. We are born with some of these bursae already in place, but others may develop in response to new or daily friction. If they become inflamed, the result is bursitis.

The protective "cushions" between bone and muscle or tendon can become inflamed through a variety of stimuli, including unaccustomed activity or exercise, ill-fitting shoes, a gouty deposit or inflammatory conditions such as rheumatoid arthritis. Germs entering the bloodstream can also cause bursitis, as can a severe bump to an area with a bursa.

Bursitis can occur in any age group but is more common in older people. One of the most common sites is the knee. Susceptible people are those who spend a lot of time kneeling down, perhaps gardening or cleaning – hence the term

"housemaid's knee". Another common site is the elbow. Students who prop themselves up with their elbows for long periods are particularly vulnerable. Sports people may suffer from bursitis of the Achilles tendon due to shoe pressure.

Treatment depends on the reason for the inflammation. If it is caused by mechanical damage, such as friction from shoes, bruising or unaccustomed exercise, the best treatment is simply protection of the area and rest. Applying ice and taking anti-inflammatory drugs may help speed up the healing process and reduce inflammation. If there is no improvement after three to four days, you should visit your doctor, who may give you an anti-inflammatory injection.

INFECTION AS A CAUSE

Bursitis due to infection is treated somewhat like a boil under the skin. If the infection is mild, a dose of antibiotics may be all that is needed. However, an advanced infection may require surgery, under either a general or local anaesthetic, to drain the pus from the infection. This gives the body a chance to deal with the rest of the infection in its own way. The wound may take a few weeks to heal. Later on, you may need another small operation to cut away the bursa if it has thickened too much from the infection and there is a risk of it recurring. ∎

BURSITIS OF THE KNEE

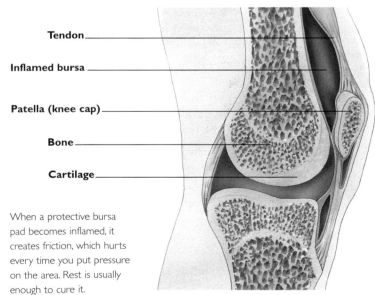

Tendon

Inflamed bursa

Patella (knee cap)

Bone

Cartilage

When a protective bursa pad becomes inflamed, it creates friction, which hurts every time you put pressure on the area. Rest is usually enough to cure it.

SEE ALSO
Chronic pain   64–65
Osteopathy   230–232
Chiropractic   234–235

CAUTION

Back pain accompanied by fever or urinary problems or that is not relieved by lying down might be due to causes other than muscles and joints. Seek medical advice if it persists.

Most types of back pain are not serious and correct themselves before you feel the need to go to the doctor. Sometimes, the cause is specific, with the pain located in a particular region of the back.

Back pain

One of the most persistent of common ailments, symptoms of back pain range from mild to excruciating, from short term to chronic. Lower back pain – or lumbago – is responsible for millions of lost working days, not to mention its depressing effects on morale and mood. Poor posture or awkward movements are the most common cause.

The human spine is made up of 26 bones called vertebrae. Each is connected to the other by a series of small joints, muscles and ligaments and by intervertebral discs (pads of cartilage). The discs separate the vertebrae and prevent them from rubbing against each other, and they also act as shock absorbers.

All vertebrae have a canal running through them. Above the waist, the canal contains the spinal cord. Nerves from the spinal cord branch off, leaving the spinal column between each pair of vertebrae and spreading deep into the muscles and joints of the body. Nerves also branch off from the spinal cord and continue into the canal below it. Nerves running out of the spinal column control movement and posture and regulate involuntary processes such as digestion. Those running into the spinal column bring in our sense impressions, including the sensation of pain.

To allow movement in all directions while maintaining a strong upright stance, parts of the vertebral column are more flexible. For example, bones in the neck allow the head to rotate and nod up and down, while bones in the lower back accommodate bending forward, backward and sideways at the waist. As a result, these areas are more prone to injury.

COMMON BACK INJURIES

One typical form of back pain is caused by strains of a muscle or tendon or sprains of a ligament supporting the spine, which are usually caused by bad lifting practices or overzealous exercise. If structures are torn or inflamed after severe injury, there will be pain, but sometimes pain is also caused by trapped or irritated nerves.

A muscle spasm is, by far, the most common cause of acute backache. One

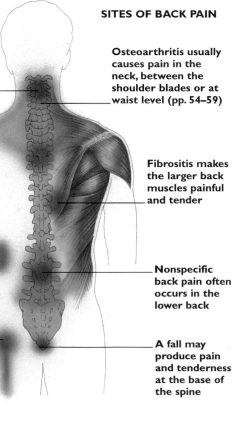

SITES OF BACK PAIN

Whiplash affects the back of the neck

Osteoarthritis usually causes pain in the neck, between the shoulder blades or at waist level (pp. 54–59)

Fibrositis makes the larger back muscles painful and tender

An infection of the kidney can give pain in the loin (pp.146–47)

Nonspecific back pain often occurs in the lower back

Sciatica sends pain shooting from the buttock down the back of the leg and into the foot

A fall may produce pain and tenderness at the base of the spine

typical injury in this category is whiplash. Because the neck is flexible and the head heavy, sudden acceleration or car stops of the kind that occur in a road traffic accident cause the neck to jerk violently back and forth, overstretching the muscles in both directions. Muscles and ligaments may be damaged and torn, and the victim may need the support of an orthopaedic collar for a period of time. However, sudden or clumsy movements of the neck or back can cause a muscle spasm that will be painful, even without inflammation or tearing. When this happens, the muscles surrounding the damaged area can seize up, a reflex action that is intended to prevent further strain or injury. This stiffens the affected part of the back and causes further pain.

Wear and tear on the small joints that stack the vertebrae on top of each other may cause the development of arthritis in the spine. Back pain from this cause is usually worse when you are sitting or standing for any length of time, but gentle stretching and strengthening exercises can be helpful.

TYPICAL CAUSES

Triggers for back pain are many, but the cause is usually simple – any movement or series of actions that places abnormal strain or loading on the spine. Back pain may arise from one sudden overload such as from a fall that jars the spine or from lifting a heavy box. Or the cause may be unaccustomed or cumulative stress; for example, repeatedly stretching over a desk at an awkward angle, carrying a heavy suitcase or bending to sandpaper a skirting board. Kidney infection can also spark off pain in the side of the back.

You will be more prone to back pain if you habitually sit or stand awkwardly or slouch. Bad posture shifts your weight into the wrong muscles, and over the years they tense up while others get weaker. These factors can set the scene for muscle and tendon strains, pinched nerves and disc damage.

WHO IS AT RISK?

Simple back pain can affect anyone at any age. Nurses, manual labourers, office employees or homeworkers are all at risk,

PROLAPSED – OR SLIPPED – DISC

If the casing of one of the discs in the spinal cord splits, some of its soft centre can protrude from the casing and press on the adjacent nerves. This injury – known as a prolapsed, or slipped, disc – can be caused by a sudden strain, such as lifting a heavy object or stretching awkwardly in a sport, and it most often occurs in men under 50 years old.

A prolapsed disc can cause sudden sharp pain felt along the path of the nerve that lasts for weeks, for example, in sciatica. It can be treated with anti-inflammatory drugs but may require surgery if the nerve is trapped.

Vertebra

Spinal nerve

Normal disc

Prolapsed disc: the soft centre bulges out and presses on a nearby nerve

Spinal cord

CAUTION

A large disc herniation that causes severe nerve pressure can interfere with the bowel and bladder functions, produce sensory loss in the legs and feet and may paralyze muscles. Urgent specialist help must be sought.

often because of bad lifting practice: bending over to pick up a heavy object, particularly if it is accompanied with twisting of the body, often triggers back pain. Even children consistently carrying a heavy satchel on one shoulder can strain their backs. Those who are excessively overweight are more frequent sufferers, as are pregnant women because their body has to cope with changes in weight and balance.

Players of sports such as golf, tennis and squash can be particularly prone to back pain because of all the twisting and turning they do. Rowers, rugby players and martial arts enthusiasts are even more susceptible because their activities involve not only swivelling but also heavy loading. No matter what sport you play, failing to warm up and overextending yourself for your level of fitness is asking for back trouble.

People with serious medical conditions such as rheumatoid arthritis, osteoporosis, ankylosing spondylitis (inflammation of the spinal ligaments) and secondary cancer of the bone can experience severe

back pain. Muscle tension associated with mental stress, depression and continual anxiety can also cause backache.

TREATING PAIN EARLY ON

Most attacks of acute back pain settle in a week or two. It can be difficult to identify an exact cause, even for a specialist. A muscle injury causes pain at the time of the injury; in this case, ice packs may help. A muscle spasm usually builds up more slowly and will probably be helped by applying warmth. If there is much initial muscle spasm in the early stages – the first 12 to 24 hours – it is best to rest in a comfortable position and take mild painkillers such as over-the-counter anti-inflammatory drugs.

Bed rest used to be recommended for back pain, but it is now known to be counterproductive because muscles tense up and eventually get weaker. Research suggests that, after an initial rest, back pain will probably resolve itself more quickly if you resume gentle activity and gradually increase what you do. Physiotherapists, osteopaths and chiropractors

TIPS TO PREVENT BACK PAIN

It is much better to prevent back strain in the first place than to go through the painful and lengthy process of setting it to rights. There are simple ways to look after your back.

Do not bend over or twist your body when lifting a heavy object (or gardening). Instead, squat down with a straight back, then lift the object using your legs.

Distribute heavy loads such as shopping or suitcases evenly between both hands. You can also carry items in a rucksack. Avoid using one large, heavy suitcase – the weight will pull your spine off balance.

usually recommend simple stretching exercises in the short term to help get the back moving again and walking, cycling and swimming to help strengthen the muscles in the medium term. Swimming is especially useful because the water supports the weight of your body and prevents you from putting excessive strain on the muscles.

TONING UP

As soon as your back feels better, ask your doctor or physical therapist to advise you on exercises to tone up muscles in both your back and stomach. It is important to do both sets of exercises, because if you strengthen back muscles without building up the abdominal muscles as a counter-balance, your back may be pulled out of alignment. If you really must return to normal activity while you still have pain, aids such as corsets may temporarily take strain off the injury and provide support.

Most simple back pain recovers within a month, but if in that time you are not substantially better, get medical advice. Physical therapy and exercises are all that is usually needed to help. Even prolapsed discs tend to recover spontaneously, although it can take several months. In a severe case, surgery may be necessary to relieve pressure on a nerve. Tests are reserved for severe or unusual types of back pain. They include X-rays and CT scans to look more closely at the bones and tissues.

LONG-TERM CARE

Any practitioner you go to for treatment will want to know the details of your pain. It is a good idea to keep a record of the type of pain (for example, dull or sharp), where it is located, when it started, what might have caused it, whether you have been ill previously and whether you have had difficulty passing water, digestive disorders or gynaecological problems before the pain started.

In the long term, a programme of exercise or physical therapy is advisable. Massage (see pp.206–09), manipulation, heat treatment and hydrotherapy (see pp.236–37) can all be helpful for persistent mechanical back pain. ■

When sitting in a chair, make sure your back is well supported, particularly at work. Sit up straight, with your lower back resting against the chair's back.

Do not push a large heavy object in front of you with your arms – this puts great strain on the back. Instead, lean your back against the object and use your legs to do the pushing.

SEE ALSO

Strains	42–43
Repetitive strain injury	44
Back pain	48–51
Osteopathy	230–232
Chiropractic	234–235

Shoulder and neck pain

The powerful muscles in the shoulders provide great flexibility, but they can make the area susceptible to injury. Aches and pains in the neck and shoulders can also be caused by poor posture or disease.

One of the most common types of shoulder problem is "rotator cuff" injury, in which one or more muscles in the complex group that surround the shoulder joint become strained or bruised in a fall or become tense and painful through overuse. There are several bursae in the joint, as well as tendons, which can become irritated, and the lining of the shoulder joint itself can also become inflamed and swollen.

Neck pain is often caused by muscle strain from bad posture or tension rather than a specific injury. Conditions such as osteoporosis (see p.179) and osteoarthritis (see pp.54–59) can also cause it.

A physiotherapist, chiropractor or osteopath will be able to tell which

structure is involved and suggest a treatment programme. Treatment for almost all shoulder and neck pain follows a similar pattern. If it is a soft tissue injury, pain generally resolves itself without treatment after a few days of rest and painkillers. Follow the RICE procedure (see p.41) for an acute muscle strain, and use a sling if you find it difficult to avoid using your arm. Anti-inflammatory drugs such as ibuprofen can help if the pain is sharp. When the pain has eased start gentle exercise to avoid the stiffening that often occurs after injury and underuse.

If the pain is prolonged beyond three to four days, your doctor may suggest a steroid injection to relax the tendon. If the neck or shoulder pain is a long-term problem, physiotherapy, osteopathy or chiropractic treament may be helpful.

POLYMYALGIA RHEUMATICA

This condition, with symptoms of pain and stiffness in the shoulders, neck, back and arms, has long been the bane of many older women. Affecting three times more women than men, it is a strange condition in that there is little physical evidence of a problem in the muscle, although it has been linked to arterial disorders.

Pain is often severe on waking or after sitting for some time. There is also usually a general lack of feeling well, low-grade fever, anaemia and loss of appetite. However, the condition responds quickly and dramatically to steroid therapy. ∎

EASING STIFFNESS

If bad posture or awkward sitting causes stiffness, try applying heat from a hot water bottle. A hot bath, liniment rub or massage can also help loosen the muscles. A doctor may recommend drugs that relax the muscles, or you may need to use a neck collar for support for some days. Physiotherapists can often help relieve neck pain through manipulation.

SEE ALSO
Arthritis   54–59

Gout

Typically, gout has been thought of as a disease of those who overindulge in rich food and alcohol. These do not help the symptoms, but they are not the main cause of this painful condition, which is a type of arthritis.

CAUTION

If gout is left untreated, the uric acid crystals may spread to other joints and tissues, as well as damage the kidneys and trigger the formation of kidney stones. If you think you have this condition, seek medical advice promptly.

The internal mechanism of the joints can be affected by gout. A joint is made up of bones contained inside a capsule. The tissues of this capsule manufacture a lubricating fluid – called synovial fluid – which helps the joint move smoothly. The fluid also feeds the tissues inside the capsule such as the cartilage that separates the bones. Gout is triggered when too much uric acid is produced by the body and uric acid crystals form inside the capsule.

Gout often strikes the big toe first. If left untreated, it causes excruciating pain that may persist for days or weeks. Attacks recur with increasing frequency until the condition is constantly present. The crystals may spread to other joints such as the knees, elbows and knuckles, as well as to tissues. They may be deposited in the skin – the outer ear is prone to this.

Small crystals of uric acid form inside the joint capsule when the kidney does not excrete the chemical fast enough. The crystals, magnified 30 times below, irritate the tissues, causing inflammation and pain.

About 75 percent of gout is caused by an inherited abnormality that prevents the proper elimination of uric acid, explaining why gout tends to run in families. Gout is more common in men and rare in women before the menopause and in children.

Eating certain protein-rich foods, particularly ones high in purine – such as organ meats, fatty fish, shellfish, spinach, asparagus and most dried beans – can raise uric acid levels in the blood and trigger the crystallization process, as can dehydration in hot climates, illness, excessive tiredness or injury. People with kidney disease may have high levels of uric acid. However, not everyone with apparently high levels of uric acid will suffer from gout, and some people may develop it at normal blood levels.

DIAGNOSIS AND TREATMENT

Doctors base diagnosis on blood tests that measure uric acid levels and the analysis of fluid from the inflamed joint for crystals. These help rule out other joint problems such as rheumatoid arthritis or infection.

Treatment is usually with nonsteroidal anti-inflammatory drugs (NSAIDs), as early as possible. Colchicine, a drug produced from crocuses, is used if stomach problems prevent the use of NSAIDs. If you have frequent attacks of gout or high levels of uric acid, you may be offered a preventive drug called allopurinol, which lowers the blood levels of uric acid. Dietary change may be an important part of treatment. ∎

Arthritis

More than 100 different diseases that cause pain, swelling and limited movement in the joints and connective tissue throughout the body are referred to as arthritis. It is usually chronic, meaning that it is unlikely to go away, but effective treatments enable many people with arthritis to lead full lives with relatively little pain or disability.

The main symptoms of arthritis are joint pain, stiffness, inability to move a joint normally and sometimes swelling that last more than two weeks. Specific causes are not yet known for most types of arthritis and theories vary. The two most prevalent forms are osteoarthritis and rheumatoid arthritis.

OSTEOARTHRITIS

A common degenerative joint disease, osteoarthritis occurs when the cartilage that cushions the ends of the bones in a joint deteriorates. This causes pain and loss of movement as bone rubs against bone. The disease usually affects middle-aged and older people. Symptoms can range from mild to severe and occur in the hands and in weight-bearing joints, such as the hips, knees, feet and back, but normally only one or two of these sites are affected.

Although increasing age is a leading risk factor, research has shown that osteo-arthritis is not an inevitable part of aging and that a variety of factors contribute to the condition. Being overweight, for example, may lead to osteoarthritis of the knees, while people who have experienced joint injuries through sport, repetitive movements in their job or accidents also have an increased risk. However, normal physical activity does not cause arthritis – you cannot wear joints out. Family history appears to play a role in the development of osteoarthritis, and allergic reactions to certain foods may possibly contribute to the pain and damage.

One theory on the overall cause of osteoarthritis is that cartilage cells release an abnormal form of enzymes, which cause cartilage breakdown and joint destruction. Another theory is that some people are born with excessive enzyme production, defective cartilage or slight imperfections in the way their joints fit together. These abnormalities can cause the cartilage to break down as a person grows older.

Diagnosis is based on the history of symptoms and the physical examination. X-rays are used to confirm diagnosis: most

HEALTHY JOINT

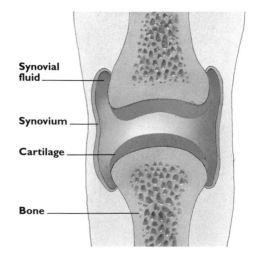

Synovial fluid

Synovium

Cartilage

Bone

people over the age of 60 show evidence of osteoarthritis, but for unknown reasons only one-third have symptoms.

RHEUMATOID ARTHRITIS

You should not confuse rheumatism, which simply means muscular pain, with rheumatoid arthritis, the more severe and disabling form of arthritis. In this disease the joint lining, known as the synovium, becomes inflamed because of an abnormal reaction of the immune system. The inflammation alone causes pain, warmth, stiffness, redness and visible outer swelling, but the inflamed joint lining can also invade and damage bone and cartilage. This causes the affected joint to lose its shape and alignment and results in loss of movement, increased pain and, in some cases, destruction of the joint.

Rheumatoid arthritis is a systemic disease, meaning it can affect many joints as well as other organs. It usually begins in middle age – but can start earlier – and affects three times more women than men. The root cause of rheumatoid arthritis is not yet apparent. What is known is that for some reason the body's immune system starts to perceive healthy joint tissue as "foreign" and attacks it, causing the inflammation and subsequent joint damage. It is thought that inflammatory cells released by the body's immune system produce an enzyme that digests bone and cartilage.

Researchers suspect that a virus may be the trigger for rheumatoid arthritis in people who have a genetic, inherited predisposition to the disease. Around 80 percent of adult sufferers have a protein known as the "rheumatoid factor" in their blood. However, this can also be present in people who do not develop the disease. About 10 percent of people who develop rheumatoid arthritis experience a spontaneous and complete recovery up to two years after its diagnosis.

Doctors base diagnosis on the pattern of symptoms, medical history, physical examination and tests, including those that indicate the presence of inflammatory activity and the rheumatoid factor. Early in the disease, people may notice general fatigue, soreness, stiffness and aching. Pain usually occurs symmetrically in the same joints on both sides of the body and starts in the hands or feet. However, rheumatoid arthritis can also affect wrists,

JOINT WITH OSTEOARTHRITIS

JOINT WITH RHEUMATOID ARTHRITIS

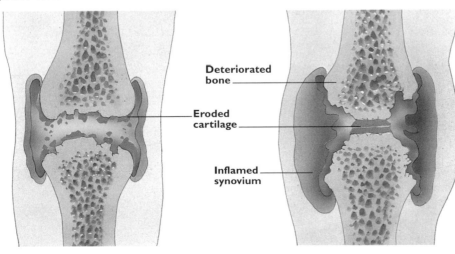

Deteriorated bone

Eroded cartilage

Inflamed synovium

In a healthy joint (facing page) cartilage cushions the ends of the bones, and a membrane known as the synovium lines the cavity of the joint and lubricates it with synovial fluid. If cartilage deteriorates over the years, the result is osteoarthritis, in which the bones rub painfully together. In rheumatoid arthritis, the joint swells because the synovium thickens and secretes excess fluid.

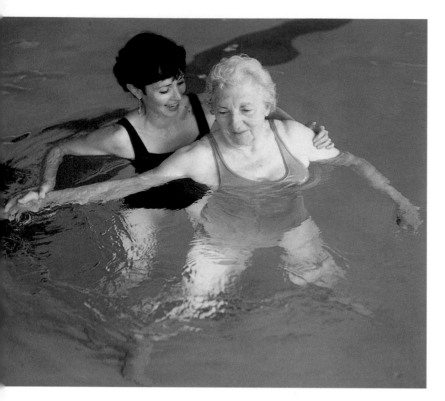

Hydrotherapy is a good symptom reliever for arthritis. Excercising in the swimming pool allows the water to take your body weight, so you can stretch joints without putting pressure on them.

elbows, shoulders, neck, knees, hips and ankles. Other symptoms include lumps called rheumatoid nodules, which develop under the skin in areas that receive pressure such as the elbows.

TREATMENT

Although there is not yet a total cure for arthritis, much can be done to reduce its impact on everyday life. The key to treatment is early diagnosis and a plan tailored to individual needs. The focus is on reducing swelling, relieving pain and stiffness and maintaining normal joint function. Most treatment programmes for arthritis include a combination of medication, exercise, heat and cold therapy, rest, joint protection techniques and, sometimes, surgery.

Drug therapies for arthritis are divided into two categories: those that ease symptoms and those that work on the disease itself. The role of drugs in

osteoarthritis is predominantly to relieve symptoms during inflammatory flare ups.

Painkillers such as aspirin and nonsteroidal anti-inflammatory drugs (NSAIDs) such as ibuprofen are the most common drugs recommended. These reduce inflammation and so lessen pain, swelling and stiffness. You should be careful if you are taking one of these medications as stomach problems, such as ulcers, are a common side effect. Corticosteroid injections also reduce inflammation, and muscle relaxants can help to prevent pain from spasms and may be used along with physiotherapy.

HELP FOR RHEUMATOID ARTHRITIS

Painkillers, NSAIDs and corticosteroid drugs decrease pain, stiffness and swelling in people who have rheumatoid arthritis. There is also a variety of drugs available, which, if given early on, may slow its progress or lessen damage. These drugs include sulphasalazine, gold, penicillamine and chloroquine (which is more often used to prevent malaria).

Little is known about how these drugs work, and it can take some time to find the best drug and the ideal way of taking it. Drugs that block the body's immune system response, such as azathioprine and methotrexate, can help. These powerful drugs are particularly useful in severe and disabling conditions where their benefits outweigh potential side effects.

Rheumatic rubs and liniments such as wintergreen or tiger balm can give temporary relief from pain. So, too, can heat lamps, hot-water bottles and the time-honoured practice of hydrotherapy. Rubbing on creams that contain anti-inflammatory ingredients around the inflamed joints and tendons can also provide temporary relief.

LIVING WITH ARTHRITIS

Regular exercise can help keep joints flexible. Combined with a healthy diet, it can also keep weight down, which will prevent extra stress on weight-bearing joints. Be careful to avoid injury or undue strain by using supports such as wrist or knee bands or built-up shoes.

Occupational therapists can help find ways to adapt your life to your abilities. These include using walking sticks and accessing the huge range of gadgets to help with everyday tasks such as opening tins or turning on bath taps.

There are other treatments available. For example, studies of an extract from the New Zealand green-lipped mussel are encouraging. Both types of arthritis (but especially osteoarthritis) sometimes respond to acupuncture, especially if the treatment takes place early in the development of the disease. There is some scientific evidence suggesting that low-antigen diets (which are difficult to stick to because they exclude many of the foods we take for granted in our society) can in the long run be of great benefit for some patients with rheumatoid arthritis. Some research suggests that capsules of fish oil may help reduce inflammatory processes.

The weather can affect the symptoms of arthritis. Warm settled weather makes sufferers feel better, while cool damp weather, with many changes in barometric pressure, is uncomfortable for some with arthritic joints. It is thought that this is because the fluctuations in atmospheric pressure affect the pressure inside the damaged joint, squeezing exposed nerves.

SURGICAL REPAIRS

In some cases of severe arthritis, surgery may be performed to repair the joints. For most people with this condition, the relief of pain is the major reason for surgery. It may also be necessary to improve movement and the ability to use the joints, or it may simply make deformed joints look better, especially those in the hand.

There are three main types of surgery for arthritis. Osteotomy is an operation in which the bone next to a painful joint is cut then refixed in a slightly different position. It is often used for knee and foot problems. Synovectomy entails removing the synovium (joint membrane) if it is so inflamed that it stops the joint working or damages tendons or ligaments. An operation known as arthrodesis involves grafting, nailing or wiring two parts of a joint together so that it cannot move but no longer hurts. This is sometimes used to lessen the pain of a joint already restricted in movement.

Hand surgery is difficult and delicate. Surgeons can carry out many operations on the hand, including tendon release and repair, decompressing trapped nerves, fusing a painful wrist and replacing small

CAUTION

Complete cures do not exist for any type of arthritis, but there are many unproven treatments available. Following the old wives' remedy of wearing a copper bracelet won't cure your arthritis, but it may provide anti-inflammatory properties from the small amounts of copper absorbed by the skin and it won't harm you. However, you should avoid any untested invasive remedies – ones that call for swallowing or injecting. If in doubt about using a form of treatment, you should consult your doctor.

TAKING EXERCISE

Finding the right balance between resting an arthritic joint and exercising it can help you manage arthritis. While inflamed joints need rest during a flare up, too little movement allows them to stiffen and muscles to become weak.

- A general rule of thumb is to take a break from exercise while inflammation is at its worst, but to be active when it is not.

- You should try to put all your joints through a full range of movement at least once a day.

- Non-weight-bearing exercise in a swimming pool is ideal for arthritis sufferers, and physiotherapists can teach special exercises that maintain and improve strength, movement and function of joints.

- Physiotherapists may also offer heat or cold treatments or massage for temporary pain relief.

In the hip of a patient with rheumatoid arthritis (right), the cartilage and bone are worn away. During a hip replacement operation, surgery replaces the femur and socket in the pelvic bone with artificial implants (far right). This restores the mobility of the hip.

An artificial hip joint consists of a metal ball part that fits into a plastic hip socket.

joints. Maintaining function of the fingers is always the main concern.

For people with rheumatoid arthritis, one of the most useful operations is the removal of damaged joints at the base of the toes, which often allows the sufferer to walk again without pain.

JOINT REPLACEMENT

A more complicated surgical procedure involves removing the joint and replacing it with an artificial one. The art of joint replacement has become increasingly sophisticated both in technique and material technology, and the results are often highly successful. Hips and finger joints are the most popular candidates for replacement, but shoulders, elbows, and ankles can also be renewed.

Hip replacement is so successful that it has overtaken all other surgical procedures for hip problems. It is done when there is severe pain or disability that does not respond to other treatment. Replacing a hip can return a person to completely normal mobility.

The principles of replacement are the same whether it is a hip or a finger. The surgeon removes the socket and the ball of the joint (in the hip the natural head of the thigh bone or femur) and glues or screws a plastic socket into the hollow. He tops the natural femur with a short, angled metal shaft. The shaft ends in a smooth ball made of hard polythene or a metal alloy, which fits snugly into the socket. Depending on where in the body replacement joints are positioned, they can usually work successfully for a minimum of 15 years.

Knee replacement surgery is not yet reliably successful. The knee is the hinge that provides motion between the thigh and the lower leg. During a total knee replacement, the surgeon replaces the end of the femur, or thigh, bone with a metal shell. He also removes the end of the tibia (lower leg bone) and replaces it with a plastic piece with a metal stem. Depending on the condition of the kneecap portion of the joint, he may also add a plastic "button" to replace it. ∎

OTHER JOINT DISORDERS

Condition	Description	Who it affects	Symptoms	Treatment
Ankylosing spondylitis	Inflammation that causes the bones of the spine to fuse together.	Mainly young adult males – strong genetic tendency.	Back pain and increasing disability.	Drugs to reduce inflammation or suppress immunity, physiotherapy and exercise.
Systemic lupus erythematosus (Lupus)	Inflames and damages joints and other connective tissues throughout the body.	Autoimmune disorder affecting mostly women, especially those of childbearing age, but also some men.	Symmetrical arthritic pain in fingers, knees, elbows and ankles. Fever, fatigue, hair loss and "butterfly" rash across nose and cheeks.	Steroids and immuno-suppressive drugs.
Paget's disease	Pelvis, leg bones, lumbar spine and skull can become softened, enlarged and deformed because of rapid growth and dissolving of the bones.	Rare before the age of 40, but becomes more common in older people. Men affected more than women. There may be a genetic component.	Sometimes aching pains; often no symptoms other than visual deformity.	Calcitonin or disodium etidronate relieve pain, regulate the laying down and dissolving of bone and can reduce nerve damage from enlarged bones.
Polymyalgia rheumatica	Unknown causes. Tests on muscle and antibodies are often normal. Blood shows abnormalities in sediment levels and 40 percent of sufferers have detrimental changes in the arteries.	Affects women three times more often than men. It is uncommon before 50 years of age.	Persistent stiffness, worse on waking, in shoulders, back and neck so severe that person may not be able to get out of bed. Fever, headache, loss of appetite, malaise and temporary blindness.	Dramatic and sustained relief with steroid tablets.
Reiter's syndrome	Occurs 1–3 weeks after a chlamydia or other venereal infection or an attack of bacterial dysentery.	People who are genetically vulnerable to the infecting agent. The most common cause of arthritis in young men.	Joint inflammation usually in the knee or ankle, fever, discharge from penis or urethra and conjunctivitis.	Painkillers, NSAIDs (nonsteroidal anti-inflammatory drugs). Recurrences are common.
Psoriatic arthritis	Linked to the skin condition, psoriasis.	Six percent of people with psoriasis. Affects men and women equally, between 10–30 years old. Those with psoriasis affecting their nails are at a greater risk.	Differs from other forms of arthritis because the entire finger or toe becomes swollen rather than just a joint.	Painkillers, NSAIDs (nonsteroidal anti-inflammatory drugs). Sulphasalazine in severe cases.

CAUTION

As a rule, headaches go away on their own. The time to seek medical advice is if you develop a new kind or pattern of headaches, if the pain is unusual or if it starts suddenly. Seek professional advice immediately for a headache with the symptoms of meningitis (see facing page).

Headaches

There are few people who can claim never to have had a headache – it is one of the most common of everyday ailments. There are a multitude of causes for headaches and, once you know what sets off yours, you can avoid the triggers. A headache is usually nothing more than an inconvenience – only a tiny proportion indicate a serious disorder.

A headache does not come from the brain itself but is caused by spasms in the muscles of the head and neck. The most common cause of these muscle spasms, and of an estimated 90 percent of nonmigraine headaches, is tension.

Characterized by a tightening or pressing sensation, like a band strapped around the head, tension headaches often occur at the end of the day or when stress levels are high. They are caused by one of the body's automatic reactions to stress – sustained contraction of muscles in the face, scalp, neck and shoulders. Unlike a migraine (see pp.62–63) – and, therefore, one way of telling the two apart – the

pain of a tension headache usually affects both sides of the head and is fairly constant, although increased stress and tiredness can make it worse. A headache can linger with a dull ache and a feeling of general discomfort for an hour or two, or for as long as several days.

Headaches can be caused by physical as well as mental tension. Just as other muscles in the body become stiff and sore from exertion or awkward use, so do those in the head and neck. This type of headache is common among people who have to maintain a single position at work, such as typists and production line and computer workers.

A further cause of head pain is known as "referred pain", where the problem is in another part of the body, such as in the eyes, ears (see pp.130–31), sinuses (see pp.132–33), teeth (see pp.86–87), a misaligned jaw or strained spinal muscles (see pp.42–43). Although treatment will concentrate on the root cause of the condition, over-the-counter painkillers can be taken to ease the headache until the cause itself has been resolved.

HEADACHE TRIGGERS

Various types of trigger are thought to account for the remaining 10 percent of headaches. Low blood sugar caused by hunger or exercise, stuffy, smoky or humid atmospheres, fumes from pollution

TENSION HEADACHE

A tension headache is commonly caused by stiff muscles in the head or neck. The pain may be localized or spread around the scalp.

Area of pain

Muscle

Muscle

Muscle

Area of pain

or fragrance, changes in barometric pressure or temperature, too much or too little sleep and side effects from prescription drugs can all be culprits. Many women suffer with premenstrual headaches. Hangover headaches after drinking too much alcohol are thought to be caused by a combination of chemicals, low blood sugar and oxygen, dehydration and high carbon dioxide.

Food intolerances (see pp.274–75) and food additives can also trigger headaches. One chemical, monosodium glutamate, or MSG, a flavour enhancer often used in oriental cuisine and in many processed foods and sauces, has been given its own headache category – "Chinese restaurant" syndrome. If you have headaches triggered by this chemical, also avoid foods with "natural flavouring" on their labels.

CLUSTER HEADACHES

Unlike other types, cluster headaches affect men more frequently than women. Although a cluster headache is often mistaken for a migraine, this type of headache is in a category on its own.

Typically, there is pain behind one eye that wakes the sufferer in the early hours of every morning for up to two months. The pain intensifies after a few minutes, and the affected eye goes red and tearful and the nostril on the same side becomes either blocked or runny. Attacks last from 20 minutes to two hours. As well as being worrying, cluster headaches can drastically impair the sufferer's life. However, the anticonvulsant drug carbamazapine can be successful in treating the condition.

FINDING A CURE

The cure for most headaches is not found in a bottle of pills, but in detecting and eliminating the source of the problem. If you are enduring headaches frequently,

keep notes of the circumstances in which they arrive to help identify the cause. The key to banishing your headaches could be anything from stress-busting techniques (see pp.12–15 and pp.76–77) that help deal with tension to correcting your posture at work.

Simple over-the-counter painkillers, such as aspirin, paracetamol or ibuprofen, may be effective in dulling the pain long enough for the root cause of the headache to subside. Tension headaches are not "cured" by painkillers, but they may respond if the medicine allows tense muscles to relax. You should seek help from your medical practitioner if recurrent headaches are interfering with your life or state of mind – there may well be a simple solution.

Contrary to popular belief, headaches are seldom a symptom of serious illness; for example, they are not an early sign of a brain tumour. Although extremely high blood pressure, a rupture in a blood vessel in the brain or increased pressure inside the skull may all bring on a severe headache, you should remember that these situations rarely occur. ∎

CAUTION

Never give aspirin to a child 12 years of age or younger: it has been linked to a dangerous condition known as Reye's syndrome. Treat a fever or aches and pains with paracetamol.

RECOGNIZING MENINGITIS

Meningitis is an inflammation of the brain lining caused by a viral or bacterial infection. It is a rare illness, but bacterial meningitis can be fatal if not treated early. One of the key symptoms is a gradually developing, then constant headache felt throughout the head, which worsens when you bend forward. It is accompanied by fever, vomiting, sensitivity to light and a stiff neck.

Typical symptoms in a baby include being difficult to awake, high-pitched crying, vomiting and blotchy skin. For further details on meningitis in children, see page 183. If you suspect that you have or a member of your family has meningitis, it is important that you contact your doctor immediately or go to the casualty department of a hospital.

Migraine

Roughly 1 in 10 people suffers from migraine, which is a complex condition with a wide range of symptoms. Women are up to three times more likely to be affected than men, and as many as five percent of children endure migraines, too. Well known triggers are chocolate, cheese and oranges, but a lack of food, stress and hormones are other culprits.

An interpretation of the "aura" phase of a migraine is shown in this painting by a migraine sufferer. Some sufferers see flashing lights or shimmering specks or have blind spots for 5–20 minutes. For those who experience such auras, it usually signals that the headache will start within an hour.

Migraine attacks can be triggered by one or a combination of factors, which vary widely between individuals. The root cause of migraine is elusive. Some experts suggest that it is a vascular problem, started by the constriction of arteries supplying blood to the brain. Others believe that a neurological problem set off by abnormal brain activity may cause the arteries to close down.

Recent studies have focused on the levels of certain chemical messengers, known as neurotransmitters, in the brain, which control the brain's functions. Serotonin (5HT) is one of them. Many medicines that have been effective in preventing migraine attacks are known to block the actions of these particular chemical messengers.

THE PHASES

A migraine attack usually comes in five distinct phases. First of all, many migraine sufferers experience a premonition or warning of an attack, sometimes as much as 24 hours beforehand. These signs can include yawning without being tired, feeling fuzzy-headed, hunger, craving sweet foods or carbohydrates (often chocolate), thirst, muscle heaviness and mood changes. Some people feel on top of the world and full of energy, others are tense, irritable and depressed. Next may come the aura stage, which brings the visual symptoms of lights before the eyes sometimes associated with migraine.

The headache phase usually starts within an hour. The key difference between a migraine and a headache triggered by other causes is that the pain of a migraine is usually restricted to one side of the head. The pain develops into a throbbing, which can feel as if the head is about to burst, and is typically accompanied by feelings of nausea and extreme sensitivity to light, smell or noise. Some people feel completely muddled, unable to remember simple things such as their own telephone number. Others manage to work through an attack with the help of pain relievers.

The fourth phase is resolution of the attack, when the symptoms slowly fade away after 2 to 72 hours. About half of migraine sufferers find relief in sleeping or resting in a darkened room. Others vomit or weep profusely, but find that they feel better almost immediately after doing so.

Phase five is the aftermath: despite the relief of pain, many sufferers feel "washed out" and find they need to rest for a day or so after the attack.

TREATING MIGRAINE

Medicines can help during a migraine attack. Simple over-the-counter painkillers such as paracetamol, ibuprofen and aspirin can stop a migraine in its tracks. However, they have to be taken early in the cycle to be effective in preventing the migraine because the digestive system, which slows down during an attack, may be too slow to absorb them.

A new type of prescription medication known as 5HT antagonists can be highly effective, even when an attack is well underway. Some doctors prescribe strong painkillers and antinausea drugs to speed the action of other drugs.

If frequent migraines are significantly disrupting your life, your doctor may recommend that you take a medication, such as a beta-blocker, serotonin blocker or even an antidepressant, every day to try to prevent attacks. How these medicines work in relation to migraine is unclear, but there is some evidence that they can break the cycle.

Some types of complementary therapies, such as acupuncture and osteopathy (see pp.230–32), may help treat both acute attacks and ongoing cycles.

The most efficient way of thwarting a migraine is to discover and avoid the triggers that affect you (see box, right). However, if an attack is triggered, being alert to the warning symptoms means that you can take drugs to prevent it from fully developing. ∎

HOW A MIGRAINE OCCURS

Constricted artery

Expanded artery

For migraine sufferers, a trigger, such as chocolate, red wine or tiredness, sets off the chain of events in the body that causes a migraine. The arteries at the base of the brain constrict (above left), then expand (above right). At the same time chemicals are released and the pain of a migraine begins.

TRACING YOUR TRIGGERS

One of the most effective methods of preventing a migraine is to know what can trigger it and avoid those factors. Keep a record of your daily life over a period of months. Your diary should include a record of events next to the hour of the day; for example, what you eat and drink, what medication you take and your bowel movements. Write down the weather conditions, extra travel or exercise, your mood and your social and work activities. Note the time of each phase of your migraine when one occurs. The following is a list of common triggers:

- Anxiety and stress, emotional upsets, excitement and depression.

- Physical or mental tiredness.

- Environmental conditions: heat, cold, light, noise, odours.

- Delayed or missed meals, dieting.

- Certain foods, including chocolate, fried foods, citrus fruit, cheese, coffee, tea, nuts and monosodium glutamate.

- Alcohol, especially red wine.

- Menstruation.

- Change of routine (holidays, shift work).

- Too little or too much sleep.

- Travel or exercise.

- Prescription drugs such as the contraceptive pill and antihypertensive medication.

Chronic pain

Any persistent pain that lasts longer than six months is called chronic pain. It may be due to an active disease such as arthritis, cancer or a nerve injury. It can also be a long-term result of a condition that has apparently healed. Chronic pain can even be caused by emotional tension. Whatever the cause, there are often effective means to relieve it.

Acute pain occurs when nerve endings called nociceptors are stimulated by chemicals released from inflamed or damaged tissues. These messages tell you that something is wrong; for example, you have trodden on a pin, you are too close to a fire or you have an injured muscle, an inflamed appendix or a cut finger.

Persistent pain is more complicated. Nociceptors will certainly be involved if there is an active tissue-damaging disease; for example, pressure on the nerve from a prolapsed disc or destruction of a bone by a malignant tumour. However, some types of pain persist even where tissues have apparently healed or, more confusingly, where there has never been any obvious tissue damage in the first place.

Drug treatments for acute pain include nonsteroidal anti-inflammatory drugs (NSAIDs) and painkillers. Certain types of persistent pain may be helped by anti-convulsants and antidepressants, but the long-term management of most chronic pain requires not only medical solutions but also a holistic approach, including psychological and lifestyle factors. Physical therapy may have a role in helping people with persistent joint or muscle pain.

TAKING EXERCISE

An effective non-drug way to combat pain is physiotherapy and exercise. Balancing a combination of rest and exercise is an important step in coping with any chronic condition. The common instruction for acute pain in situations such as a flare-up of arthritis or a muscle strain is rest, which is sensible to avoid aggravating the injury and to let healing take place. In long-term pain, however, rest alone can do more harm than good. Exercise is vital: it prevents muscles from wasting, weakening or tensing up, which otherwise can cause further pain and strain. Muscle movement also encourages the production of endorphins, our natural

PAIN AND THE GATE CONTROL THEORY

When nociceptors, or pain receptors, are stimulated (see above) they send signals via a pain pathway. They travel along a sensory nerve to the spinal cord, then the brain, where pain is perceived. Normally, pain is registered only if it rises above a certain level.

Whether or not pain is perceived will depend on "pain gating" in the spinal cord and the brain. Various factors control the pathways. One of these is endorphins, the human body's natural painkillers, which can be found in the brain, spinal cord and nerve endings. They can establish how much the "gates" open or close. The level of endorphins circulating in the body is affected, for example, by mood and exercise and by previous experience of pain. One explanation for some types of chronic pain is that once a pain pathway has been laid down, it is more easily set off again, even after the original problem heals. For some reason the "gates" along the pain pathway stay open. Psychological, as well as physical, treatment may help.

painkillers. Athletes, for example, are often unaware of an injury until after they finish competing because of the surge of brain chemicals, including endorphins, triggered by exercise and competition.

Doctors, physiotherapists, osteopaths and chiropractors can advise on the type and level of activity and how to gradually build up a routine. Occupational therapists can give advice about work and household tasks.

LEARNING TO RELAX

Another essential tool for self-help relief is relaxation. Chronic pain can set off a vicious circle of stress, tension, fear, anxiety, more pain and more stress. Like any stress reaction, this has a generally detrimental effect on health, reducing circulation, increasing heart rate, tensing muscles and disturbing digestion and sleep patterns – all of which further impairs the ability to cope with pain.

Deep physical and mental relaxation helps to break the cycle. Relaxing allows tension and toxins to flow out of the muscles and organs, encourages the production of endorphins and gives the body an opportunity to use its own healing powers. Profound relaxation usually involves a combination of rhythmic breathing and progressively relaxing the body by tensing and loosening each muscle group. Some people like to visualize a tranquil scene or a time when they have been entirely relaxed and happy. Relaxation tapes are available. Visualization – sometimes called self-hypnosis – can also be a tool to implant positive thoughts that help to control the pain in day-to-day life.

Complementary therapies for chronic pain management include cognitive psychotherapy. Acupuncture may help some kinds of chronic pain. Acupressure, massage (see pp.206–09) and aroma-therapy (see pp.192–95) may help you to relax, raising endorphin levels and increasing your pain tolerance.

NERVE TREATMENT

Pain relief without drugs can be provided by transcutaneous electrical nerve stimulation, or TENS. A small machine sends electrical impulses via electrodes to the part of the body that hurts. It may give relief by triggering endorphins or by blocking the transmission of the sensation of pain to the brain. Research shows that it can relieve chronic pain in one-third of people, depending on the cause. ∎

VISUALIZATION

Try this technique to help you relax. Choose a quiet room where you will not be disturbed for 10–20 minutes.

- Lie down, or sit comfortably in a straight-backed chair with your feet flat on the ground, and shut your eyes. Begin by slowly and deliberately raising your eyebrows and tensing your forehead muscles for a count of five, then relax them. Repeat.

- Go through the same procedure for each part of your body, tensing then relaxing in turn the muscles in your scalp, face, jaw and neck, shoulders, one arm and hand then the other, rib cage, abdomen, upper and lower back, legs and feet.

- Now breathe deeply, feeling your abdomen rise and fall with each in-breath and out-breath.

- After a few minutes, picture in your mind's eye a lovely calm scene such as a meadow by a river or a beach with gentle waves. Listen to the sounds around you – the birds singing or the noise of the water – and smell the flowers or the salty air. Feel the sun's warmth spreading through your body. Now imagine the sun moving to focus its rays on the particular part of you that hurts. Feel its warmth bringing comfort and ease to that spot. Rest quietly, enjoying the tranquil experience.

- When you are ready, slowly open your eyes and gradually ease yourself back into movement.

CAUTION

Some children will have convulsions whenever their temperature is high, but this does not mean they will develop epilepsy in later life. Nonetheless, when any child has a first convulsion, seek further medical advice and let your doctor know of any subsequent episodes. Convulsions can be a symptom of meningitis in babies (p.183), so it is particularly important to get advice from a doctor.

Epilepsy

During an epileptic attack or seizure, a person can lose consciousness for anywhere from only a few seconds to several minutes. Epilepsy is a common disorder of the brain that causes recurring seizures, which are alarming to witness and confusing for the sufferer afterward. It can now be almost completely controlled with drugs.

Epileptic attacks or seizures occur when the brain's activity is briefly disturbed, scrambling its networks of messages and upsetting its normal control of the body. The brain consists of millions of nerve cells, or neurons, which regulate our every activity – thinking, feeling, seeing and moving muscles.

Well-ordered patterns of electrical activity pass from one nerve to another in lightning-fast networks, all dependent on the action of chemical messengers known as neurotransmitters, which control all brain function. In an epileptic attack, an upset in the brain's chemistry causes some neurons to fire more quickly than usual and completely out of synchronization. The result is a seizure or convulsion.

Of the several forms of epilepsy, the most common are tonic-clonic (in which the sufferer loses consciousness), complex partial and absence seizures. Tonic-clonic seizures, in particular, can be extremely frightening to watch, but they rarely cause any damage to the brain. Once the seizure is over, the person gradually returns to a normal state of mind without suffering any ill effects. For other types of seizure, see the chart on the facing page.

WHEN DOES EPILEPSY STRIKE?

In children under the age of five, fever can cause brief seizures – known as febrile convulsions – which are similar to tonic-clonic attacks, but are not epilepsy. You can reduce the risk of febrile convulsion by trying to lower the child's fever as soon as it appears. Sponging or bathing with lukewarm water and giving paracetamol may help. However, in children over five years of age, you should consider the possibility of epilepsy with the occurrence of any seizure.

Roughly 1 in 200 adults suffers from epilepsy and 70 percent of these have their first seizure before the age of 20. Those who have epilepsy when they are young often experience a reduction in the intensity and frequency of their seizures as they grow older, with attacks sometimes disappearing completely.

WHAT TRIGGERS A SEIZURE?

Some people inherit a trait that gives them a lower threshold for seizures. It may also mean they are susceptible to circumstances that would not cause an attack in people without the tendency. For example, some individuals are sensitive to disturbed sleep patterns. If they experience either a lack of sleep or too much, they may have a seizure.

Other triggers include excess alcohol, emotional stress and a high temperature when ill. Sensitivity to light, such as the flickering rays that come from watching television at close quarters, video games, a flash from a camera, disco lights or

RECOGNIZING SEIZURES

Type	Area affected	What happens	Aftermath
Tonic-clonic seizure (formerly "Grand mal")	Involves the whole brain.	The body becomes stiff all over. The person loses consciousness and falls to the ground, jerking and shaking. She may make strange sounds, dribble or be incontinent and the face can turn blue from lack of oxygen. She may vomit or bite her tongue and can injure herself if she hits nearby objects.	The seizure normally stops after several minutes. The person will usually feel confused and drowsy as she recovers. She may have a headache or sore muscles from the violence of the contractions, and she may want to sleep for a few hours.
Simple partial seizure	Abnormal electrical activity comes from only one area of the brain. Does not alter consciousness.	Person stays alert, but experiences symptoms such as jerking, twitching, pins and needles, nausea or disturbances of sight, smell or taste, depending on the area of the brain that is affected.	Usually lasts several seconds and then goes away with no ill effects.
Complex partial seizure	Originates in one of the temporal lobes of the brain, which are responsible for many different brain functions. Alters consciousness.	Person appears dazed or confused and detached from her surroundings. She may act strangely, for instance, plucking at her clothes, smacking her lips, swallowing repeatedly or wandering around as if drunk.	Person may feel disorientated and remember nothing of the seizure.
Absence seizure (formerly "Petit mal")	Unknown. Most common in children, who may have repeated attacks.	Person stares blankly and loses contact with surroundings for a few seconds but rarely falls. Eyes may roll back or eyelids flutter.	Child sufferers are often accused of neglecting schoolwork and daydreaming. It can take time for someone to realize that there is a specific medical problem.
Atonic seizure	Unknown	Sudden brief loss of muscle tone and consciousness, causing person to go limp and fall to the ground.	Lasts only a few seconds and person usually feels well immediately afterward.
Myoclonic seizure	An inherited form of epilepsy.	Sudden and severe jerks of certain muscles or the entire body. Brief; may look like a sudden forward flexing or nodding of the head. If consciousness is lost, it is only for a few seconds.	No known after effects.
Status epilepticus	Rare, mostly occurs in people with brain disease, but can be brought on by sudden withdrawal or irregular use of anti-epilepsy medication.	A series of major seizures that happen without any recovery in between. Urgent medical treatment is necessary to stop the seizures and clear the airway.	Person is usually hospitalized for recovery.

dappled sunlight filtering through trees, is commonly thought to be a seizure trigger. However, light sensitivity only affects fewer than five percent of people with epilepsy.

Many women report that their seizures are linked to their menstrual cycle and usually cluster around the time of a period. Hormonal changes that occur in puberty can also affect the frequency or pattern of attacks.

DOS AND DON'TS DURING A SEIZURE

If someone is having an epileptic fit, follow the advice given here to help make her safe and comfortable until the fit is over.

Do
- Loosen any tight clothing around the neck.
- Protect the person from injury by removing sharp or hard objects nearby.
- Cushion the person's head if she falls.
- Help breathing by gently placing a fallen person in the recovery position (p.300).
- Stay with the person until she has fully recovered.
- If it is a complex partial seizure, gently guide the person away from danger if necessary and speak quietly to reassure her.
- If it is an absence seizure, quietly tell the person when she recovers what has happened and fill in any missed information.
- Call an ambulance or doctor only if a seizure lasts more than a few minutes or if one tonic-clonic seizure follows another without the person regaining consciousness.

Don't
- Attempt to restrain the person or try to stop the jerking. You cannot stop or shorten a seizure.
- Try to force anything in the person's mouth or between her teeth. Attempting to open the mouth may break teeth and damage the tissues in the mouth and throat.
- Try to move the person unless she is in danger.
- Give the person anything to drink.

Epilepsy can result from a variety of other causes, too, such as an infection, head injuries, low blood sugar, a stroke or alcohol or prescription drug use. Once a person is susceptible, an attack can be sparked out of the blue by a number of trigger factors.

DIAGNOSIS AND TREATMENT

Epilepsy is hard to diagnose. It cannot be identified from one seizure; it is rare that your doctor will see you having a fit; and there are many reasons other than epilepsy for a brief loss of consciousness or fit, including stress, fever, drugs, poisoning and stroke. About 1 person in 20 has a seizure similar to an epileptic attack at some time in her life.

If you have a seizure, it is likely that you will not remember what happened afterward. You should ask people what occurred or take someone who has witnessed it with you to your doctor. If the doctor suspects epilepsy, there are several tests she can use to investigate the situation further.

An electroencephalogram (EEG) involves putting electrodes (small signal receivers) on the scalp to record the brain's electrical activity. The trouble is an EEG can only tell what is going on in your brain at that moment, not what happens during an attack – unless you happen to have one while attached to the machine. However, it can help the doctor to decide what type of epilepsy you have and what might be the most appropriate treatment. Sometimes portable EEG machines are used to take recordings while you go about your daily life.

The more sophisticated tests include computerized tomography (CT scanning), which involves taking X-rays from different angles and using them with a computer to produce pictures of "slices"

The brain patterns recorded by an EEG help to determine what type of epilepsy a sufferer has. The waves here are characteristic of tonic-clonic seizure, one of the most common forms.

of the brain, and magnetic resonance imaging (MRI), which creates a similar image of the brain without using radiation. Both can reveal whether there are areas of damage in the brain that could account for the seizures. A blood test can also eliminate other conditions that could be responsible, such as kidney malfunctions or low blood sugar.

Although medication cannot cure epilepsy, about 80 percent of people with the disease can reduce or completely control their seizures with drugs. There is a wide choice of anti-epilepsy drugs, and they work in many different ways. The newest forms function by curbing certain neurotransmitters, which calm excessive electrical activity in the brain, or by raising the seizure threshold. In general, seizures can be controlled with just one drug taken regularly.

Addressing lifestyle factors, such as adequate sleep, stress management, diet and limitation of alcohol, can also help in managing epilepsy. For a small percentage of people, surgery can help.

A DIET FOR CHILDREN

Some doctors, especially in the United States, suggest that eating a restricted "ketogenic" diet can help reduce seizures, particularly in children. The diet is extremely rich in fats and oils, but low in proteins and carbohydrates.

The unusual combination creates a condition in the body known as "ketosis", which can increase the seizure threshold. Calories and liquid are also restricted in ketogenic diets. The process requires close medical supervision, careful preparation and a great deal of commitment to be successful. However, some children have greater seizure control with this diet than with conventional drug therapies.

LEARNING TO RELAX

About 30 percent of people with epilepsy have an increased number of seizures during times of stress. Complementary therapies such as yoga, meditation and massage can help them to relax.

Acupuncture can also be effective in reducing stress and anxiety. Research in aromatherapy suggests that the essential oils of ylang ylang (the flowers of a tall tropical tree) and the herbs camomile and lavender are particularly beneficial for people who suffer from epilepsy. ■

An EEG records the electrical activity of the brain through differences in readings from electrodes attached to the scalp. The resulting waveforms are either printed out on to a moving strip of paper or computed and averaged.

CAUTION

Do not stop taking drugs for epilepsy except on your doctor's advice. Stopping suddenly may trigger several dangerous attacks.

SEE ALSO
Heart disease   **35–39**
Recovery position
              300–301

Stroke

Roughly every five minutes, someone in the developed world has a stroke. Yet it is estimated that half of all strokes could be prevented by reducing common risk factors.

A stroke occurs when the blood supply to the brain is suddenly cut off, severely damaging or destroying areas of brain tissue. The result is that body functions controlled by those parts of the brain may be lost. Older people are more susceptible, although strokes can occur in younger age groups, too.

The most common cause is a blood clot blocking an artery in the brain. This is known as an ischaemic stroke. Clots are generally triggered when the artery wall is damaged by atherosclerosis – a build up of fatty plaque, which both hardens and narrows the arteries. Clots form either where scabs develop over a patch of damaged artery or when a clump of plaque is flicked off into the bloodstream. The second cause of stroke is a cerebral haemorrhage, or a brain "bleed". This occurs when an artery in the brain leaks. It may be caused by high blood pressure or by a weak spot in the artery wall, which is known as an aneurysm. These strokes may require urgent treatment or surgery to stop the bleeding. Strokes caused by blood clots are usually painless, but those that occur from bleeding may cause a severe headache.

The after effects of a stroke depend on where and how much permanent damage has been done to the brain. They commonly include weakness or paralysis on one side of the body, twisting of the face, loss of balance, disturbed vision, slurred speech, incontinence and difficulty in swallowing. Many sufferers also find it difficult to coordinate movement, and some become confused, are less stable emotionally, are unable to understand words or are forgetful.

THE RISK FACTORS

Many of the factors that increase the risk of a stroke are the same as those for heart disease, so taking some preventive action can have a double reward. High blood pressure is the most important known risk factor for strokes. About 50 percent

REDUCING SALT IN YOUR DIET

Sodium from salt is a key factor in maintaining the body's fluid balance and blood pressure. There is controversy about just how crucial a role excessive salt consumption plays in raising blood pressure, but the consensus is that cutting back is a good idea.

Research suggests that even as little as half a level teaspoon (3 g) of salt a day can lead to high blood pressure in susceptible individuals. Average salt consumption is 1½ teaspoons (9 g) a day in most developed countries and experts recommend reducing this to a teaspoonful (6 g).

Over 75 percent of the salt we consume is hidden in prepared foods, so aim to become "salt aware". Many packaged foods contain large amounts of sodium even though they do not taste salty, so you should always read the labels. Watch for the words "soda" (which refers to sodium bicarbonate, or bicarbonate of soda), "sodium" and the symbol "Na". Canned soups and Chinese takeaways are particular salt traps.

It is also important to break the habit of cooking with too much salt or adding it at the table. Salt substitutes or low-sodium salt products are available which can help you adjust, or try using herbs for a new range of flavours.

HOW A STROKE OCCURS

Artery feeding the brain

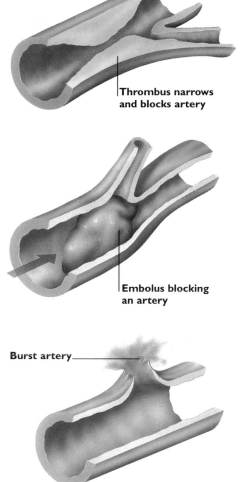

Thrombus narrows and blocks artery

Embolus blocking an artery

Burst artery

A cerebral thrombosis occurs when a thrombus, a blood clot that builds up on the wall of an artery in the brain, blocks the circulation. It accounts for 40–50 percent of strokes. A cerebral embolism – a blockage caused by an embolus, or travelling clot – is responsible for 30–35 percent of cases. The remaining 15–25 percent of strokes are caused by a cerebral haemorrhage – when blood from a burst artery flows into the brain.

of strokes are linked to it. A 40-year-old person who has high blood pressure is 30 times more likely to have a stroke than someone with a normal reading. Because high blood pressure carries no symptoms of its own, an annual check is worthwhile for those who are over 40 years of age. Reducing your salt intake (see box, facing page) is one way that you can help keep your blood pressure healthy, but in some cases medicines may be necessary to reduce and control its level.

A low-fat, high-fibre diet helps to maintain a healthy weight and prevent atherosclerosis. It is also important to avoid heavy drinking. Excessive amounts of alcohol can have a dramatic effect on blood pressure. Smoking is another risk factor because of its effects on blood flow and artery health. Stopping smoking can dramatically reduce the risk of a stroke.

Keeping up regular exercise can also be beneficial. This does not have to be running marathons or intensive workouts in the gym – brisk walking, dancing, swimming or even energetic household and garden jobs should be enough if you practise them regularly. Part of the benefit comes from improving circulation and eliminating toxins more efficiently, but exercise also helps to keep weight down.

SECONDARY CAUSES

Other factors that increase the risk of a stroke include having diabetes and high levels of stress. Stress is not a trigger, but it can adversely affect blood pressure and blood clotting processes. Being pregnant and taking oral contraceptive pills are also risk factors. Women who have high blood pressure or who smoke heavily might seek an alternative method of contraception. Hormone replacement therapy taken after the menopause, however, may reduce the risk of a stroke. The oestrogen that it contains helps to keep the arteries healthy.

CAT (computerized axial tomography) scanning produces cross-sectional images of the brain by combining X-rays and a computer. The patient has to lie on a table that is slid into the machine before the X-rays are taken. The results are then examined on a computer screen.

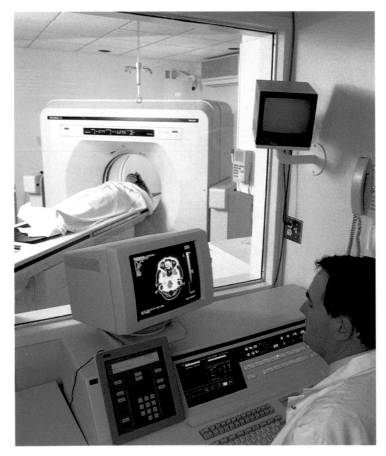

COMBINED RISKS

The trouble with the risk factors for strokes is that they do not simply add up, they multiply. If you smoke, you run double the risk of a stroke of a nonsmoker. If you smoke and have high blood pressure (a common combination), you have six times the risk. If you have these two risk factors and do not exercise, you run 16 times the risk of suffering a stroke. The good news is that reducing a couple of the factors – say, smoking and extra weight – can make a huge difference to your risk levels.

RECOVERY

Two-thirds of people who suffer a stroke survive, and if they act to reduce their risk, may well never suffer another one. Some people recover completely, while others recover but retain a lasting disability of some kind.

Although brain cells that die will not recover, those that have been affected by local swelling can heal and start working again. In addition, parts of the brain which are unaffected can be persuaded to take over some of the work of irreparably damaged cells, sometimes to a remarkable extent. With help, too, someone who has suffered a stroke can adapt to their particular loss of function and find new ways of performing tasks. Progress depends on the severity of the stroke and the motivation of the individual. Most of the recovery occurs in the first couple of weeks, but some people continue to improve for months afterward.

TREATMENT

Medical care starts with tests to investigate the type and extent of the stroke. This may involve CAT (computerized axial tomography) scans or MRI (magnetic resonance imaging), which give images of the brain tissue and injury. The doctor may also do other tests to determine the cause of the stroke.

There is as yet no definitive medical treatment for the stroke itself, but medication or advice may be given to reduce the risk factors. For example, the doctor may prescribe a daily dose of aspirin (150–300 mg) or warfarin to reduce the stickiness of the blood, which helps to prevent clots. He may also prescribe drugs to lower your blood pressure and recommend altering your lifestyle – for example, switching to a healthier diet and exercising. Current research is focused on drugs that prevent blood clotting or dissolve clots (similar to those used in heart attacks) or drugs that stimulate brain function after the event.

REHABILITATION

The most important aspect of all stroke treatment is rehabilitation. The sooner it starts, the greater the chance the patient has of making a full recovery. Current practice is to encourage movement and speech almost immediately after the stroke, whether the person is in hospital or at home. The strategy is two pronged: first, to prompt brain cells that have been only temporarily stunned by the effects of the stroke back into action as soon as possible; second, to encourage other cells to take on the tasks of destroyed ones.

Programmes usually involve specialist therapists. Physiotherapists help the person to regain posture and balance, mobility and the ability to carry out everyday tasks, such as dressing, eating and washing, through exercise and practice. Occupational therapists are responsible for providing practical ways to adapt life to living with the disabilities caused by stroke. Speech therapists can be helpful if speech has been affected.

Family and friends have a key role to play, not only in caring for the person and helping him with tasks he cannot manage, but also in motivating and giving him moral support. Many people who have had a severe stroke feel mentally and emotionally shattered because the change in their life and abilities is so sudden; however, it is crucial not to turn stroke victims into invalids. Strokes usually leave a person's intellect and memories fully intact. Positive encouragement and support to do things for themselves will do far more good than being fiercely overprotective, which can, in fact, retard rehabilitation.

Make sure, too, that if you are caring for someone who has had a stroke you have some practical and emotional support yourself, as well as opportunities to rest and relax. It can be a demanding time and sometimes almost as much of a shock to the carer as to the person who has had the stroke. ■

TRANSIENT ISCHAEMIC ATTACK (TIA)

Ischaemia means lack of blood, and transient ischaemic attacks, or TIAs, are mini-strokes caused by tiny blood clots or arterial spasms that cut off circulation momentarily. Symptoms depend on which blood vessel to the brain is blocked and which side of the brain is starved. They are similar to those of a full-blown stroke, but usually last for only a few minutes.

TIAs can be frightening, but they do not cause permanent harm. However, they are a serious warning that a more severe stroke could be on the way: if blood can make a tiny clot, it can produce a larger one. Having a TIA is also an indication of an increased risk of heart attack because it suggests that your arteries are narrowing.

Seek the advice of a doctor immediately so that you can take preventive action to reduce any further risk. This often means stopping smoking, controlling blood pressure and possibly taking aspirin to thin the blood.

Alzheimer's disease

Contrary to popular belief, dementia – forgetfulness and confusion – is not an inevitable part of the aging process. The most common cause of dementia in older people is Alzheimer's disease, which results from a process that gradually destroys the brain cells. The cause of this debilitating disorder is not fully understood.

Under the microscope, brain tissue affected by Alzheimer's disease reveals areas of tangled nerve connections and hardened plaques of an abnormal protein called beta-amyloid, which have destroyed the vital connectivity of the brain. There is also a noticeable decrease in brain volume.

Alzheimer's disease rarely occurs in people under the age of 50 but evidence suggests that 10–15 percent of people over 65 years of age are affected, and this increases to 20 percent in those in the over-80s age group.

A computer graphic of a scan shows a vertical slice through the brain. The brain of the Alzheimer's patient looks considerably shrunken and patchy compared with that of a healthy person.

HOW ALZHEIMER'S AFFECTS THE BRAIN

Alzheimer's brain

Healthy brain

WHAT CAUSES IT?

There are thought to be a number of contributing factors that may cause Alzheimer's, and these differ from one individual to the next. One genetic cause has been defined in a small number of families and is responsible for a rare type that affects people in their 40s. However, links have also been found with a gene called apolipoprotein E4 (ApoE4), and some researchers believe that this may be implicated in 30 to 40 percent of cases. Another track of research speculates that the disease may be triggered by a virus.

A third theory suggests Alzheimer's is related to exposure to aluminium. Studies on communities where there are high concentrations of aluminium in the water have also found high rates of Alzheimer's disease. More controversially, others believe that there is a link with the mercury found in dental fillings.

Whatever causes it, Alzheimer's disease begins gradually, so much so that it is often only much later after diagnosis that relatives or friends look back and recognize the pattern of the symptoms.

SPOTTING THE SYMPTOMS

Affected people can become so forgetful of recent events that they may repeat themselves in conversation and are less able to grasp new ideas. They may also appear detached or confused and perhaps more anxious about making decisions. As the disease progresses, memory loss becomes more apparent.

People with more advanced Alzheimer's disease become disorientated and are often confused about time or place, thinking day is night or becoming lost. They start having difficulty in communicating, either forgetting their own train of thought and becoming garbled or failing to understand what is said to them. They lose practical skills such as the ability to wash, dress or eat. These symptoms have obvious implications around the house. Appliances such as ovens can be left on. Sufferers can leave home on an errand and forget where they were going or lose their way back, or they can be taken advantage of when shopping or paying the bills.

Behaviour and personality may also change. An affected person may become angry, agitated, upset or withdrawn or may behave strangely. Underlying features of personality, such as a tendency to worry or be verbally aggressive, can become exaggerated. The sufferer may also be awake at night and sleep during the day.

In later stages, people with Alzheimer's may no longer recognize those close to them. They can be increasingly dependent but hard to care for, becoming suspicious, demanding and even violent.

DIAGNOSIS AND TREATMENT

It should not be assumed that every elderly person who seems confused or seriously forgetful has Alzheimer's disease. These symptoms can be caused by a variety of treatable disorders such as a thyroid malfunction, depression or atherosclerosis in the brain. Doctors will rule out the possibility of other illnesses before diagnosing Alzheimer's. Symptoms and tests of mental state will also help a specialist to make a diagnosis, and she may order a brain scan. Sometimes diagnosis can only be confirmed by brain biopsy (removing a sample of tissue for microscopic analysis) after death.

There is currently no effective treatment for Alzheimer's disease. Tranquillizers and other mood-controlling drugs may ease symptoms. Recently launched drugs delay the loss of cognitive skills in some people, but only in the short term. ■

TIPS FOR CARERS

- Keep it simple. Stick to familiar routines and use reminders to keep the person orientated in her surroundings. Leave notes on the refrigerator to remind her to eat, label the rooms (particularly the bathroom) and give clues for everyday tasks such as leaving out her toothbrush on the sink.

- Break down chores into manageable steps to allow her to do what she can herself. Help her to have as much control as possible over her life for as long as is feasible.

- Make sure the house is safe and gives a feeling of security. Remove hazards such as scatter rugs, and think about installing safeguards such as automatic cut-outs on electrical or gas equipment and reducing water temperature to avoid scalding.

- Check that you have her attention before you start talking, and make eye contact and speak slowly and clearly. Keep conversations simple and use Yes/No questions if possible. Repeat information and show as well as tell her what to do.

- Remember gentle touch and body language such as holding a hand or smiling when talking. Pay attention to the expression on her face and respond to her moods and feelings.

- Introduce all visitors by name, explaining who they are even if you think they are well known. Try to include the sufferer – it is painful to be ignored because you find communicating hard.

- Help the person to keep active and stay in contact with family and friends by arranging for her to partake in social activities such as listening to music and enjoying outings with others.

- Use gentle persuasion and coaxing. Never apply force and try not to take over tasks the person could do herself.

SEE ALSO
Your emotional life 12–13
Aromatherapy 192–195
Acupuncture 212–213

Stress

The catch-all term stress has come to mean anything that disrupts the balance in your life. However, stress in itself is not bad or dangerous. It is a natural mental and bodily reaction to challenge or change, and in moderate amounts, it can boost performance and spur you on. Problems only arise when the stress response is too great or unrelenting.

The stress response stems from the body's ancient "fight or flight" mechanism, which allowed humans to react instinctively to a threat. Adrenalin flows, your heart rate and breathing speed up and your mind races. In the past the threats were wild and ferocious animals; today they can range from a traffic jam making you arrive late for an important appointment, a work deadline, an influx of bills, children's demands, pregnancy or moving house to major life-altering crises such as redundancy, a relationship breakdown or death. In more primitive

THE FIGHT OR FLIGHT REACTION

In a stressful situation, the adrenal glands release adrenalin, which triggers a host of changes to prepare the body for "fight or flight".

Pupils dilate, or enlarge, giving greater field of vision

Lungs expand, creating greater surface area to take in oxygen

Liver releases sugars and fats into the bloodstream as fuel for muscle cells

Digestive system slows down so body does not waste energy

Immune function may be less effective making you more prone to infections

Hypothalamus in brain is activated, triggering the adrenal glands

Saliva is no longer secreted, making mouth dry

Muscles contract, ready for action

Heart rate increases, blood reaches muscles faster

Adrenal glands release adrenalin, stimulating body to prepare for action

Capillaries near the skin contract, increasing blood supply to muscles – this makes skin look pale situations when dangers were real and immediate, your adrenalin would be dissipated by literally "fighting" or "fleeing". Unfortunately, now you often have to curb the instinctive reaction – you cannot run away from problems. Physical and mental pressure can build up.

Some stresses are internal: for example, worrying about a physical illness, paying the mortgage or juggling childcare and a job. Others come from outside, such as a constantly ringing telephone, pollution or a conflict at work. Whether or not a particular event causes stress depends less on what it is than how well you cope with it. A small problem that you are powerless to change may cause a great deal more stress than a big issue that you feel well equipped to handle. What's more, daily hassles may build up and cause as much difficulty as major life changes.

RECOGNIZING SYMPTOMS

Stress affects people in many different ways. You may become short-tempered, impatient or tearful, find it difficult to think clearly or to make decisions or feel depressed and demotivated. Normal worries can loom large, and you may lose your appetite and find it difficult to relax or sleep well. Stress can make some people physically ill with headaches or muscular pains. In time this makes you run down and more vulnerable to illness.

All these symptoms can make it even more difficult to cope with everyday life and its frustrations and problems. The stress reaction also affects the chemical balance of the body and may contribute to disorders such as heart disease, asthma, psoriasis and rheumatoid arthritis.

If you feel that the symptoms of stress are getting the better of you, your body may be sending you warning signals. It is time to find ways to reduce your stress. ■

REDUCING STRESS LEVELS

■ Identify the events that are stressful to you and find ways to make them less so before they occur. Rehearse strategies for common problems and anticipate how others might respond.

■ Try not to overcommit yourself. No one can do everything – delegate where you can. Organize, prioritize and make lists. Decide what must be done the next day and leave other issues for later on. Planning ahead helps avert panic and gives you a sense of control. Treating each item separately can make the whole seem less overwhelming and help you identify the truly essential priorities.

■ Try not to store up problems in the hope that they will go away. Confronting an issue and making a decision are better than having problems festering in the back of your mind.

■ Take a break and do a little physical activity every day, even if it is only a quick walk. Exercise helps to dissipate stress hormones and refresh the brain.

■ Eat properly and healthily – do not live on rushed snacks, coffee, cigarettes and junk food. Your body needs the right fuel to keep up with your demands.

■ Learn quick tension-releasing techniques such as clenching the whole body deliberately then releasing it with a couple of deep long breaths (p.65). Set aside at least 20 minutes each day for deeper mental and physical relaxation such as yoga (pp.218–23) or meditation (pp.216–17).

■ Make time every week to do what you enjoy. See a movie, have dinner with friends, paint, read, sew – any activity that involves no compulsion or competition, just pleasure.

■ Try to develop a sense of perspective about the pressures on you and think positively about change. Instead of seeing it as a threat, look for opportunities, new experience or knowledge.

■ Seek help or advice if you feel in need of it. Share thoughts with friends, family, colleagues or specialist counsellors. If you have a particular problem or circumstance, there may be a self-help group with whom you can share experiences and strategies to help reduce the pressure.

■ Stay away from excessive alcohol or long-term sedative and tranquillizer drugs. Alcohol has a depressant effect and drugs treat the symptoms but not the cause.

Depression

Everyone feels fed up and miserable at times – this kind of depression is common and normal. Usually there is an obvious reason and the feeling fades or something jolts you out of it. However, an intensely low mood, affecting body and mind, that persists for weeks or months is called clinical depression. This is an illness – it is not a weakness to seek help.

Biochemically, depression seems to be caused by an upset in the body's chemistry, which leads to a shortage of the chemicals (neurotransmitters) that trigger communication activity between brain cells. Particularly important are a group of chemicals called monoamines, including noradrenaline, serotonin and dopamine.

A distressing circumstance such as being lonely or a death can trigger depression. It can also result from a physical illness. Viral infections, including influenza, glandular fever and chronic fatigue syndrome (myalgic encephalomyelitis, or ME), are often associated with depression. Having a life-threatening disease such as cancer or suffering from a chronic illness such as multiple sclerosis can cause it. Certain drugs, including the contraceptive pill, steroid drugs and beta-blockers can trigger depression, as can alcohol.

About 1 in 10 people who suffers from serious depression also experiences periods of feeling wildly elated and hyperactive. This is known as manic depression.

WHO IS AT RISK?

Women appear to suffer from depression more than men. This may be because they admit their feelings more than men do or because doctors are more likely to diagnose women as having depression. It can be linked to hormonal changes that take place with menstruation, pregnancy and menopause. Some women feel depressed before their period. Severe depression may occur after childbirth.

There are many treatments available (see chart, facing page). Antidepressants are commonly used for clincal depression, but they may take a week or two to have an effect. You may need to try several treatments before you find the right approach for you. ▪

SYMPTOMS OF DEPRESSION

It has been estimated that **30 percent** of people have clincal depression at some time in their lives. Talk to a professional if you exprience a combination of the following symptoms:

- Very low self-esteem or unaccountable feelings of guilt, shame, unworthiness or uncleanliness.

- Persistent, unaccountable aches and pains or other unexplainable physical symptoms, including constant tiredness and low energy.

- Disturbed sleep, especially if you wake up early and cannot go back to sleep.

- Loss of appetite or sex drive.

- Unaccountable restlessness or anxiety.

- Mood swings, a noticeable change in mood at different times in the day or unexplained highs and lows in your level of energy or emotions.

- Constant feelings of dejection or suicidal thoughts.

THERAPY AND DRUGS FOR DEPRESSION

Type	How it works	Advantages	Drawbacks
Psychotherapy and counselling	Includes talking over feelings or worries with a trained therapist to uncover the root cause of depression, which the sufferer may not be able to recognize or face.	Talking can help sort out feelings. Having someone else's undivided sympathetic attention can bring relief and help the person feel better about herself.	Requires time and commitment.
Cognitive therapy	Teaches patient to avoid negative patterns of thinking that fuel the depression.	(See above)	(See above)
Monoamine oxidase inhibitor (MAOI)	An antidepressant drug that ensures important chemicals stay in the brain cells longer.	Sometimes works where other drugs do not.	Reacts with meat and yeast extracts, cheese and red wine, causing violent headaches and rapid rises in blood pressure.
Tricyclic antidepressants	A large group of anti-depressant drugs, divided into those that work by stimulating the brain and those that sedate it.	This wide range of drugs is well researched and familiar to doctors and an effective option can be found for most people.	An overdose can be dangerous. Can cause dry mouth, blurred vision, constipation, sweating, low blood pressure, weight gain and sexual dysfunction.
Selective serotonin reuptake inhibitor (SSRI)	This antidepressant drug increases the serotonin held in the brain cells.	Can suit people overly sedated by tricyclics. Fewer side effects and no weight gain. Less toxic in overdose.	Side effects include nausea and indigestion.
Lithium	Displaces sodium in the body's cells, but exactly how this treats depression is unknown.	Effective in severe and manic depression. Can be used instead of ECT to prevent bouts of depression.	Fine balance between correct and toxic dose. Side effects include shaking hands, weight gain, dry mouth and tiredness.
L-tryptophan	Dietary supplement turned into serotonin by the body, increasing levels in the brain.	Used to boost other antidepressants or alone in cases of mild depression.	None
Hypericum extract	Research suggests that this herbal extract can be useful as an antidepressant.	Can be effective in mild to moderate depression.	May increase the side effects of antidepressant drugs if taken together. Taken alone, there are no obvious side effects.
Exercise	May stimulate certain chemicals in the brain.	Can be as effective as tricyclics in mild to moderate depression.	Requires time and commitment.
Electroconvulsive therapy (ECT)	Treatments of electrical current passed through the brain to alter the brain's chemical messages.	Used in severe depression if other treatments do not work. Can return people to normal but most need drugs.	Immediate confusion. Memory problems can last a few months. May have long-term effects on intelligence or memory.

Sleeping disorders

Sleep allows the body to replenish, rest and repair itself. So severe insomnia – whether it is persistent difficulty in falling asleep or awakening too early – can affect your whole sense of wellbeing.

Individual need for sleep varies widely – from 4 to 10 hours a night. Older people often need less sleep because the body's processes slow down and the need for long repair periods at night is reduced. Alternatively, if you are under stress or ill, your sleep requirement may increase.

Insomnia is usually a symptom of another problem – sleep is as sensitive to your mood as your appetite is. Anxiety, pressure or tension about a situation at work, school or in the family makes

relaxing difficult. There is always the tendency to keep turning over the problem in your mind – a process guaranteed to banish sleep. Emotional crises, such as bereavement or relationship problems, or a painful illness also make it difficult to relax and drift off to sleep. A person suffering from depression will often find sleep elusive. He frequently wakes up early, giving him plenty of time to worry. As an added burden, having a few sleepless nights creates anxiety about not sleeping, compounding insomnia.

BREAKING INSOMNIA PATTERNS

The most important step in treating insomnia is to find the real cause. If this is worries or pressure left over from the day, relaxation techniques such as breathing exercises, visualization and gradual muscle relaxation (see p.65), as well as trying to develop a calming routine before bedtime (see box, left), will help.

It may be beneficial to keep a sleep diary for a couple of weeks, noting information such as how long you think you have slept, what time you went to bed, how many times you woke up and when, and how refreshed you felt in the morning. This can help you understand your own pattern of sleep and identify particular reasons why sleep comes less easily to you. It will also be helpful if sleeplessness begins to affect your daily life and you need to consult your doctor.

Medication to help you sleep is widely recognized to be of use only in short-term

CHECKLIST FOR RESTFUL SLEEP

■ Make sure your bedroom is well ventilated and quiet and you are not too hot or too cold in bed.

■ Get up and go to bed at the same time every day – it helps to establish day-time and night-time patterns.

■ Avoid napping during the day.

■ Drink warm milky beverages to trigger brain chemicals that make you sleepy, but avoid those containing caffeine such as coffee, tea, cocoa and cola. Although alcohol can make you sleepy, it usually wakes people in the middle of the night as the effect wears off.

■ Develop a calming bedtime routine: avoid work, big meals, intense discussions and watching television late at night.

■ Take a walk or some form of exercise in the late afternoon or early evening.

■ Set aside a time early in the evening to go through the day and plan for tomorrow, rather than doing it at bedtime.

■ Save the bedroom for sleep-related activities – entering it should not make you think of work, bills or appointments.

In severe cases of sleep disturbance, the patient may be invited to visit a sleep lab, where she will be attached to machines to monitor her sleep patterns.

times of crisis or emotional stress. Taking sleeping pills over long periods reduces the body's tolerance to them and the dose will have to be increased to achieve the same effect. This results in addiction and damages both mental and physical health.

SNORING AND SLEEP APNOEA

As many couples know, snoring is the cause of much sleeplessness, although often not for the snorer himself. The sound associated with snoring is caused by air vibrating the tissue known as the soft palate. Anything that prevents normal nose breathing – from a cold or being overweight to clinical conditions such as enlarged adenoids and nasal growths – can spark off snoring. It is more likely to occur if the sleeper lies on his back because the mouth tends to drop open and the tongue to slide back, constricting the flow of air.

Various gadgets are available to stop snoring, from simple clips for the nose to keep nasal passages open to – for serious cases – masks through which oxygen is pumped. More simply, some people sew a hair brush to the back of the snorer's pyjamas to encourage him to sleep on his side. Surgery is performed in rare cases.

Occasionally, snoring can lead to the more serious condition sleep apnoea, in which the breathing of a sleeping person stops spontaneously many times during the night, causing him to awaken constantly. Although the sleeper may not be aware of continually waking up, sleep can be disturbed and the body is robbed of oxygen, and as a result, exhaustion and irritability can disrupt daytime life.

Sleep apnoea may be caused by an obstruction of the airway or, more seriously, by a failure of the nerve impulse that drives breathing. It is most common in overweight men between 30 and 50 years old. Treatment usually involves losing weight, night-time artificial ventilation or, in severe cases, surgery to either remove the tonsils or adenoids or shorten the soft palate. ∎

SEE ALSO
Depression   78–79
Your best weight
           258–259
Losing weight   260–261

Eating disorders

Although eating disorders are often defined as illnesses of eating too little food, in the developed world ill health is more frequently caused by overindulgence in food.

The two main disorders associated with eating too little – anorexia nervosa and bulimia – are not primarily about food, but are symptoms of underlying emotional and psychological distress. Although 9 out of 10 sufferers of anorexia nervosa are young women, these disorders do sometimes occur in men, too. The illness usually begins with the everyday dieting that is so much a part of teenage life, but anorexics slim long after they reach a desirable body weight. They become excessively thin, elusive about discussing the amount of food they eat and often refuse to eat in public. Some anorexics may also exercise vigorously, take slimming pills or laxatives and withdraw from social life.

Bulimia usually affects a slightly older age group and is rooted in similar fears. Instead of starving, however, a person with bulimia goes on eating "binges". She secretly eats huge amounts of fattening foods that she would not normally allow herself to eat, such as cakes, chocolate and biscuits, then makes herself sick or uses laxatives. Afterward she often feels guilty and depressed. Unlike anorexics, the weight of a bulimic usually stays within normal ranges.

WHY SLIM EXCESSIVELY?

There are many different therories about what causes anorexia nervosa and bulimia. Some suggest that these two eating disorders are rooted in the current "thin is beautiful" fashion in Western countries. Others believe that dieting may be a way for those who feel insecure to attempt to exert control in their life, gain attention or postpone growing up. In some people, anorexia or bulimia may be triggered by an upsetting event, such as the break up of a relationship, or by comfort eating during depression.

Both conditions can have serious medical consequences. Anorexics become hyperactive and restless and menstruation stops. They may develop stomach pain, severe constipation, dizzy spells and

A person who becomes anorexic will continue to slim long after she has reached a desirable weight, because of a distorted perception of her shape and an exaggerated fear of becoming fat. For people with anorexia, life is dominated by weight and avoiding food.

swelling of the stomach, ankles and face. The constant vomiting of bulimia can cause ulcers, stomach and bowel disorders, throat irritations and hair loss, while the continual wash of stomach acid erodes tooth enamel. The body's mineral balance is also upset, damaging the heart and kidneys. Both conditions are characterized by mental anguish, low self-esteem and fatigue, and they can be fatal.

Therapy for treating anorexia and bulimia usually involves psychological investigation and psychotherapy or medication for the underlying problems. The sufferer may have to address these psychological issues before she can make a slow return to normal eating patterns.

OBESITY

There has been much speculation about whether the tendency to become over-weight is a genetic problem. Animal studies have found that mice that have too little of the hormone called leptin chronically overeat. However, although it is known that obesity can run in families, no "obesity gene" has yet been identified in humans and, after all, families usually eat the same kind of food and often have similar attitudes to physical exercise.

A person becomes overweight when food intake exceeds energy expenditure over a prolonged period of time and the excess calories from the food are stored as fat. The "simple" answer to reducing fat is to eat less than you need so that the body starts using its stores. But, as anyone who has already tried knows, cutting down food intake is easier said than done.

Weight gain usually takes place over several years, yet many people expect fat reserves to drop off in a few weeks. The most effective and healthy way to lose weight and keep it lost is not starvation dieting, but a long-term strategy that combines a moderately low-fat and high-fibre diet with increased physical activity. (For advice on nutrition, healthy eating and losing weight see pp.238–91.)

DRASTIC MEASURES

There are drug treatments to aid weight loss but these have two key drawbacks. If you do not change your eating and exercise habits at the same time, the weight returns as soon as you stop taking the drugs. Most also have potentially serious side effects.

Generally speaking, doctors consider prescribing drug treatments, such as appetite suppressants or those that increase energy expenditure or block the digestion or absorption of fats, only for the dangerously overweight. Such drugs should still be combined with significant changes in lifestyle. ∎

CAUTION

If your child seems to be obsessed with dieting or preoccupied with food and is either losing a lot of weight or making frequent visits to the bathroom, she might be anorexic or bulimic. Both of these conditions require medical help before there are serious consequences.

THE DANGERS OF OBESITY

Too much body fat can have detrimental effects on the body – and some of them can be serious:

■ The cardiovascular system is put under strain, contributing to high blood pressure and heart disease (pp.35–39).

■ People who are obese have twice the risk of having a stroke as do lean people.

■ The storage of excess fat can enlarge the liver.

■ Adult-onset diabetes (pp.102–07) can be triggered by even a moderate weight gain.

■ The more obese a man is, the higher is his risk of developing cancer of the prostate, colon and rectum.

■ The more obese a woman is, the greater is her risk of developing cancer of the breast, uterus and cervix.

■ Excessive weight can put strain on the back, hips and knees.

■ Obesity is often seen as a social stigma, which can lead to psychological problems of low self-esteem.

CAUTION

*It is best to accept tran-
quillizers only as a short-
term emergency measure.
They can become addictive
after only two weeks' use
and can cause side effects
and withdrawal symptoms
as painful as those they
seek to cure.*

Anxiety and panic attacks

*In moderation, anxiety helps you perform tasks better and more rapidly.
However, if anxiety occurs needlessly or is overwhelming or persistent,
seek advice. Anxiety can make life miserable.*

The everyday reactions of the stress
response can stimulate the body and
mind to face challenges (see pp.76–77),
which is useful in the appropriate place.
Unfortunately, in about 1 in every 10
people it causes a troublesome anxiety
or phobia (a type of anxiety, see facing
page) at some point in his life.

Sometimes the cause is obvious – an
examination looming, a conflict with
the boss, a family problem to solve, the
menopause – and once the tension is over,
the anxiety subsides. At other times, an
event can be so upsetting and threatening
that it causes anxiety long after it is over.
This is known as post-traumatic stress
syndrome and often occurs after a life-
threatening situation such as a car crash,
fire or violent attack.

In most cases, however, a person may
not be aware of what is causing his
anxiety. There are various theories for why
this happens. For example, some people
tend to be more easily made anxious
about things. And, there may have been
past events, not necessarily remembered,
which contribute to a deep feeling of

unease. Whatever the cause, such people
will tend to misinterpret situations that
are not necessarily fear-inducing in
themselves. Psychologists think helping
the person explain and reassess that
situation using cognitive/behavioural
therapy will help clear the anxiety.

Tranquillizer drugs are effective at
relieving acute anxiety and the doctor may
prescribe them for a brief period for some
types of extreme anxiety. Learning how
to relax and reduce stress can also be a
great help if you are prone to anxiety.

PANIC ATTACKS

Some people experience sudden surges
of anxiety known as panic attacks. Any or
all of the unpleasant symptoms of anxiety
occur simultaneously and in an extreme
form, together with an acute sense of fear.
Attacks can last up to an hour and cause
immense distress, not only from the
symptoms but also because sufferers are
afraid they will make a fool of themselves
by passing out or vomiting. Panic attacks
usually occur for no apparent reason,
unlike the panic associated with a phobia.

Treatment for panic attacks usually
involves cognitive/behavioural therapy
with a specialist. He will try to help the
person understand the thoughts and
feelings that can trigger and perpetuate
the panic and teach coping strategies.

Some antidepressants can be used to
prevent panic attacks. They can also be
used to treat a type of anxiety that is a
symptom of depression (see pp.78–79). ■

HOW TO RECOGNIZE ANXIETY

Emotional signs are constant worry and fear, irritability, feeling
tired but sleeping poorly and an inability to concentrate or
organize. Physical symptoms include hyperventilation, irregular
heartbeats (palpitations), breathlessness, sweating, diarrhoea, dry
mouth, tightness in the chest, nausea, dizziness and muscle pain.

SEE ALSO
Your emotional life 12–13
Anxiety and panic attacks
84

Phobias

An intense, irrational fear when there is no real reason for it causes a type of anxiety known as a phobia. Unlike a panic attack, the phobic only suffers anxiety when faced with the subject of his fear.

Someone with a phobia often begins to worry that he will be humiliated if others see his reaction and often tries to avoid situations he suspects might trigger the phobia, which only reinforces it. Avoidance of fear can mean the person's life becomes dominated by precautions.

HOW TO BEAT PHOBIAS

Phobias are common, but if you are phobic of a common object or situation that causes you to avoid familiar objects or everyday activities, then it is important to get help. Phobias are usually treated with "behavioural" therapy. This involves gradually exposing the person to the subject of his fears, analysing what is happening and what he thinks will occur, and reprogramming these expectations. Psychotherapists might help you use the following strategies:

■ Calming strategies: for example, breathing control, tensing and relaxing your muscles or imagining a pleasant scene such as lying on a beach (see p.65).
■ Cards to be referred to when you panic: these will help you learn how to cope with the sensations. You'll be asked to write down how you feel when frightened: "I can't breathe" or "I think I might faint."
■ Exposing yourself to your fear: at first, this will be with someone you trust. You'll be told to stay with your fear as long as possible, using your strategies. Afterward, you should note how you feel and rate the fear on a scale of 1 to 10. Talk about it and record what you aim for next time. ■

Crowds – many people's nightmare – can trigger ochlophobia, agoraphobia, social phobia (fear of humiliation and embarrassment) and claustrophobia. Such fears are often associated with dread that something horrible will happen.

NAMING FEARS

Phobias come in many guises and there are names for most of them:
Agoraphobia: fear of open spaces, of being alone or of public places.
Claustrophobia: fear of confined or enclosed spaces.
Ochlophobia: fear of crowds.
Hydrophobia: fear of water.
Acrophobia: fear of heights.
Arachnophobia: fear of spiders.
Gatophobia: fear of cats.
Nyctophobia: fear of the night.

SEE ALSO
Good eating habits
262–263

Tooth and gum disease

*A tooth consists of an outer enamel coating, a middle layer of dentine –
which is harder than bone but softer than enamel – and the inner pulp
containing sensory nerves sensitive to heat, cold, pressure and pain.*

The two most common diseases of the
mouth are dental caries (decay) and
gingivitis – inflammation of the gums.
Tooth decay is caused when dental plaque
builds up and erodes holes in the enamel
and underlying dentine. Plaque is a
mixture of dried saliva, food debris and
bacteria, and it forms where the teeth
meet the gums.

If you do not regularly clean your teeth,
plaque hardens into a chalky crust, which
not only helps to gather more of the same
but also traps bacteria close to the teeth
and gums, where they cannot be removed
even with vigorous brushing. These
bacteria produce acid by breaking down
food residues, particularly from items
containing processed sugars. It is this acid
that eats into the enamel and dentine to
create cavities in the teeth.

A cavity reduces a tooth's protection
and makes it sensitive to stimuli such as
cold, heat and sweet foods. If neglected,
it can deepen and allow infection to reach
the pulp. Infection here can cause pain
and inflammation and damage the fine
blood vessels and nerves on which the
survival of the living tooth depends. If
the pulp is destroyed, the tooth dies.

GINGIVITIS

A build up of plaque or old impacted
specks of food around the neck of the
teeth can cause gingivitis. The gums swell,
turn bright pink and become tender. They
also bleed easily after eating or brushing
and, in severe cases, if the tissue starts to
die, breath smells bad. Smoking makes
gum disease worse. If gingivitis is not
treated by plaque removal and regular
brushing and flossing, it can damage the
socket membrane and loosen the tooth –
a condition called periodontitis.

PREVENTION

These tooth and gum conditions can
be easily avoided or relieved by having
a dental check-up every six months and
taking good care of your teeth in the

Once infection enters a
cavity and seeps into the
pulp, it can spread down the
root canal and into the
bone socket of the tooth,
where pus collects and
causes an abscess. This can
cause severe toothache and
tenderness when chewing.
Extracting the tooth solves
the problem, but drilling into
the abscess to release the
pus can save the tooth.

THE TOOTH

Cavity
Enamel
Pulp
Dentine
Gum
Bone socket
Root
Root canal
Abscess

times between. Efficient tooth brushing after meals and regular flossing prevent plaque accumulating and nip the whole process of tooth decay in the bud. So, too, does attending to any small cavities early on by having a dentist put in a filling. This can save the tooth.

SUGAR INTAKE

Fluoride, either added to the water or in toothpaste, helps to remineralize and strengthen the tooth enamel. However, it cannot protect teeth against a steady stream of acid produced by frequent sugar intake, such as the 14 lumps present in one can of a fizzy soft drink.

Artificial sugars – even those extracted "naturally" from fruits – are the worst culprits. They come in many forms, including dextrose, glucose, fructose, sucrose and maltose. These sugars attack the teeth every time they enter the mouth. Limiting the number of times a day sugar swills around the mouth by restricting sweet foods and drinks to mealtimes reduces the risk of decay.

STARTING EARLY

Tooth decay begins in early childhood. It is estimated that in Great Britain about four percent of two year olds have cavities in their baby teeth. The story is the same with second teeth: four percent of six year olds have decay in teeth that have just started to break through. By the time they are 15 years of age, 68 percent of children have some decayed teeth that need filling after the decayed sections are drilled out.

To prevent children from becoming part of these statistics, start healthy teeth routines early in life. Avoid giving sweet drinks to babies and toddlers at bedtime, during the night or for lengthy periods as comforters because they leave sugar in contact with the teeth for too long. Begin

FLOSSING TEETH

Use 10 cm (4 in) of floss between fingers

Wrap the floss around your index or middle fingers

You should floss your teeth to remove plaque and food particles from the gaps between teeth. Using a 45 cm (18 in) length of dental floss, gently push the floss between the crevices at the base of the teeth. Rub the sides of each tooth with a gentle sawing action.

brushing babies' teeth as soon as they begin to break through the gums.

For older children and adults, good dental habits include replacing sugary snacks and sweets with fruits and crisp vegetables, and substituting water and milk for fizzy drinks. ■

HOW TO KEEP YOUR TEETH CLEAN

■ Thoroughly brush your teeth twice a day with a toothpaste, using small gentle movements from side to side.

■ Make sure that you clean each part of your teeth – the front, back and tops of the teeth and the sides of the back teeth.

■ Choose a toothbrush that can reach into the difficult corners and change it about every three months.

■ Floss your teeth once a day, preferably after eating your evening meal.

■ Built-up plaque known as tartar can be removed by a dental hygienist or dentist in a process called scaling, which involves chipping away the material with a sharp miniature pick. It is possible to keep your teeth truly clean only if they are scaled every six months, or more often if recommended by your hygienist or dentist.

Constipation

Because people have different bowel habits, what is constipation in one person may be normal for another. If your rhythm of bowel activities changes, you may have constipation if the symptoms include more infrequent stools than normal, straining, hard painful stools or an uncomfortable bloated feeling in the back passage or abdomen.

Lack of fibre in the diet and situations that distract people from paying attention to the need for a bowel movement are key causes of constipation.

Fibre is found in fruit and vegetables and bran (the husks of grains). It is not digested but passes into the large intestine or colon where it works like blotting paper, drawing water into the stool. This bulking agent absorbs waste products left over after the nutrients have been extracted from food, and it also increases the number of helpful bacteria in the colon. Bulk and bacteria together make the stools larger, softer and easier to pass.

AVOIDING CONSTIPATION

The easiest way to avoid constipation is to alter your diet: consume wholemeal rather than white bread, plenty of fresh fruit and vegetables and a breakfast cereal that includes bran, washed down with at least three pints of fluid during the day.

Try to establish a regular routine for going to the toilet and act promptly on any urge to move the bowels. Remember that there is plenty of variation between individuals. Often there is no need to worry if a gap of a day or two passes without a bowel movement.

Children in particular need a good toilet routine and lots of fluid, especially during minor illnesses. A painful bowel movement can make children avoid going, setting off a vicious circle.

LAXATIVES

If increasing your fluid and fibre intake does not work, occasional use of a gentle laxative such as Epsom salts can help. However, regular use of laxatives, particularly senna and cascara, can overstimulate the bowel and eventually make it inactive. Dietary measures are a much healthier long-term answer.

If constipation does not respond to simple treatments or if your bowel habits change suddenly for no obvious reason – especially if you are over 40 years of age – see your doctor. This is particularly important if constipation is accompanied by pain, weight loss or blood in a stool. The problem may be related to a much more serious condition such as an inflammation or tumour. ∎

CAUSES OF CONSTIPATION

Apart from not eating enough fibre, psychological and external factors can cause constipation. Shift work, emotional upsets and unpleasant toilet facilities can make people ignore the body's signals for bowel movements. If moving the bowels is left too long, the stool dries out and becomes hard. Not drinking enough liquid can have the same effect. If this continues, the bowel becomes packed with dried stools, which are uncomfortable and even more difficult to pass.

Haemorrhoids

Commonly called piles, haemorrhoids are varicose veins in the anal canal. Many people have haemorrhoids at some stage, but they usually only cause discomfort if they protrude from the anus.

Straining during constipation can cause haemorrhoids, as can the persistent passing of hard stools, which can damage the lining of the anal canal and the normal protection of the veins. Restricted flow of blood in the area is another cause, which is why the condition is common in pregnancy. They are not caused by sitting on damp ground or radiators.

METHODS OF TREATMENT

Treatment is not necessary unless the haemorrhoids are prolapsed (protruding) or if they cause irritation, inflammation and bleeding or mucus discharge. In younger people, an increase in dietary fibre can relieve constipation and allow blood vessels to return to normal. Various ointments and suppositories (small pellets of medication that are inserted into the anus) are available without a prescription. These ease discomfort, but are not a cure.

If treatment is necessary, common approaches are to inject the haemorrhoid with a sclerosant – a chemical that shrinks the vessel – or to "band" it with an elastic band to cut off the circulation. Both may cause discomfort and bleeding, which clear up in several days. In serious cases, an anal stretch operation that breaks up the haemorrhoid or a haemorrhoid-ectomy, an operation in which the haemorrhoid is removed, may be needed. Both are done under general anaesthetic.

If haemorrhoids are large, they are less likely to respond to simple treatments. In serious cases, neglect can lead to anaemia because of blood loss. Haemorrhoids do not lead to cancer, but any rectal bleeding needs a medical check. ∎

TYPES OF HAEMORRHOIDS

The considerable network of blood vessels in the anal canal have no valves to regulate the flow, so the weight of blood bears down on the lowest vessels, which tend to stretch. Piles higher in the canal are internal haemorrhoids. Lower ones are external haemorrhoids, and these are prolapsed when they extend from the anus. At first a prolapsed haemorrhoid may retract on its own, but later on you may need to push it back in after defecating. Eventually, it may refuse to go back in.

Anus

Internal haemorrhoid

Anus

External haemorrhoid

CAUTION

If symptoms of diarrhoea do not clear up after a few days, visit your doctor.

Diarrhoea

There is little need to describe the symptoms of diarrhoea. Most people have experienced a bout of "tummy trouble" at some point and vividly recall the loose runny stools and desire to stay close to a toilet.

Most diarrhoea is short lived and uncomfortable rather than serious. However, young children and the elderly can become dangerously dehydrated, which may require medical help, especially if diarrhoea is accompanied by fever, sickness or lack of appetite.

Sudden diarrhoea can have many causes, from unfamiliar foods to bowel infections (gastroenteritis), anxiety or antibiotics. Physically, it can be triggered when too much fluid passes from the bloodstream into the bowel – this is what happens in bowel infections. Anxiety or infection can prompt the bowel to shift its contents too quickly and too little fluid is passed back into the bloodstream.

In older children and adults it usually passes in a couple of days and requires minimal treatment. Drink plenty of fluids and observe good hygiene. Infectious diarrhoea, caused by organisms such as *Escherichia coli*, salmonella and *Giardia lamblia*, can be serious and are usually spread by poor hygiene, so wash your hands before preparing food and eating.

You can buy antidiarrhoeal drugs over the counter, but they are best used only if you are not going to be within reach of a toilet. Rehydration fluids containing essential salts and electrolytes are also available to help prevent dehydration.

MORE SERIOUS CASES

Babies can develop diarrhoea from lactose (milk sugar) intolerance or when they switch to solid food. Keeping fluid intake up by using formulas with good vitamin and electrolyte contents can help. It is best to check with a doctor before trying over-the-counter remedies because the risk of dehydration is high in babies.

Diarrhoea that persists over a long period of time may be more serious and should be reported to a doctor. Although it is often caused by irritable bowel syndrome (a disturbance of the bowel rhythm that often involves diarrhoea, constipation and bloating), other less common causes of diarrhoea are inflammatory conditions of the digestive system such as Crohn's disease and ulcerative colitis, which may need treatment. Coeliac disease, an intolerance to gluten, results in severe diarrhoea. Less obvious food intolerances (especially to lactose) are other possible causes. ∎

WHAT TO EAT AND DRINK

■ During a diarrhoea attack, try to avoid food for 24 hours.

■ Make sure you stay well hydrated by drinking small amounts of mineral water, weak black tea or herb tea (avoid coffee) at half-hourly intervals. Homemade rehydration fluid can be made from 250 ml (9 fl oz) of fruit juice or bottled water mixed with a pinch of salt and a teaspoon of sugar.

■ As symptoms subside, eat small amounts of bland food such as boiled rice, plain unsweetened live yoghurt, dry toast and vegetable soups.

■ Gradually return to a normal diet. Eat only sparing amounts of meat and cheese, which are difficult to digest, and bulky foods.

Nausea and vomiting

Being sick is the body's way of rapidly removing toxic substances, but it can also be linked to other conditions that have little to do with the stomach. Vomiting is usually preceded by feelings of nausea.

CAUTION

■ *Sudden, forceful persistent vomiting, called "projectile vomiting" needs immediate medical attention.*
■ *Severe persistent vomiting may be due to a tumour or brain inflammation (encephalitis) as a result of viral infections such as chicken pox, mumps and measles.*
■ *Vomiting blood requires quick medical attention.*

To vomit, the diaphragm – the muscle between the abdomen and chest – suddenly moves down. The abdomen squeezes in, while the sphincter (the stomach valve, which normally only lets food go down) relaxes. This forces the stomach contents up the oesophagus and out of the mouth. The epiglottis prevents vomit from entering the trachea to the lungs.

The process of vomiting is triggered by a brain mechanism that is aptly known as the "vomit centre". This receives information from the digestive tract, from other parts of the body and from blood.

The symptoms of nausea include sweating, excessive salivation, paleness and dizziness. However, feeling nauseous does not necessarily mean that you will vomit. The symptoms may pass with some fresh air or a sip of water.

THE VOMITING REFLEX

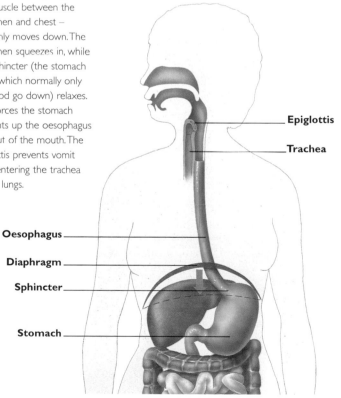

Oesophagus
Diaphragm
Sphincter
Stomach

Epiglottis
Trachea

CAUSES AND TREATMENTS

Vomiting is often a sign of some other problem. For example, if you overindulge in fatty foods or alcohol, your stomach may need to expel some of its contents, or it may want to rid itself of toxins made by bacteria or chemicals in contaminated food. Problems in the digestive system, such as a peptic ulcer, gallstones, hepatitis or a tumour, can cause vomiting. Changes in hormone levels during pregnancy (usually between the 6th and 14th weeks), diabetes, migraine and anxiety may cause vomiting, too.

Motion sickness develops when the balance organ in the inner ear is over-stimulated by movement. Disorders of the balance organ such as Ménière's disease and viral infections can also cause dizziness and sickness. Drugs are available that prevent motion sickness only if they are taken before travelling.

There are acupuncture points that may ease nausea of all kinds and wristbands for applying pressure to them are available. Drugs that control vomiting (antiemetics) may be prescribed if vomiting is severe and persistent or to help patients undergoing treatment such as radio-therapy, which can cause vomiting.

It is important to track down the cause of severe, persistent vomiting. In young children it should prompt a call to the doctor. Otherwise, vomiting is harmless. Let the body do what comes naturally, and follow the advice on what to eat and drink in the box on the facing page. ■

SEE ALSO

Diarrhoea	90
Nausea and vomiting	91
Travellers' problems	122

CAUTION

Most bacteria are killed by adequate cooking, so heat food thoroughly. Do not use the same utensils for meat and other foods.

Food poisoning

The cause of food poisoning can be bacteria, parasites or viruses, poor personal or kitchen hygiene and, occasionally, toxic chemicals.

The most common symptoms of food poisoning are diarrhoea and vomiting, but you may also have a fever, stomach pain and blood in your stools. Most food-borne infections are short lived and resolve without medical attention.

You should take plenty of liquids and, in severe cases, rehydration solutions containing essential salts can aid recovery. The risk of dangerous dehydration is greater in the particularly old or young, and medical advice should be sought. ∎

WHAT CAUSES FOOD POISONING?

Bacteria	Found in	Symptoms	Duration
Campylobacter	Contaminated unpasteurized milk and raw poultry.	Bloody diarrhoea, vomiting, stomach ache and fever.	Occurs up to a week after infection.
Salmonella	Contaminated raw meat, poultry, sausages and eggs.	Diarrhoea and vomiting.	Starts 12 to 24 hours after infection; brief, but organisms excreted for up to six weeks.
Escherichia coli (E. coli)	Intestinal bacteria in cattle can contaminate raw meat.	Bloody diarrhoea and kidney problems, particularly in elderly.	Occurs 6 to 72 hours after infection.
Staphylococcus aureus	Septic spots or cuts on food handlers.	Severe vomiting and diarrhoea.	Begins 2 to 6 hours after infection; clears in 12 hours.
Clostridium perfingens	Contaminated meat.	Severe vomiting.	Occurs 12 to 24 hours after infection; short lived.
Bacillus cereus	Contaminated rice.	Severe vomiting.	Begins 2 to 12 hours after infection; short lived.
Listeria	Soft cheeses, fish, shellfish, pre-cooked foods, undercooked poultry. Pets can be infected.	Include fever, conjunctivitis, swollen glands, rash. Most cases are mild; infection is serious in pregnancy.	Starts 7 to 30 hours after infection.
Hepatitis A	Food and water containing human faeces. Poor hygiene.	Fever, loss of appetite and energy, yellow skin, inflamed tender liver.	Starts 6 weeks after infection; recovery takes months.
Shigella (Bacterial dysentery)	Contaminated water and food.	Stomach pain, vomiting, watery diarrhoea, aching, fever, then stools with mucus and blood.	Occurs 1 to 7 days after infection; lasts about a week.
Clostridium botulinum (Botulism)	Rare. Inadequately cooked or preserved meat.	Weak muscles; disturbed vision, swallowing and speech; paralysis.	Occurs 4 hours to a week after infection; can be fatal.

Indigestion

The symptoms of indigestion occur when the stomach is upset, often by eating too quickly, by eating rich, fatty or spicy foods or by putting strain on the stomach from being overweight or pregnant.

Among the most common sensations of indigestion are pain or discomfort in the upper stomach, an uncomfortable feeling of fullness or bloating – even after you have eaten only a modest meal – and belching. Heartburn (see p.94), which is a painfully tight, burning sensation behind the breastbone that is caused when digestive juices rise out of the stomach, is also typical. Smoking, stimulants such as alcohol, too much stress and high anxiety levels all encourage the symptoms because they prompt the stomach to produce more, and stronger, acid.

ACUTE INDIGESTION

Indigestion can last from a few hours to a few days. Over-the-counter antacid medications available at pharmacies and supermarkets can help alleviate the immediate symptoms. However, if indigestion lasts for more than two weeks, you should visit your doctor. It may be due to a medical condition such as hiatus hernia, acid oesophagitis, peptic ulcer or gastritis. Gastritis is an acute irritation and inflammation of the lining of the stomach, which is commonly caused by anti-inflammatory drugs such as aspirin or by too much alcohol.

HOW TO AVOID INDIGESTION

Prevention is, as usual, the best cure. To avoid indigestion, eat frequent small meals instead of one or two large ones a day and chew food thoroughly before swallowing it. Try to eat in a relaxed environment and do not rush through your food. Avoid fatty or spicy foods or those that trigger your symptoms.

Aim to cut out any stimulants – do not drink coffee or alcohol, especially if you can identify these as triggers for your indigestion, and try to stop smoking. Substitute paracetamol for aspirin and avoid nonsteroidal anti-inflammatory drugs (NSAIDs) if possible. ▪

ALL ABOUT FLATULENCE

Flatulence often causes embarrassment because people believe that they pass wind more often than others. In fact, healthy people typically pass wind from the anus 3–10 times a day, but the average can be as much as 40 times a day with a person still being healthy. Episodes may increase with age. The human body can expel 400–2000 ml (14 fl oz–2½ pt) of gas daily.

Where does all the gas come from? Nitrogen and oxygen come in swallowed air, while other gases such as carbon monoxide are produced by the huge range of chemical reactions that constantly take place in the intestines, making them a veritable gas works. The huge population of bacteria is essential to good health, but it produces gas as it helps process undigested carbohydrates and proteins.

Gulping food, drinking a lot with meals, chewing gum, smoking and being tense all increase the amount of air you swallow and wind you produce. A high-fibre diet produces more gas than one low in roughage, but it also has more health benefits. However, avoid overdoing notorious gas producers such as beans, Brussels sprouts, cauliflower and onions. Sorbitol, a sweetener commonly used to replace sugar, is also a gas producer. Smelly wind does not necessarily denote sickness, but your preferences – spices, beer, fruit juices and white wine can all be culprits for malodour.

Reflux and heartburn

Acid indigestion, reflux and heartburn are all terms that describe what happens when the acidic digestive juices of the stomach reach the wrong place – the oesophagus.

Reflux occurs when, for some reason, the one-way valve that allows food to enter the stomach from the oesophagus (the gullet, or passageway, in which food travels from the mouth to the stomach) becomes weakened. Eventually, the stomach contents and acids manage to wash up into the oesophagus.

The characteristic symptom of reflux is a burning sensation in the chest and throat, or "heartburn". It often occurs immediately after swallowing alcohol, fruit juice, hot fluids or hot fatty foods, or after meals, especially if you lie flat or bend over. Food or fluid may also come back into the mouth, particularly at night, and provoke a feeling of choking.

Being overweight or pregnant is a common cause of reflux because it increases the upward pressure on the valve, as does wearing tight clothes.

Smoking cigarettes and drinking too much alcohol increases the production of stomach acid, as well as weakens the valve. A hiatus hernia can also cause reflux.

Because the oesophagus does not have the same protective lining as the stomach, repeated washing with acid can damage its tissue, which becomes inflamed and even ulcerated. This is called oesophagitis. In the long term oesophagitis can scar and narrow the oesophagus and cause difficulties in swallowing.

WHEN TO SEEK TREATMENT

Simple measures (see box, below left) often resolve reflux problems. If these fail, drug treatments range from those that neutralize the acid or protect the surface of the oesophagus to stronger medicines that reduce or block the production of stomach acid. Drugs are usually taken only intermittently.

If your doctor suspects that you are developing oesophagitis, she may recommend an endoscopy, in which a narrow flexible tube containing a light and "eye" is passed down your throat to see if there is any reddening, ulceration or narrowing. In serious cases, it is possible to repair the weakened valve with surgery.

The term "heartburn" suggests a link with heart disease, but there is none apart from the similarity of pain. Angina, or heart pain, usually begins suddenly with exercise and may spread into the arms (usually the left one). If you have any doubts, telephone your doctor. ∎

EASING REFLUX SYMPTOMS

- Eat a small evening meal at least a few hours before going to bed so that there is plenty of time for it to digest.

- Raise the head of the bed 15–20 cm (6–8 in) on blocks or use pillows to help keep acid and food down in the stomach.

- If you need to, try to lose weight.

- Avoid alcohol, excessive caffeine, chocolate and fats.

- Do not smoke.

- Avoid tight belts and clothes.

- Avoid bending down too much or lying flat after meals.

Peptic ulcers

The treatment of peptic ulcers has been revolutionized by the discovery that they are almost always caused by a bacterium called Helicobacter pylori (H. pylori).

A peptic ulcer is a sensitive raw patch, similar to a mouth ulcer, but it develops either in the lining of the stomach (a gastric ulcer) or in the part of the intestine immediately below the stomach (a duodenal ulcer). It forms when the acids that digest food break through the mucus that normally protects the stomach lining and eat into the tissue.

The symptoms are severe burning, abdominal pain, usually felt at the top of the stomach and sometimes going through to the back. The pain is eased by eating but returns once the stomach empties. Symptoms can be accompanied by vomiting and are often worse at night.

It used to be thought that producing too much stomach acid – by smoking, drinking, eating rich foods or having a high-stress lifestyle – caused ulcers. The only cure was to try to neutralize the acid or protect the stomach lining by eating bland foods or taking acid-blocking drugs, so that the ulcer could heal. However, almost all ulcers recurred.

Helicobacter pylori is now known to irritate and weaken the lining of the stomach and let acid infiltrate. It is thought to be the cause of 90 percent of peptic ulcers and has also been suggested as a cause of gastric cancer. Most of the remaining 10 percent of ulcers are caused by the stomach's reaction to nonsteroidal anti-inflammatory drugs (NSAIDs), such as aspirin, often used to ease the pain of conditions such as arthritis.

TREATING AN ULCER

The discovery of *H. pylori* means that most ulcers can now be completely cured. Treatment involves a one to two week course of two antibiotics and a drug that reduces acid production. This both allows the antibiotics to work and weakens the *H. pylori* which, unlike almost all other bacteria, thrives in acid conditions.

Doctors can test for *H. pylori* infection by using a blood or breath test. Because so few ulcers develop without the bug in residence, many doctors will simply diagnose an ulcer from the symptoms and prescribe the cure without testing. For those with ulcers produced by NSAIDs, drug therapies to ease symptoms, such as antacids, alginates and acid blocks, are the mainstay of treatment. ∎

About half the people in the industrialized world are infected with *Helicobacter pylori,* and even greater numbers in developing countries have it. Doctors are uncertain how the bacteria are transmitted. In many people they cause no symptoms at all, but almost everyone with an ulcer has *H. pylori.* The bacterium shown here has been magnified 7700 times.

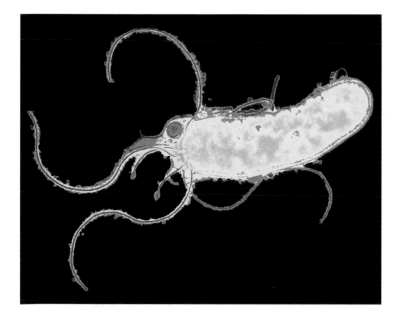

Hernias

When an organ or other type of tissue protrudes through a weak area of muscle or other tissue a "hernia" forms. Hernias can be found in a variety of places, but the two most common locations are in the groin, where inguinal and femoral hernias develop, and at the diaphragm, where a hiatus hernia occurs.

The term hernia usually applies to a bulging of the intestine through the abdominal wall. Inguinal and femoral hernias are formed when the lining of the abdominal cavity pushes outward and forms a small pouch. Pressure in the abdomen gradually makes this pouch bigger and sooner or later a loop of bowel slips into it. What you see and feel when this happens is a painful swelling in the groin. If not treated, it can grow bigger and more painful as successive bowel loops slip into the pouch.

Inguinal hernias occur in men. The swelling tends to move into the scrotum, down the inguinal canal, through which the testicle descends early in life. In femoral hernias, which are most common in obese women, the swelling moves into the upper leg. Both form because of a weakness in the abdomen and the muscles of the groin. This weakness can be present from birth, but more often it is the result of a strain, perhaps caused by a chronic cough, straining to go to the toilet or pass urine or by lifting heavy objects.

TREATING A GROIN HERNIA

Surgery is the first-line treatment to put the bowel loops back into the abdominal cavity, remove the pouch and repair and strengthen the surrounding muscle, either with strong stitches or a patch of nylon material. You will have to avoid strenuous activity for about a month after surgery to avoid stressing the repair, but after that most people recover completely.

If surgery is not possible for reasons of age or other medical conditions, a doctor will push the bowel back into place from the outside. You will then need to wear a truss – a pad strapped against the weak area to stop the pouch protruding again.

Ignoring a hernia can cause serious problems. The bowel can become trapped, causing vomiting and severe abdominal pain. If swelling cuts off the blood supply to the area, the hernia may become "strangulated". In either case emergency surgery will be necessary.

HIATUS HERNIA

When a hernia occurs involving the stomach, it is known as a hiatus hernia. Normally the stomach lies below the diaphragm – the muscular sheet that separates the abdomen and the chest. The stomach is connected to the oesophagus (the passage linking the mouth to the stomach) by a one-way valve, or sphincter, which allows food to pass down but stops digestive stomach acid rising. In a hiatus hernia, a small loop of the stomach slides up through the diaphragm, usually as a result of a type of strain. This stops the valve from working properly and allows the stomach's acidic contents to move up into the oesophagus.

SITES OF COMMON HERNIAS

FEMORAL HERNIA

INGUINAL HERNIA

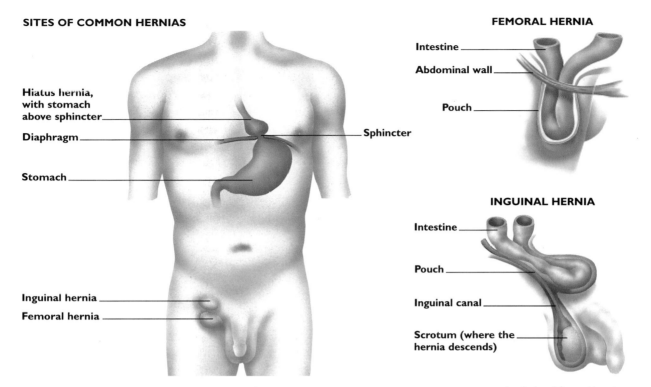

Hiatus hernia, with stomach above sphincter

Diaphragm

Stomach

Sphincter

Inguinal hernia

Femoral hernia

Intestine

Abdominal wall

Pouch

Intestine

Pouch

Inguinal canal

Scrotum (where the hernia descends)

The most common symptom of hiatus hernia is the severe burning pain in the chest and throat known as heartburn, which worsens after a meal or on leaning forward or lying down. The pain can be so severe that it is sometimes mistaken for a heart attack. Hiatus hernia can also make it difficult to swallow. Over time, the constant flush of acid into the oesophagus can damage its lining and cause ulceration, bleeding and, more rarely, cancerous changes in the tissue.

Hiatus hernia is common in middle-aged women, and in overweight people and smokers. It can also be caused by heavy lifting, sneezing or coughing.

TREATING A HIATUS HERNIA

The severity of your symptoms will determine the treatment. If you have mild symptoms, you may simply be advised to avoid large meals and fatty foods, tight clothes and bending from the waist. You may also be advised to lose weight or to raise the head of your bed a few centimetres (inches) to avoid lying flat. Giving up cigarettes is another key factor because smoking increases the production of acid.

If this does not improve matters, you may be prescribed medicines. Antacids neutralize stomach acid and reduce irritation. Alginate liquid is taken after meals and floats on the surface of the stomach contents, protecting the oesophagus. Your doctor may suggest drugs to reduce the amount of acid produced. They have to be taken continuously and are only prescribed when severe symptoms outweigh the possible side effects. Although symptoms should improve within a few weeks, they may return if you do not correct the original cause such as being overweight or smoking. Alternatively, you may be offered surgery, in which the stomach is returned back to the appropriate place. ∎

Inguinal and femoral hernias are visible as a bulge, which may feel heavy or tender. These hernias may appear gradually or form suddenly. Although a hiatus hernia is not visible, it can be suspected from the feeling of "heartburn", and it will show up on certain types of X-rays.

Irritable bowel syndrome

This common digestive disorder affects up to 20 percent of adults in the developed world and is second only to the common cold as a cause of absenteeism from work.

Although irritable bowel syndrome (IBS, or nervous colitis) does not produce serious long-term complications, it can compromise the quality of life. Symptoms vary: they commonly feature abdominal pain and spasm, feelings of bloating or fullness, excessive flatulence and stomach grumbling, a sensation of incomplete emptying of the bowels and persistent diarrhoea or constipation, or an alternating pattern of both. Some sufferers find that their symptoms are relieved by going to the toilet, but others do not. All symptoms cause embarrassment, anxiety and distress.

Exactly what causes irritable bowel syndrome is not fully understood. What is known is that sufferers develop a more sensitive – or irritable – bowel than usual and become unduly responsive to what might be normal events such as the passage of gas or certain foods in the bowel. This sensitivity affects rhythmic muscle contractions that move digesting food through the intestines. It may send bowel muscles into spasm, which brings the process to a halt and results in constipation. Or it may send the muscles into overdrive, propelling the contents through at an abnormally fast rate.

WHAT TRIGGERS IT?

The sensitivity appears to be triggered by any one of a range of factors, depending on the individual. About half of sufferers develop the disorder after a bout of gastroenteritis or food poisoning. Others find symptoms appear after childbirth or a stressful life event such as divorce or job loss. Some complementary practitioners

THE DIGESTIVE SYSTEM

The process of digestion starts in the mouth, where saliva and chewing begin to break down food, continues in the stomach and is completed in the intestines. Nutrients are absorbed through folds in the wall of the small intestine. Waste products pass into the rectum, the last part of the large intestine, and are expelled from the anus. Irritable bowel syndrome occurs when the muscle contractions in the intestines go out of sync.

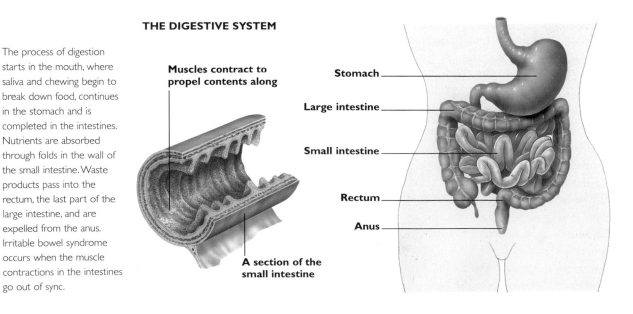

Muscles contract to propel contents along

A section of the small intestine

Stomach

Large intestine

Small intestine

Rectum

Anus

believe that altered bowel bacteria or a yeast infection can be a root cause.

Once sensitized, any irritant can trigger a bout. The irritant can be spicy, high-fat foods, too little or too much dietary fibre, alcohol, coffee, smoking, menstruation or emotional upset.

There is a link with stress: research shows that the condition is more common among those who suffer from anxiety or depression or lead stressful lives. It is not always clear whether stress causes, or results from, the disorder. For example, a sufferer might worry about whether the symptoms are a sign of a more serious illness or anticipate problems in a restaurant. This concern may trigger a bout, and a vicious circle is set up.

CONTROLLING THE DISORDER

Diagnosing irritable bowel syndrome can be difficult because it has a complex combination of physical and psychological factors, and it shares symptoms with a number of other digestive conditions. It may be confused with inflammatory bowel disease (IBD), the term used to describe Crohn's disease and ulcerative colitis. Your doctor may suggest tests such as endoscopy (an internal examination with a flexible fibre optic wire) to rule these out. The disorder also has symptoms similar to those of food intolerances, such as to lactose (milk sugar) or wheat, but these are different problems.

When considering treatment, remember that irritable bowel syndrome does not progress to serious complications. Weigh up the pros and cons, particularly of taking drugs for the condition. If you have infrequent or mild attacks, simply knowing more about the disorder may relieve anxiety and help you cope with the symptoms. Following some of the tips in the box (right) may also help. Research

shows hypnotherapy brings relief to some, while dietary changes work for others. Other complementary treatments include peppermint oil, which relaxes the digestive system, aloe vera juice and live yoghurt.

In more severe cases, doctors may prescribe antispasmodics, laxatives or diarrhoea-controlling drugs. Psycho-therapy or antidepressants may reduce symptoms if the disorder is linked to depression or anxiety. ∎

EASING IRRITABLE BOWEL SYNDROME

To reduce symptoms, try adjusting your eating habits:

- Keep a food, drink and activity diary to see if you can identify specific foods, additives or events that trigger your bouts.

- Eat smaller, more frequent meals.

- Avoid high-fat, fried, rich or spicy foods. Additives such as monosodium glutamate (MSG) and the artificial sweetener sorbitol may also be troublesome.

- Use fibre carefully. If you suffer from constipation, increasing intake may help, but studies show high-fibre diets can make up to 50 percent of sufferers feel worse. Increase or decrease fibre intake gradually, eating foods such as fruit, vegetables, pulses and cereals. Be careful with Brussels sprouts, cauliflower and beans – known troublemakers.

These changes in your lifestyle can also ease symptoms:

- Learn as much as you can about the disorder and your own triggers – knowledge will help you to feel more in control.

- Stress symptoms of all kinds may be related to irritable bowel syndrome so make a checklist. It might include overwork, poor sleep, juggling family and job, too much caffeine or no exercise. See what you can do to change them.

- Learn a relaxation technique that suits you. Try complementary therapies such as massage (pp. 206–09), yoga (pp. 218–23) and aromatherapy (pp. 192–95).

- Do not smoke.

- Take a little exercise every day (pp. 10–11) to help the circulation and reduce levels of stress chemicals.

Other digestive disorders

Some bowel conditions, for example, diverticular disease, are caused by a physical abnormality. Others, such as Crohn's disease and ulcerative colitis, are associated with factors such as infection and food intolerance.

Bowel disorders often share symptoms, making diagnosis difficult, so prepare a precise list of your symptoms for your doctor. Diagnosis may include using colonoscopy to examine the lining of the colon. A long thin flexible cable of fibre optics with a tiny lens at its tip is inserted into the anus and guided up the colon. A sigmoidoscopy uses a similar but shorter tool to monitor polyps or small growths on the bowel lining. The doctor may take a snip of the lining for inspection at the same time. Or he may use a barium enema X-ray: white barium liquid is piped into the intestine to highlight its shape.

If he thinks the problem is in the upper tract, he may ask you to swallow the liquid so that an X-ray can be made, or he may do an endoscopy, with the flexible cable and lens inserted via the throat. ∎

POSSIBLE BOWEL CONDITIONS

Condition/Cause	Symptoms	Risk factors	Treatment
Crohn's disease Can affect any part of the gastrointestinal tract, causing inflammation, ulceration and scarring deep into the intestinal wall. **Cause** Unknown. Theories include genetic susceptibility, lingering measles, infection by *Mycobacterium para-tuberculosis* or certain foods that weaken the intestine wall and allow normal gut organisms and chemicals into the tissue.	Abdominal pain and wind; diarrhoea (sometimes with bleeding); bowel obstruction causing vomiting; fever; tiredness; and weight loss from the difficulty of absorbing nutrients and fear that eating may worsen the symptoms. Periods of good health alternate with lengthy flare-ups. Sometimes a leak (fistula) may break through the inflamed gut, causing serious infection.	Depending on the individual, common infections such as colds, influenza or gastro-enteritis, drugs such as antibiotics and aspirin, certain foods such as milk products or cereals and stress (see pp.76–77) can trigger a flare up. Smoking usually makes Crohn's disease worse.	No cure: the aim of therapy is to extend remission. Steroids and azathioprine are used to decrease acute inflammation, and sulpha-salazine or mesaline are used long term to prevent inflammation. In severe flare ups, liquid diets can prevent malnutrition and ease symptoms. Badly diseased sections of bowel may be removed, but the disease often recurs in nearby tissue.
Ulcerative colitis Inflammation and ulceration affecting the lining of the colon and rectum. **Cause** Unknown, but theories are similar to those for Crohn's disease (see above).	Frequent, urgent need to pass stools with blood and mucus, diarrhoea in severe cases, abdominal pain and tiredness. Periods of good health alternate with acute flare ups. May cause skin lesions, eye inflammation, joint pain and liver disorders.	Similar to Crohn's disease: stress, anxiety, particular foods or general poor health may trigger relapse. Surprisingly, nicotine (best taken in patches or gum) can ease symptoms.	Drug therapy similar to Crohn's disease. In severe cases, or if precancerous cells are found, the colon is surgically removed and replaced with an internal or external "pouch".

POSSIBLE BOWEL CONDITIONS continued

Condition/Cause	Symptoms	Risk factors	Treatment
Diverticular disease Disorder of the intestines. **Cause** Unknown. Intestinal muscles thicken and develop a highly contracted, folded structure. The muscle change also narrows the colon.	Pain in the left lower abdomen, distended stomach, irregular bowel habits with pelletlike stools and, sometimes, small amounts of blood.	Low-fibre diets, large meals and rich fatty foods may provoke symptoms.	Increasing fibre in diet to ensure stools are soft and easy to pass. However, some individuals benefit from decreasing fibre. Anti-spasmodic drugs relax colonic muscles.
Diverticulitis Inflammation of diverticula (intestinal pouches). **Cause** May develop in later life from low-fibre diets, which cause small hard stools that change the pattern of intestinal contraction. Infection or infiltration by food chemicals causes inflammation.	Sore abdomen in area of inflammation, fever and nausea.	Diverticula are dangerous if they rupture, causing abscess or infection within the abdomen (peritonitis), or if they perforate into another organ. Scarring after infection may also narrow the bowel.	Antibiotics and, in severe cases, a temporary liquid diet. Urgent surgery is necessary if there is a rupture or perforation.
Coeliac disease Damage to lining of upper intestine. **Cause** Sensitivity to gluten (a protein in cereals) causes hairlike cells, called villi, on the lining of the intestine to flatten. This impairs nutrient absorption from food. Often appears when children start solid food.	Loss of weight or failure to grow, appetite loss, large pale soft and more frequent stools, swollen stomach, pale skin, tiredness and irritability. Also associated with itchy blistering skin eruptions on knees, elbows, buttocks and back called dermatitis herpetiformis.	Sufferers often have nutritional deficiencies because food nutrients are not well absorbed. Many people may have gluten sensitivity that is not recognized because they have few symptoms.	Can be cured with the permanent removal from diet of all foods containing wheat, rye or barley. Because sufferers usually feel so much better, this seems a small price to pay.
Polyps Small growths protruding from the lining of the bowel. **Cause** Largely unknown, although a small number of people have an inherited condition known as familial adenomatous polyposis.	Most polyps cause no symptoms. Occasionally they may bleed easily or secrete a mucus, which is seen in the stool. However if not removed, some types may develop into cancer.	There are two main types of polyp: those that are unlikely to develop into cancer and those that may become malignant. The latter are known as adenoma.	Polyps are removed with a colonoscope – a tube with a wire snare at its tip, which is looped over the polyp base, then flushed with an electric current to separate the growth from the lining. Tests identify the type of growth.
Gallstones Crystal-like lumps containing cholesterol, which form in the gallbladder. **Cause** Occur in pregnant women, obese people, diabetics and women taking the oral contraceptive pill.	Severe pain in the upper right abdomen, which may extend to the back; bloating, wind, and nausea. If a stone blocks the gallbladder, it can cause pain and inflammation and possibly jaundice.	Gallstones can cause an infection of the liver and, in severe cases, lead to liver failure. They can migrate and block the intestines, and they can also cause cancer of the gallbladder.	Drugs can dissolve small stones, or ultrasound may be used to break them up. The stones may have to be removed by surgery and, in severe cases, the gallbladder may also be removed.

Diabetes

Already a common condition, diabetes is on the increase in many industrialized countries. The number of sufferers has tripled between the mid-1980s and mid-1990s, and the rise is set to continue. It is no coincidence that this upward trend is paralleled by a corresponding increase in obesity.

Commonly known as diabetes, diabetes mellitus is a disorder that occurs when there is a malfunction of the pancreas. The digestion of carbohydrates produces a simple sugar called glucose. This circulates in the blood and enters the body's cells, which then convert the glucose into energy. Insulin, a hormone produced by the pancreas, prevents this blood sugar from rising too high.

In diabetics, the pancreas cannot make any insulin or only produces insufficient levels of it. In the absence of insulin, the result is an abnormally high level of glucose in the blood. The body cannot use or store it all, and the excess causes symptoms (see facing page). There are two principle types of diabetes: non-insulin-dependent diabetes (or NIDDM) and insulin-dependent diabetes (or IDDM).

NON-INSULIN-DEPENDENT TYPE

Non-insulin-dependent diabetes is the most common type of diabetes, affecting as many as 75–85 percent of all diabetics. It occurs when the body produces too little insulin or when the body is unable to properly use the insulin that is produced. It usually appears after the age of 40, which is why it is also called maturity-onset diabetes.

Because this type of diabetes develops slowly, it often goes undiagnosed. It is estimated that for every non-insulin-dependent sufferer who has been diagnosed, there is someone else whose diabetes has been overlooked.

TREATMENT

The non-insulin-dependent type of diabetes is usually the less serious form; nevertheless, it is important to treat it. Some 20 percent of sufferers are able to manage their condition with diet alone. Foods that need to be restricted, or avoided, include sugar and other refined carbohydrates, such as white flour, pasta

This slice of a cell of an islet of Langerhans has been colour enhanced and magnified 4800 times. The red and white spots are secretory granules. The islets of Langerhans, found in the pancreas, are responsible for secreting the hormones insulin and glucagon, which control blood sugar levels.

THE PANCREAS: A MULTI-FUNCTIONAL ORGAN

Head of pancreas

Pancreatic duct

Tail of pancreas

Duodenum
(leading to
the small
intestine)

The pancreas, located behind the stomach, secretes digestive enzymes (which travel to the duodenum via the pancreatic duct) to help break down food. The hormone insulin is made by another type of pancreatic tissue, the islets of Langerhans.

and rice. These are easily digested and turned into glucose, so they quickly raise the blood sugar level. Unrefined foods, such as wholemeal flour, brown rice and fresh fruit and vegetables, take longer to break down and will not have the same effect on the level of blood sugar.

About half of sufferers must also take pills. There are four types, which work in different ways. One helps the pancreas to produce more insulin; another helps the body to make use of the insulin that is produced; a third type slows down the speed at which the body absorbs sugar; and the fourth type increases insulin sensitivity. Several pills may have to be taken in combination. About 30 percent of sufferers also have to supplement their dietary treatment with insulin injections.

PREVENTION

Non-insulin-dependent diabetes is much more likely to develop in people who are inactive and overweight. It is largely preventable, particularly if you keep to a

WHAT ARE THE SYMPTOMS?

If you suspect that you may have diabetes, it is important to make an appointment with your doctor staight away. You will be given a blood and urine test to check your sugar levels.

Symptoms develop in all untreated insulin-dependent diabetics, but they develop in only one-third of those who have the non-insulin-dependent type and are also less severe. As a result, there are many people suffering from a mild form of the disease who are unaware of it until the onset of complications. The symptoms of both types are the same and include:

- excessive thirst and a dry mouth
- increased appetite
- a need to urinate frequently
- fatigue
- weight loss in insulin-dependent diabetics
- blurred vision
- boils
- tingling and numbness in the hands and feet
- genital itching

CAUTION

Complications as a result of diabetes are more likely to occur if the diabetes has not been well managed and controlled. It is important for a diabetic to follow dietary and other health-related instructions given by her doctor.

reasonable weight. Your body mass index should not rise above 25 (pp.260–61). Cutting down on the amount of fat in your diet is the easiest way to keep your weight down. Keeping active is another important way to control your weight, and it will also reduce your risk of high blood pressure and heart disease.

If you smoke, you should cut back sharply on your tobacco intake or, preferably, stop smoking completely. Smoking doubles the risk of diabetes.

INSULIN-DEPENDENT DIABETES

Insulin-dependent diabetes usually begins early in life and is often inherited. The child of someone suffering from diabetes has a 1 in 20 chance of developing the disease. This type of diabetes develops when there is very little, or no, insulin in the body because the cells in the pancreas that make it have been destroyed. Unlike the other type, this form of diabetes develops quickly – usually in a matter of just a few weeks.

The aims of treatment are threefold: they are to prolong life, to relieve

An insulin-dependent diabetic should monitor her blood sugar levels every day. A finger is pricked to allow a drop of blood to fall on to a test strip. The strip is then inserted into a machine that provides a digital reading of the blood sugar levels.

symptoms and to prevent long-term complications from developing. It is important that the condition is treated with self-injections of insulin as soon as it has been detected. Insulin may be obtained from animals; there is also a human type that is made artificially.

SUPPLYING THE INSULIN

Injections of insulin have been used to control diabetes since its discovery in 1921 and, since then, there have been various attempts to administer it in a more user-friendly way than by injection. Insulin cannot be given as a pill, however, because it is destroyed – either by the digestive juices in the stomach or by the pancreas – before it can get into the bloodstream. The possibility of supplying it with nasal sprays and skin patches is being investigated.

There are two types of insulin: a clear, quick-acting, short-term one and a cloudy longer-acting one. The first type is typically used during the day and taken before meals to counter the rise in blood sugar when food is being digested. The second type is usually used at night to maintain a stable base level of insulin, which will control symptoms until the morning. The two types can be combined in a single shot, which is given twice daily. Depending on the kind of insulin being used, up to four injections every 24 hours are necessary.

There are various ways of injecting insulin: with a traditional syringe, one of the newer-style pens, a state-of-the-art jet injector or a portable pump. However, none of the newer methods has proved to have a significant advantage over the traditional syringe.

In the pens, the insulin is contained in disposable cartridges that are used much in the same way as they are in writing pens. Some of the pens are disposable. The jet injectors (used mostly in the United States) shoot insulin under the skin, using a strong jet of pressurized air.

Portable pumps can be useful during pregnancy, when close control of blood sugar is important, and in the minority of diabetics whose blood sugar level is prone to sudden, sharp fluctuations. The insulin is infused through a narrow, flexible tube that runs from a holster carrying the insulin pump to a point in the skin, usually in the torso.

If too much insulin is injected by mistake, it is essential for the diabetic to eat some type of food that is high in sugar as fast as possible in order to raise the level of blood sugar. If she fails to do this quickly enough, a hypoglycaemic attack is likely to occur. While insulin injections are the cornerstone of treatment of insulin-dependent diabetes, they should be combined with other self-help measures (see p.107).

BLOOD SUGAR LEVELS

Most diabetics learn to recognize the symptoms of low blood sugar. Nevertheless, it is important to monitor the level regularly and accurately with blood or urine tests. Either of these can easily be done at home.

To take a blood test, a sample of blood is placed on a chemically treated testing strip. One type of strip is placed in a machine which provides a reading of the result for you. Another type of strip changes colour, and by comparing this against a colour chart you can determine the level of glucose in your blood.

A urine sample can also be tested with a "dip stick", which operates in a similar way to the blood-testing strips that change colour. But this method is less reliable because it does not always reflect

---

WEIGHT AND EXERCISE

Non-insulin-dependent diabetes has increased dramatically in recent years. Although there is a hereditary factor, the reason is probably due to the increase in obesity and the decrease in activity in industrialized countries. In fact, the World Health Organization (WHO) estimates that since the 1960s adults are using an average of 20 percent less energy.

This type of diabetes is most common after the age of 40 because it is in middle age when people tend to become more sedentary and to put on weight. Around 80 percent of sufferers are overweight. Body fat places a strain on the pancreas. The more fat that is carried, the more insulin the pancreas has to produce to maintain a normal level of blood sugar. This in turn can cause the body to store more fat, perpetuating the cycle.

Physical activity is also important in maintaining good insulin function. When the muscles are working hard, they use glucose from the blood for energy, reducing any excess. All adults should be doing the equivalent of 20 minutes' aerobic exercise three times a week.

---

the blood sugar level at the particular moment the test is performed.

These tests are usually carried out at certain set times of the day: before each main meal, at bedtime, before and after exercise and at the first signs of a hypoglycaemic attack. They are taken more frequently during periods of illness.

HYPOGLYCAEMIC ATTACK

If either form of diabetes is not properly controlled, the blood sugar level may fall. The body will react by having a hypoglycaemic attack (often referred to as a "hypo"), which can cause weakness, confusion and irritability, sweating, seizures and even loss of consciousness. This warns the diabetic to take immediate action to raise blood sugar.

A hypoglycaemic attack can occur if too much insulin has been given, a meal has been missed or delayed, alcohol has been

---

CAUTION

Certain over-the-counter medicines can affect blood sugar levels. If you have diabetes, always check with a doctor or chemist to make sure that a medicine is safe for you to take.

CAUTION

It is difficult for some diabetics to feel any sense of pain in their feet, which are prone to infection. If you have diabetes, you should inspect your feet daily for any signs of cuts, blisters, bruises or sores, as well as dry skin and ingrown toenails. Always wear comfortable shoes.

drunk without eating food, an insufficient amount of carbohydrates has been eaten or exercise has been over-strenuous. Diabetics should avoid these circumstances by following the dietary rules for diabetics and by exercising sensibly.

At the first signs of a hypoglycaemic attack (see below), the diabetic should eat something sugary. Many diabetics carry with them sweets or glucose tablets – glucose is absorbed into the blood quickly. A spoon of honey or treacle can be taken if at home. These foods give the body an instant sugar boost. They should be followed by others that release sugar more slowly: bread, breakfast cereals, biscuits or fruit are all good examples.

COMPLICATIONS

In both types of diabetes, treatment must be maintained or complications can develop. These fall into two groups. The first of these affects the body's small blood vessels, which can cause problems in the eyes, nerves and kidneys. If the retina at the back of the eye is damaged, it can result in retinopathy, in which the tiny blood vessels of the retina swell and leak. Excess pressure of the fluid in the eye can cause glaucoma. In either condition, there are few symptoms other than a gradual deterioration in vision. If left untreated, retinopathy and glaucoma can eventually lead to blindness. Cataracts, in which the lenses of the eyes become cloudy, are also more common in diabetics. They can cause increasingly blurred vision.

The second type of complication affects the body's large blood vessels to the heart, brain and legs. Damage to the blood vessels leading to the heart and brain can result in serious conditions such as heart disease and stroke. Poor blood circulation to the legs and feet can cause ulcers and, at worst, gangrene.

MEDICAL TESTS

Long-term complications are extremely common. They are experienced at some time or other by as many as 75 percent of all diabetics. Therefore, it is important for all sufferers to have regular medical tests throughout their lives.

Eye examinations can help detect early damage to the retina. Kidney disease, which affects more than one-third of all diabetics, can be detected with urine analyses. Because diabetics are twice as likely as others to have high blood pressure, which increases the risk of heart disease and stroke, regular blood pressure tests are important.

You should report to your doctor if you experience any loss of sensation in your lower limbs. Men should also report any problems experienced having an erection. Both of these may indicate that there has been some degree of damage to the nerves or blood vessels.

SIGNS OF A HYPOGLYCAEMIC ATTACK

The symptoms of an impending hypoglycaemic attack differ between individuals; however, the most common signs are:

- sweating
- tingling lips
- palpitations
- forgetfulness
- unsteadiness
- anxiety and irritability
- blurred vision
- going pale

DIABETES IN CHILDREN

There is some evidence that the incidence of insulin-dependent diabetes is increasing among children. The cause of this is not understood, but some experts suspect that sociological factors (such as a decline in breast-feeding, which provides some immunity to the baby) may trigger an existing, inherited susceptibility. The rise in incidence is a cause for great concern: the longer the period in which a person has diabetes, the greater is the risk of complications arising in later life.

Any child who is diagnosed with diabetes should be referred to a team of paediatric specialists. They will develop a programme of care for the child and will monitor progress carefully.

Parents of a young diabetic should remember that a child cannot be relied upon to control her condition on her own. It is much more difficult for a child to decline sugary foods or to avoid vigorous exercise. She may also be less inclined to drop what she is doing to take action when a hypoglycaemic attack threatens. It is essential, therefore, that your child's carers, both at home and at school, are informed of her condition and are completely aware of all her dietary and medicinal needs.

DIABETES IN PREGNANCY

Careful management of diabetes is especially important in pregnancy. Pre-mature births, congenital malformations and stillbirths are all more common in diabetic mothers. But most of these can be avoided by good diabetic control during pregnancy, from conception through to the birth itself.

The key to a successful pregnancy in a diabetic is good control of the condition before conception. This should then be maintained throughout the pregnancy,

---

SELF-HELP FOR HANDLING DIABETES

- Eat regular meals and snacks, based around starchy carbohydrates (bread, potatoes, pasta, rice and cereals).
- Cut down on sugar, salt and fat.
- Eat plenty of fruit and vegetables.
- Exercise regularly and try to maintain a stable weight.
- Limit alcohol consumption and always take food with alcohol.
- Have regular eye, kidney and blood pressure examinations.
- Take your medicine with you when you go away from home.

---

with more frequent than usual blood sugar monitoring.

Hypoglycaemic attacks occur most frequently in the first three to four months of pregnancy, in the last few weeks (when they usually occur at night), and around the time of delivery. However, they are unlikely to harm the baby, as long as they are treated immediately.

Some women develop diabetes when they are pregnant. This is known as "gestational diabetes". It is most often detected in the second half of pregnancy. The risk of developing it is greater if a woman smokes, is overweight before she gets pregnant, is over 35 years of age or has diabetes in her family. Even an increase in weight of around 7 kg (15 lbs) increases the risk of diabetes in pregnancy by two-thirds. Smoking more than five cigarettes a day before conception can also increase the risk by nearly 50 percent. Gestational diabetes disappears once the baby is born, but it can be a sign of diabetes developing in the future in up to three-quarters of women affected.

Babies of women who suffer from diabetes during pregnancy also have a higher risk of developing obesity and diabetes themselves in later life. ∎

CAUTION

Use of concentrated steroid creams and ointments can thin the skin and may even cause eczema to return in a worse form. Always follow the package instructions and ask your doctor's advice before using one.

The key characteristics of contact eczema are intense itching, red scaly patches and small fluid-filled blisters, which burst, leaving the skin moist, "weeping" and crusty.

Eczema

A group of different skin complaints all fall under the umbrella term eczema. Although eczema is most common on the hands, ears, feet and legs, it can affect any part of the skin.

The typical symptoms of eczema are itching scaly patches on the skin and blisters. They may be triggered when the immune system responds to an allergy or to an irritation or injury to the skin; however, the causal factor is often unclear. Histamine is released, which dilates the blood vessels in the skin and allows the area to be flooded by certain white blood cells known as lymphocytes. This process affects the skin by making it swollen, red, hot and itchy.

Eczema can be roughly divided into two categories: "contact" eczema, which is caused by irritants, and "atopic" eczema, which is associated with allergies.

CONTACT ECZEMA

When the skin is repeatedly exposed to substances that interfere with its protective oils, contact eczema results. Detergents, shampoos or industrial chemicals, sunscreens, constant washing and drying, or cold or dry conditions are all culprits. Damage accumulates over time and prompts the inflammatory reaction that causes eczema.

Eventually, the skin can become hypersensitive to the trigger substance and only a minor exposure to it can set off a widespread reaction, which can affect even unexposed areas. This explains why some people seem to suddenly develop allergies to substances they have handled without any problems for many years.

Contact eczema can also occur when a person is sensitive to the touch of a particular substance. Common culprits are cosmetics, latex found in rubber gloves and metals such as nickel or chromium, which are often used in watch casings or underwear fastenings. Other triggers include dyes and inks, sticking plasters, plants (particularly primulas), and wool. Repeated exposure can increase this sensitivity and lead to asthma or other acute allergic problems.

ATOPIC ECZEMA

Also associated with allergy, atopic eczema occurs in people who have an inherited genetic trait called "atopy". It makes people more susceptible to allergens in the environment, particularly house dust mite excreta, animal fur and pollens. The allergens do not have to touch the skin to set off an immune system reaction, which in some people manifests itself as eczema and in others causes asthma and hayfever. Atopic people are more prone to all three diseases and 50 percent of children who develop atopic eczema go on to have asthma – although many grow out of both as they reach puberty. Atopic eczema can also be triggered by allergies to foods such as milk, wheat or eggs.

GETTING HELP

Treatment for eczema involves isolating and removing the cause, whether it is a contact or atopic problem. With atopic eczema, the trigger can be more difficult to track down because the problem may have nothing to do with the skin. You may require the assistance of an expert dermatologist. You can help isolate the problem by keeping a record of your symptoms, what you eat and drink, your activities and the weather.

Although medications that treat the skin directly – known as topical therapy – do not cure eczema, they do play a vital role in easing the excruciating itching and embarrassing scaling. They also help to curb scratching, which is hard to resist but makes the condition worse and increases the risk of infection. Steroid ointments can reduce inflammation and give rapid relief from itching. If itching prevents sleeping, sedative medicines may be a temporary remedy.

Applying a dressing on top of the medication can help deter scratching. You should also avoid wearing irritating materials such as wool and rough synthetics; cotton is the most comforting material to wear next to your skin.

It is important to keep the skin moist. A wide variety of lotions, emollients and oils are available on prescription and over the counter, and they often contain ingredients that moisturize the outer layer of the skin, soothing it and encouraging healthy regrowth. You may need to try several preparations to find the one that suits you best, because they may contain preservatives that can irritate some people.

Oral medication with antihistamines or other anti-itch drugs is occasionally used to help break the "itch-scratch-itch" cycle. In severe cases, a short course of oral steroids or potent immuno-suppressant drugs, such as cyclosporin, may be prescribed, but only after the doctor and the patient have taken into consideration the potential side effects.

OTHER FORMS OF ECZEMA

Contact and atopic are not the only forms of eczema. Seborrhoeic eczema is a crust of thick brown-yellow greasy scales or crusty red patches on the scalp, behind the ears, on the eyebrows or in skin folds. Known as "cradle cap" in babies, it usually clears up of its own accord before the child reaches two years of age. It is more persistent in adults but antidandruff shampoos often seem to help.

Nappy rash is usually contact eczema as a result of damp nappies or an irritant reaction to stools or urine. Don't let a baby with this condition get too hot, which will only aggravate the skin, and make sure that you allow only cotton clothing in direct contact with the skin.

Varicose eczema is caused when varicose veins reduce the supply of oxygen and nutrient-carrying blood to the area. Compression stockings may reduce swelling, and corticosteroid ointments can provide some relief.

Skin-to-skin eczema is a contact form produced by sweaty chafing. It occurs mostly in people who are overweight. ■

ATOPIC TRIGGERS

Natural
■ House dust mite droppings

■ Tree and grass pollen

■ Fungal spores

■ Animal hair, skin flakes and dried saliva

■ Feathers and kapok

■ Grain dusts

Manmade
■ Washing powders, fabric softeners and detergents with enzymes

■ Perfumed skin creams, shampoos and sun screens

■ Over-the-counter medicines

■ Industrial chemicals such as inks, oils and paints

■ Food additives such as tartrazine

Food
■ Cow's milk

■ Egg protein

■ Nuts

■ Shellfish

■ Wheat and rice

Psoriasis

A fault in the skin cell production line can lead to psoriasis, a skin condition characterized by dry reddish patches covered with silvery scales. Once it occurs, psoriasis may return intermittently throughout life.

In psoriasis, too many skin cells are generated. These cells live a high-speed life, racing up through the upper layers of skin to the surface in five or six days. They then amalgamate with dead cells, causing raw red patches. The cells eventually shed in masses of scales.

What causes this malfunction is not known. Roughly 40 percent of cases occur in people with a family history of the condition. Nonconventional theories suggest that it is caused by the negative effects of stress on the immune system or by an immune disorder that stimulates unnecessary chemical production. Some complementary practitioners believe that liver overload – caused by anything from an unhealthy diet to exposure to environmental pollutants – could be the problem, forcing the body to expel its toxins and poisons via the skin.

A sore throat, stress, wounds or injuries, hormonal changes from the contraceptive pill, pregnancy or menopause, alcohol, drugs – such as beta-blockers, steroids, antimalarials or lithium – and sunlight can set off psoriasis, although the trigger is not usually obvious.

REDUCING THE SYMPTOMS

Treating psoriasis can be problematic. There is no cure, so the symptoms – not the cause – are treated, and what works for one person may have no impact on another. Your doctor may prescribe a topical therapy (applied to the skin) that contains coal tar, dithranol, steroids or the vitamin D-based calcipotriol. The downside is that many of these are sticky, smelly and stain, and steroids have side effects with persistent use.

In severe cases, "phototherapy" using UVA and UVB lamps can be effective. Sometimes this therapy is combined with a drug called psoralens in a treatment known as PUVA (psoralens plus UVA). Because of the dangers of skin cancer, you should take the advice of a specialist before using phototherapy – and be aware that normal sunbeds do not use the correct wavelength of light and may harm the skin rather than heal it.

Drug treatments for psoriasis, such as methotrexate (which works by killing excess cells), retinoids (which slow cell production) and the immunosuppressant cyclosporin A are very potent and only considered in extreme cases. ∎

New cells are created in the epidermis layer of the skin. They normally take about a month to mature and reach the surface of the skin, where they die and flake off. This process is accelerated in psoriasis, and the skin erupts in flaking lesions.

OVER-PRODUCTIVE SKIN

Psoriasis lesions

Cells pushed to surface

Epidermis

Dermis

CAUTION

Never try an elimination diet where certain foods are omitted from a diet and then reintroduced – without first consulting your doctor. In some people, a severe reaction to an allergen can occur.

The rash shown below was caused by an allergic reaction to the antibiotic penicillin. Whatever the allergen, acute urticaria usually lasts no more than a few hours. Identifying and avoiding individual triggers are the keys to preventing recurring attacks.

Urticaria

A rash sometimes triggered by an allergy, urticaria starts with irregularly shaped, raised red weals that eventually become white or yellow with a red rim. Depending on the trigger, the rash may sting or itch.

Although urticaria can occur anywhere on the body, it commonly shows up on the legs, arms and torso. The rash may come and go over several hours, with some patches clearing and disappearing while new ones arrive.

Urticaria is usually an allergic reaction to milk, eggs, shellfish, strawberries, nuts or yeast; to an additive or preservative in certain foods; or to a drug such as aspirin, penicillin or opiates. Other cases can be triggered by vegetation such as stinging nettles or temperature extremes.

An allergy prompts the immune system to make an antibody known as IgE, which releases the chemical histamine into the lower layers of the skin. Histamine dilates the tiny blood capillaries of the skin, which leak fluid into the surrounding tissue and cause it to swell into the rash.

People with asthma, eczema or hayfever are more susceptible to urticaria. Many of these people have an "atopic" tendency, a genetic predisposition to allergy.

For some people, identifying what they are allergic to is easy – they come out in red blotches if they eat a specific food such as shellfish. Preventing an outbreak simply means avoiding the trigger.

If you are allergic to something more general, such as a food preservative or additive, it can be much more tricky to track down. Skin-patch tests – where a small amount of a suspected allergen is placed on the skin – may help narrow the field. Another method is to keep a detailed diary of what you eat and drink and of your symptoms. It can highlight a pattern and identify the trigger.

WHEN TO SEEK TREATMENT

For most people, a rash comes and goes within a few hours. Calamine or aloe vera lotions can soothe the itching and an oral antihistamine, which can be bought over the counter, can help shorten the attack. Be careful – some antihistamines can make you sleepy, particularly if you drink alcohol at the same time.

For an unfortunate minority, urticaria can become a chronic condition that recurs continuously for months, even years. When this happens, your doctor may prescribe regular antihistamine medication or, in extremely severe cases, a course of steroids may be necessary.

It is important that you make sure any new doctor you visit knows that you are susceptible to urticaria. She can then avoid giving you drugs such as opiates and salicylates that could trigger an attack. ▪

Acne

Although spotty adolescents often feel that they have been singled out by fate, the truth is that over 70 percent of teenagers suffer some degree of acne, at a time when they are often the most self conscious. However, there have been great advances in understanding what causes this skin condition and how to treat it.

Common acne – or *acne vulgaris* – occurs when hair follicles become blocked by an excess production of sebum, the oily substance that keeps the skin supple. The skin's normal bacteria may multiply excessively in the plug of sebum, making the follicle infected and inflamed and producing any of a variety of acne blemishes.

Sebaceous glands are largest and most dense on the face – where there are about 600 per square centimetre – and upper back, neck and chest. Therefore, these are the common sites for acne eruptions.

TYPES OF BLEMISH

Blackheads form when the plug of sebum is exposed to the air, while whiteheads develop when the plug is trapped below the surface of the skin. Occasionally, the inflammation process is more exaggerated and hard, painful red nodules or pus-filled cysts may appear. Spots such as these can leave behind deep pits and scarring of the skin after they heal.

Although sebum glands produce more oil in some people than others, the most well-known trigger for an increase in sebum production is the onset of puberty.

The sebaceous glands make sebum, a moisturizing oil that comes out of the hair follicle to the skin surface. Too much sebum can clog the follicle, forming a whitehead below the surface or a blackhead if exposed to the surface. The colour of a blackhead comes from exposure to air, not dirt.

HOW A SPOT FORMS

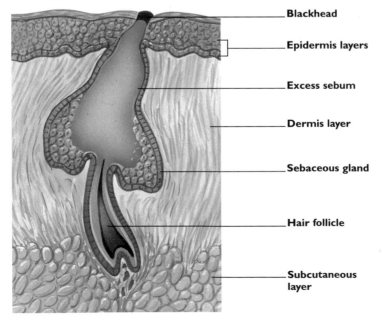

- Blackhead
- Epidermis layers
- Excess sebum
- Dermis layer
- Sebaceous gland
- Hair follicle
- Subcutaneous layer

ACNE ROSACEA

A variant of acne, acne rosacea is a skin inflammation that causes red cheeks and nose, prominent broken blood vessels and, from time to time, swelling and pus spots. It usually appears after 30 years of age and is more common in women and people who flush easily.

The root cause of acne rosacea is unknown, but flare ups can be triggered by sun exposure, alcohol, caffeine and cheese. In the long term, the condition can cause the nose to become enlarged and distorted. Antibiotics are the best treatment.

This is accompanied by an increase in sex hormones, including testosterone. Although teenage boys are most prone to develop acne, the small amount of testosterone produced in girls can also spark off the condition.

Acne can develop later in life, and some women have bouts of it just before their period as their hormones change. Some contraceptive pills, particularly those with progestogen, can also cause acne.

COMMON MISCONCEPTIONS

Contrary to popular wisdom, eating greasy foods, chocolate and sweets has nothing to do with acne. Nor does greasy hair, which is often also prompted by hormonal changes, although acne can develop at the hairline or under a fringe if the hair is preventing the normal escape of skin oils. Sexual activity, or lack of it, does not alter acne in any way.

Some complementary therapists believe that acne is caused when the body's waste disposal systems – the liver, kidney and bowel – are under stress because of an unhealthy diet or environmental pollutants. These introduce toxins into the body, which are transported to the skin for disposal.

TREATING ACNE

Mild acne can be treated with creams or lotions that work by removing sebum and unblocking the pores. Most contain benzoyl peroxide, which both reduces the infection in the skin and causes the top layer of the skin to rub off, unblocking the pores. Other creams have antibiotics to combat infection or preparations based on synthetic vitamin A, which are most effective in blackhead-type acne.

If topical treatment fails, oral antibiotics may be prescribed for periods of up to six months. These kill bacteria and reduce sebum production and inflammation in the follicles. It is important not to stop antibiotic therapy suddenly, because this can cause acne to flare up. Reduce the medicine gradually. In women, oestrogen-containing contraceptive pills may be used to counteract the testosterone; however, ironically, some may trigger acne.

In extremely severe cases, retinoid drugs that reduce oil production and dry the skin may be prescribed. These are taken as a last resort because they can cause liver damage. Severe scarring from acne can be improved with "dermabrasion" therapy, in which the top layer of the affected skin is removed. However, with modern treatments, such lasting damage and drastic measures should be preventable. ■

TIPS FOR A HEALTHY SKIN

■ Wash the affected areas twice daily with a normal soap or cleansing bar. Do not become obsessive – more frequent washing only removes the surface oil, which can encourage oil production.

■ You should treat an outbreak of acne before it has a chance to get worse. Use an over-the-counter acne treatment, such as one containing benzoyl peroxide, as soon as you notice the first blackheads or whiteheads.

■ Moisturize your skin, especially if you are using drying treatment creams.

■ Go out in the sunlight as often as possible, remembering to take precautions against sunburn (p.119).

■ Do not pick or squeeze the spots – this can worsen the condition and lead to scarring.

■ Drink plenty of fresh water and eat plenty of fresh fruit and a variety of vegetables.

■ Avoid the following, which can make acne worse: oily or greasy cosmetics; regular contact with mineral or cooking oils; stress; hot, humid environments; and certain drugs such as steroids and, in some cases, the oral contraceptive pill.

Skin infections

Damage to the skin, hair and nails can come from bacteria and viruses, fungus and moulds, mites and insects. Most skin infections and parasites are itchy, and the inevitable scratching worsens sore areas.

Bacterial and viral skin infections are common and can prompt a wide range of symptoms from boils to rampant, sometimes fatal infections such as the rare "flesh-eating bug", necrotizing fasciitis.

Also known as tinea, fungi and mould infections, such as athlete's foot, are spread mostly through contact with affected people, but occasionally from animals or soil. Symptoms depend on the fungus strain and the part of the body affected. Some cause inflammation, redness and soreness; others, just a slight roughness or scaling of the skin. Infection is more common in people with diabetes and those with a depleted immune system. Sweating, skin moistness and friction encourage infection.

Various mites and insect parasites such as lice can infest the skin. The condition is often compounded by further injury and infection as a result of scratching. ■

A GUIDE TO SKIN INFECTIONS AND INFESTATIONS

Description	Location	Treatment	How to avoid
Boils Most often caused by the *Staphylococcus* bacterium, a boil takes hold in a hair follicle and prompts the formation of a red lump, which gradually fills with yellow pus as the infection thrives. The lump can become painful from pressure on nerves. Boils often arise in crops because of the high local concentration of bacteria. If other follicles become infected, a carbuncle, which is a multi-headed boil, can form. It can grow as wide as 5 cm (2 in) across.	Key sites for boils are the back of the neck, armpit and groin, where *Staphylococci* colonize because these areas offer an attractive moist environment for the organism to thrive. Boils sometimes develop at other sites such as in the nose. A stye is a small boil in an eyelash follicle.	To reduce the chance of infection spreading, thoroughly wash the area around a boil with an antiseptic soap. In severe cases, antibiotics can prevent further development but, once a boil has become established, it must run its course and cannot be eliminated without treating with drugs. Do not burst a boil because this can spread infection. Applying a hot compress can relieve discomfort and soften the boil, allowing it to come to a head. For a large boil, a visit to a doctor may be necessary to lance it under a local anaesthetic.	Poor personal hygiene, obesity and heavy sweating encourage boils. People with diabetes and eczema can also be prone to boils because they have lowered resistance to bacterial infection.

A GUIDE TO SKIN INFECTIONS AND INFESTATIONS continued

Description	Location	Treatment	How to avoid
Impetigo Contagious weepy blisters that burst, leaving behind honey-coloured crusts or scabs can identify impetigo, which is caused by *Staphylococcus* or *Streptococcus* bacteria.	It often starts around the lips, nose and ears, especially if there are cuts, scratches, cold sores or eczema. Touching the affected skin can spread the infection around the body and to others.	Antibiotic tablets clear infection in about 5 days. Loose crusts should be gently washed off with soap and water and dabbed dry.	Keep affected children away from school and prevent them from touching others. Boil pillowcases, towels and flannels after every use.
Warts Common, contagious, but mostly harmless growths on the skin, warts are caused by infection by the human papilloma virus (HPV). At least 30 types of HPV have been identified. Children are susceptible to human papilloma virus because their immunity is less developed. Ill health in older people also makes them susceptible.	Common warts appear on sites prone to injury such as hands, face, elbows and knees, especially in children. Plantar warts, or verrucas, on the sole of the foot can be painful when standing. Flat warts occur mainly on the wrists, hands and face. Genital warts are spread by sexual intercourse.	About 50 percent of warts disappear of their own accord within a year. However, wart paints or gels, available over the counter from pharmacies, are quick and effective. Most contain salicylic acid and should be used after a bath when the skin is soft and absorbent. Warts can be frozen off with liquid nitrogen – this is called cryotherapy.	If you have a verruca, cover it in swimming pools and public showers to avoid spreading it. You should always report genital warts to your doctor. They greatly increase the risk of cervical cancer in women and can be spread between sexual partners. Use a condom during sexual intercourse.
Molluscum contagiosum This highly contagious viral infection mainly affects children –particularly those with eczema. It forms shiny wartlike spots, or papules, which develop a dimple on the top as they grow.	The papules usually appear in groups on the genitals, thighs, face and elsewhere and can be spread around the body by scratching.	They sometimes disappear on their own. Treatments include freezing with liquid nitrogen or liquid phenol. The doctor may prescribe an ointment that can limit the spread. Children with only a few warts can soak in a warm bath, then gently scrub with a pumice stone.	Prevent an infected child from sharing baths and towels with others.
Ringworm Red, itchy scaly patches with centres that usually heal and leave characteristic scaly circles, are the symptoms of ringworm, a type of fungal infection. It can cause persistent scaling that resembles eczema on the hands and feet. If the scalp is infected, it can cause patchy hair loss.	Patches are most often on the torso, groin (known as jock itch), buttocks and armpits. Ringworm can occur on the palms of the hands and the soles of the feet, as well as on the scalp. It can also infect nails, giving them a smooth white or crumbly yellow surface.	Treat early with antifungal creams, tablets or nail paints. Most infections clear in a week or two, but continue treatment as prescribed to prevent regrowth. Nails take a year to heal. In persistent cases, skin or nail samples may be sent to a laboratory for analysis.	To protect others, use separate towels and flannels. Unaffected people in the household may minimize the risk of infection by using an antifungal dusting powder.

A GUIDE TO SKIN INFECTIONS AND INFESTATIONS continued

Description	Location	Treatment	How to avoid
Athlete's foot The skin becomes cracked and sore and often blisters and peels away when infected by athlete's foot, a type of fungal infection. Affected nails become detached or thick and discoloured. It often occurs in those who wear thick boots or shoes.	It is common between the toes, from where it can spread to the soles of the feet and the toenails.	Antifungal cream can clear up this condition.	Dry your feet carefully, and dust them with antifungal powder. Always wear cotton socks and change them daily. Wear sandals or go bare foot if possible. Disinfecting bathroom and shower floors helps prevent the infection from spreading.
Pityriasis versicolor In this condition, white, brown or salmon scaly patches up to 1 cm (½ in) wide are caused by a fungus that is normally present on the skin, but growing at an abnormal rate. It most often affects young and middle-aged adults, especially men.	The patches typically appear on the torso and arms, with no other symptoms.	Carefully treat the whole body with an antifungal shampoo. If any patches are missed, the fungus will recur. The skin may take several months to return to its normal shade.	Not contagious, but people who are prone to the condition should change their underclothes and nightwear daily and thoroughly wash them.
Scabies Caused by a parasite called *Sarcoptes scabei*, scabies is transmitted from person to person by close contact, such as sharing a bed, hugging or sitting on a knee. Eggs show up as tiny grey scaly swellings. There is itching or, later, reddish lumps, caused by an immune system reaction to a protein produced by the mites.	Female mites lay eggs just under the skin's surface, most often on the fingers and wrists, around the nipples in women and on the penis in men. The eggs may not hatch for a month, but when they do, the itching becomes severe and affects the whole body from the neck down.	Use special "scabicide" preparations over the entire body, particularly in any skin crevices. The itching may persist for up to two weeks.	Scabies is highly contagious during the "window" period between infection and when the eggs hatch. Treat anyone who has been in physical contact with an affected person at the same time, whether or not itching is present. Wash bed linen and underwear. Hang out other clothes or store in a bag for 24 hours – the mites die quickly once they are away from the body.
Lice These small insects feed on blood and cause irritation by puncturing the skin. There are three types: head lice (nits) and pubic lice (crabs), which live on body hairs, and body lice. All of them cause intense itching.	Head lice live on the scalp, are common in children and spread by close contact. Easy-to-see pubic lice infest pubic hair and are often spread by sexual contact. The rare body lice feed on skin but live and lay eggs in unclean clothing.	For head or pubic lice, apply a special lice shampoo, and use a fine toothed comb to remove the eggs from hair. Boil or dry clean clothes to kill body lice.	Ensure lice are gone by repeating treatment weekly for several weeks, and check and treat those who are in close contact with an affected person. To avoid pubic lice, do not share towels or clothes used by an affected person.

SEE ALSO
Skin infections 114–116

Calluses and chilblains

Formed of thickened hard skin, a callus develops anywhere on the body where there is regular or prolonged pressure or friction, providing a protective pad against injury. When small blood vessels just below the surface of the skin narrow in cold weather, a chilblain – a reddish-blue swelling – can form on a finger or toe.

In general, calluses appear on the feet, the part of the body that absorbs the most friction on a daily basis. However, manual labourers and athletes (such as tennis players) often develop calluses on their hands, desk workers get them from resting on their elbows and guitarists have them on their fingertips. Even pushing a pen may create a "writer's" lump where the pen presses into the finger. Calluses are not usually painful, although they do blemish the skin.

WHAT IS A CORN?

A thick callus on a toe is known as a corn, and it has a hard kernel formed in the centre. Because it often presses on the nerves below, a corn can be painful. You can use corn-removing plasters, which are available from pharmacies, to remove a corn. They consist of a foam circle with salicylic acid in the centre, which eats away the plug of dead skin. Or you can visit a chiropodist who will carefully pare away the thickened layers of skin with a scalpel. Remember that for a complete cure you must remove the pressure that caused the corn in the first place. Make sure that your shoes fit properly.

PREVENTING CHILBLAINS

The itching, burning swellings called chilblains arise after exposure to the cold. They most often occur on fingers and toes but can also appear on other parts of the body such as the buttocks. To keep internal organs warm in cold weather, the body curtails the amount of blood sent to the extremities such as the hands and feet. This drop in blood circulation reduces the skin's supply of oxygen and triggers chilblains. People with poor circulation are particularly susceptible.

Chilblains generally cure without treatment. The best prevention is to wear warm clothing, particularly on your legs, hands and feet. Take regular exercise to stimulate your blood flow and do not smoke, which reduces blood circulation in the skin. Scratching chilblains makes them worse and slows the healing process, so try to resist the temptation. ∎

If a corn – a type of callus on the toe – causes any discomfort, you can soak the affected area in warm water to soften the skin, then rub off the dead skin with a pumice stone.

CAUTION

If removing a tick, be careful not to separate the body from the head:

■ *Use tweezers to grasp the head as close to the skin as possible. Pull gently – do not twist or use force.*

■ *You can smother the tick with petroleum jelly or nail polish remover to deprive it of oxygen and make it withdraw. The drawback of this technique is that it can take several hours for the tick to be affected.*

■ *Use heat from a lit match or cigarette to make the tick back out.*

When an insect such as a mosquito bites, it does so to have a meal of blood. However, when it pokes its specially designed proboscis through the skin, it deposits saliva or faeces near the puncture. These cause an allergic reaction, which can produce a painful and itchy or weepy rash.

Insect bites and stings

Bites from insects affect people to differing degrees: some complain that their blood seems to draw insects from miles around; others do not seem to be bitten, or react, at all.

Most bites cause only temporary irritation and clear up in a few days. If bitten, you should wash the area with soap and water; you can also apply a soothing lotion such as calamine or an antihistamine cream. Try not to scratch or rub the bite – this spreads the allergen.

In tropical areas biting insects transmit diseases such as malaria, sleeping sickness and typhus. If you visit one of these areas, use nets impregnated with insect repellent and cover as much of your body as you can with clothing to avoid being bitten.

STINGING INSECTS

When bees, wasps and hornets sting, they inject a venom as a defence. Inflammatory chemicals in the sting cause pain, redness and swelling. These insects often leave their sting sac in the wound. Gently scrape it out with a fingernail or knife –

do not grasp it with tweezers or your fingers because this injects more venom. Wash the area with soap and water and apply a cold compress. Painkillers can ease discomfort and the symptoms should subside within 48 hours.

One in 200 people is hypersensitive to insect venom and develops more serious symptoms, including a widespread itch, dizziness, vomiting and swelling of the face and throat immediately after being stung. In extreme cases, the person may go into anaphylactic shock. This life-threatening reaction demands immediate emergency treatment with adrenaline. Anyone who is hypersensitive to stings is well advised to carry an emergency self-injection kit with them at all times.

A technique called "hyposensitization" is sometimes used to reduce sensitivity to stings. It involves carefully injecting increasing doses of the venom to retrain the immune system's reaction.

LYME DISEASE

Ticks carrying Lyme disease can pass the disease on to people. The bite containing the disease may be unnoticeable, but a bull's eye rash – a reddened area with a clear centre up to 20 cm (8 in) wide – often appears for two to four weeks. Fever, headache, lethargy and muscle pains are symptoms, and the joints, especially the knees, become red and swollen. The severity of symptoms varies but they often recur weekly. Treatment with antibiotics is necessary to get rid of the disease. ■

WHEN A MOSQUITO BITES

Proboscis

Cross section of layers of skin

Blood vessel

CAUTION

■ Certain medications, such as diuretics and antibiotics, make the skin more sensitive to the sun.
■ Remember that when outside you can burn even if it is cloudy.
■ Rays reflected off water, snow and sand can also increase your chances of sunburn.

Sunburn

A certain amount of sunshine is good for you – the body needs it to synthesize vitamin D and a sunny day improves most people's mood. Overexposure, however, is harmful.

There are two types of ultraviolet (UV) radiation from the sun that reach the earth's surface: UVA and UVB. Too much UVB can cause sunburn and skin cancer, and UVA contributes to the premature aging of the skin. How sensitive you are to the sun depends on the amount of the protective pigment melanin in your skin. The paler your skin, the less melanin it contains and the more vulnerable you are to sun damage.

Sunburn is painful. The skin turns lobster red and may blister, and there is little you can do except apply calamine or aloe vera lotion to soothe the pain. If the burn is widespread and severe, you may feel dizzy, dehydrated and nauseous and have a headache. Stay covered up and in the shade until the skin recovers.

Overexposure to the sun can have more serious consequences than sunburn. Solar keratoses are raised red, rough scaly patches of skin that often form on the head, neck or hands of people who spend a lot of time in the sun. The patches usually remain benign, but they may be frozen off with liquid nitrogen because they can change into skin cancer.

One of the greatest risks from overexposure to the sun is skin cancer, and the incidence of this form of cancer has dramatically increased in recent years. It is thought that severe sunburn changes the make-up of the skin, although it may be years before the cancer itself develops. There is believed to be a link between severe sunburn in childhood and the development of malignant melanoma in the middle-aged years, so it is important to protect children from the sun.

Another long-term hazard of sunlight is wrinkled skin. The youthful bronzed of today become the weatherbeaten of tomorrow because excess UVA irreparably damages the elasticity of the skin.

SUNSCREENS

Most sunscreens work by absorbing or reflecting the sun's rays. They do not protect against all the components of the sun's rays and should not be a substitute for avoiding excessive exposure.

Sunscreens that block mostly UVB rays lessen the risk of acute sunburn but let you spend more time in the sun receiving aging doses of UVA. Sunscreens are often numbered from 2 to 42, which denotes their sun protection factor. The higher the number, the greater the protection. ■

WHAT ARE BLISTERS?

Blisters are nature's way of protecting an injured area of skin. They usually form as a result of burns or friction – for example, from an ill-fitting shoe. The fluid comes from the underlying blood vessels and is sterile. It cushions the damaged tissue and protects it from infection. It is better not to burst a blister but to let it heal of its own accord.

Some diseases, such as eczema and impetigo, cause blisters. Small blisters known as vesicles can accompany the rash of chicken pox, shingles and herpes simplex. Again, do not burst them as they contain virus particles that spread the infection.

SEE ALSO
Your immune system
26–27
Travellers' problems 122

CAUTION

If a child's temperature rises to 39°C (102°F) or above or he has a fit following a vaccination, call the doctor immediately or go to the nearest hospital casualty department.

Vaccinations

Also called immunization, vaccination works by artificially inducing immunity to infectious diseases. As well as protecting an individual from an illness, vaccines can eradicate that disease from society over the course of time. Being vaccinated is particularly important to vulnerable groups such as children and the elderly.

A vaccine contains a small part of the bacterium, virus or chemical that causes the disease. When the disease "trigger" is injected into the bloodstream, it prompts the immune system into producing antibodies to the illness. This confers immunity in the same way as having the disease itself does.

The British physician Edward Jenner coined the word vaccination in 1798. He used cowpox inoculation to give immunity to smallpox, then a deadly disease.

DIFFERENT TYPES OF VACCINE

There are three types of vaccine: an inactivated vaccine is produced from organisms that have been chemically inactivated; an attenuated vaccine is made of live organisms that are altered to prevent infection; and an inactivated toxin is made from a disease-causing organism, but the toxins are modified so they do not cause disease. The vaccine chosen depends on the disease it is meant to prevent.

Most children are vaccinated within the first two years of life (see box, facing page). In Great Britain, over 90 percent of children receive all the routine vaccinations. Some vaccines are given in combination. This applies to diphtheria, pertussis (whooping cough) and tetanus (DPT), as well as to measles, mumps and rubella (MMR). However, all of these can be given in single shots if any component of a multiple vaccine is contraindicated (an individual displays adverse symptoms that make the treatment inadvisable).

AFTER THE VACCINE

Many children develop a temperature after being vaccinated. This is not a cause for concern unless it rises above 39°C (102°F). Otherwise, if a child's temperature is over 37.5°C (99.5°F):

- Give the child plenty of fluids to drink.
- If the child is in bed, make sure there are not too many blankets on the bed.

WHEN NOT TO VACCINATE

Sometimes immunization is not advisable or may have to be deferred. Tell your doctor or health visitor if your child has:

- Had a bad reaction to another immunization or has had anaphylactic shock from eggs (only for an MMR vaccine)
- A high fever
- An immune-related illness (or a member of the family has one)
- Had convulsions in the past

■ Give an infant paracetamol according to the manufacturer's instructions.
■ If necessary, sponge the child with luke-warm water and allow the skin to dry.

THE DEBATE

Despite vaccination's role in reducing the number of serious infections, there are many who argue against it. There have been no scientific studies into the long-term effects, and the impact of vaccines on the immature immune system may disrupt it, leading to other illnesses in later life. The increase in some immune-related diseases has been linked to child-hood vaccination. Some vaccines do not give lasting immunity, while having the disease itself does. Many of the illnesses immunization prevents would be mild in children, but are more serious in adults, who can catch them once the vaccine wears off. ■

> **CAUTION**
>
> *Never give aspirin to a child 12 years of age or younger: it has been linked to a dangerous condition known as Reye's syndrome. Treat a fever or aches and pains with paracetamol.*

CHILDHOOD IMMUNIZATIONS

Vaccination	Age	Contraindications	Risks/side effects	Comments
Polio	2–4 months, 3–5 years, 14–19 years	Diarrhoea, vomiting or febrile illness.	None to the individual.	Small risk of infection to family members through contaminated nappies.
Diphtheria	2–4 months, 3–5 years, 14–19 years	An acute illness; reaction to prior diphtheria vaccination.	Redness, swelling where injected; slight fever; rarely, neurological reactions.	Disease rare in Great Britain, but may occur in travellers to developing countries.
Pertussis (Whooping cough)	2, 3, 4 months	Family history of fits or epilepsy.	Pallor; small risk of convulsions and fits.	Stop injections if there is a reaction after first one.
Tetanus	2, 3, 4 months and 3–5 years	Acute febrile illness.	Slight fever; rarely, anaphylactic shock if allergic.	Booster advisable every 10 years. Vaccination can be given at time of infection.
Measles	12–15 months and 3–5 years	High fever; immuno-suppressive medication; tuberculosis; egg allergy.	Malaise; fever; rash; rarely, convulsions.	Disease and its complica-tions much more serious in adulthood.
Mumps	12–15 months and 3–5 years	Acute illness; immuno-deficiency disorder.	Slight fever; rash; cold symptoms.	More important for boys as may lead to orchitis (inflammation of testis).
Rubella	12–15 months and 3–5 years	Hodgkin's disease; leukaemia; immuno-suppressive therapy; pregnancy; in child, fever.	Febrile illness; small risk of arthritis in later life.	Important for young girls, due to risks if contracted in pregnancy. Immunity may last only 5 years.
Hib (Haemophilus meningitis)	2, 3, 4 months	Any type of acute illness.	Swelling and redness where injected.	Most common at 10–11 months, with risk declining to 4 years; rare afterward.
Tuberculosis (TB)	10–13 years	None	Abscess or ulceration where injected.	Preceded by skin test to see if individual is immune.

CAUTION

The holiday spirit sometimes encourage people to take risks. Road accidents with hired cars and mopeds are the most common type of holiday accident. Always familiarize yourself with local traffic regulations and never drink before driving.

Travellers' problems

One in every 100 holiday-makers requires medical treatment when away from home and 15 percent of them are hospitalized. With the right precautions, most of these accidents and illnesses can be avoided.

Food poisoning is a common holiday hazard. Make sure that any meat, fish or shellfish you eat is well cooked. In tropical countries, do not eat raw food unless you can peel it or shell it yourself. You should avoid buffet food that has been on display for more than three hours (two hours in hot climates). If you get diarrhoea, take a rehydration fluid or drink plenty of water with salt and sugar.

Be wary of tap water in the developing world. Do not drink it, have ice cubes made from it, brush your teeth with it or rinse food in it. To ensure that water is safe, use water purifying tablets or an iodine resin water filter, or boil and cool the water. Never swim in suspect waters.

TRAVEL VACCINATIONS

If travelling overseas, you should have any vaccinations several weeks before your departure date. If you are unsure of which ones you need, you can check with the advisory board or your family doctor. These are the immunizations most often suggested: polio, tetanus, typhoid, hepatitis A and B and yellow fever, as well as malaria prevention tablets.

SUN

Never sunbathe in the midday sun in hot countries (from 11.00am to 3.00pm). To protect against dangerous UVA and UVB sun rays, apply a sun lotion with a rating of at least 15 SPF about 15 minutes before you expose your skin to the sun, then every two hours. Keep young children covered in light clothing and hats and never expose the skin of a baby under six months old to the hot sun.

OTHER PRECAUTIONS

To reduce jet lag when flying across time zones, adapt to the local hours as soon as possible. Try sleeping on the plane and, once you arrive, stay outdoors in the daylight as long as you can. Flying also causes dehydration, so drink plenty of fluids during the flight, but avoid alcohol. You should also avoid tobacco, which decreases the already-reduced supply of oxygen. The combination of flying at high altitude and heavy meals can slow down your circulation enough to make you feel dizzy, so you should avoid heavy meals.

Sexually transmitted diseases can be the result of the relaxed attitude adopted by some travellers. If you sleep with someone new, use a condom. ∎

BASIC FIRST AID KIT

If you are taking a holiday away from home, you should plan to take along a basic first aid kit. Where you go will determine what should be in it.

■ The essentials: plasters, bandage, antiseptic ointment, diarrhoea tablets, rehydration powder, insect repellent, insecticide spray, sun lotion, painkillers, astringent spray, sticky sterilized strips (for closing a wound) and indigestion tablets.

■ If travelling to the developing world or tropical countries, also take: an iodine resin filter or water purification tablets, a mosquito net, mosquito coils and a sterile syringe and needle.

SEE ALSO

Styes   124

CAUTION

Do not use eye drops designed to make the whites of the eyes stand out. They may cause blood vessels in the eyes to contract, thus draining the eyes of blood, and they can create a rebound condition in which the whites remain red, making the eyes worse than before applying the drops. They can also raise or lower the blood pressure of the whole body; possibly causing an acute attack of glaucoma.

■ Dry eyes can be caused by a tear deficiency. Artificial tears may be prescribed to relieve this condition.

■ A sore eye that feels worse in strong light may signal a corneal ulcer or inflamed iris. Seek medical help straight away.

Conjunctivitis

One person in every 50 who consults his doctor each year does so because of conjunctivitis. This is an inflammation of the conjunctiva, which is the transparent membrane that covers the front of the eye.

Conjunctivitis can be caused by bacteria, an allergy or a virus. The bacterial infection is usually caught from contaminated fingers, face flannels or towels. The virus is often associated with a cold, sore throat or childhood illness. An allergy may be caused by cosmetics, pollen or contact lens cleaning solutions.

Newborn babies can contract conjunctivitis from the mother's vagina during birth. This condition is known as *Ophthalmia neonatorum* and must be medically treated without delay. If not, the infection can spread and cause blindness in the baby.

Diagnosis is made from the appearance of the eye. If the doctor suspects an infection, he may take swabs to find the causative organism. This is particularly important in the case of a newborn baby.

TREATMENT

Any discharge and crusts on the eyelids should be removed with warm water, using a flannel that has been freshly washed in particularly hot water.

The choice of treatment will depend on the cause. Bacterial conjunctivitis is treated with antibiotic eye drops or ointment. Allergic conjunctivitis is usually treated with antihistamine eye drops. Both of these usually clear up within several days. Viral conjunctivitis tends to get better without treatment.

EYE HYGIENE

If the condition recurs, the answer is to follow scrupulous hygiene. Wash all face flannels and towels at high temperatures and make sure that each member of the family uses only her own flannel.

Proprietary eyebath solutions should never be used. Tears, the natural liquid of the eyes, are the best solution for washing eyes. An eyebath is not sterile and can contaminate the tear film and the eye.

Cosmetics such as mascara and eyeliner can contaminate the margins of the eye lid and allow organisms to collect, which predisposes you to eye infections. If you develop conjunctivitis, throw away your current cosmetics and start with new ones after the infection has completely cleared.

Contact lens wearers need to be particularly careful about eye hygiene, especially with their cosmetics. They should stop wearing their lenses while they are suffering from conjunctivitis. ■

RECOGNIZING CONJUNCTIVITIS

The symptoms of conjunctivitis are the same, whatever the cause. The eyes become bloodshot and the membrane swells. The eyes also feel itchy and may discharge a yellow pus, which may dry to a sticky crust after a night's sleep.

Bloodshot veins   **Red and swollen lid**

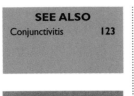

SEE ALSO
Conjunctivitis   123

CAUTION

A persistent lump on the eyelid may be a meibomian cyst. Although this is never cancerous, it may become infected and resemble a stye. It can be removed by minor surgery.

Styes

Our eyes are ringed with eyelashes, each hair of which springs from a hair follicle. When one of the hair follicles becomes infected, a painful and inflamed abscess appears.

A stye, or hordeolum, is a common eye disorder. It can be the result of an infection and can also signify a weakness of the immune system (see pp.26–27). It can, for example, occur during any debilitating illnesses, such as measles.

Styes often recur. What happens is that one clears up, usually within a week, but by then another hair follicle has become infected by the same bacteria and produces another stye. You should never squeeze a stye – this can spread the infection to other hair follicles.

RECOGNIZING A STYE

A stye usually forms near the inner corner of the eye, but it may also develop at the base of any of the eyelashes.

Abscess

TREATMENT

You can speed up the healing of the stye by applying a clean, hot compress three times a day, which should help the pus to discharge. An eyebath of eyebright or camomile may reduce inflammation.

When the pus comes to a clearly visible head, remove the eyelash with a pair of clean tweezers and wash the eye with a sterile cloth. An antibiotic eye ointment can help prevent a recurrence.

EYE HYGIENE

The key to preventing styes is scrupulous hygiene. Make sure each member of the household uses his own clean face flannel and does not share one with anyone else. Do not use proprietary eyebaths, as these are not sterile and can contaminate the tears, which are the best solution for washing the eyes.

Cosmetics, such as eyeliner and mascara, can contaminate the margins of the eyelid and allow organisms to collect, predisposing you to eye infections. If you develop a stye, throw away your current cosmetics and start again with new ones after the infection has completely cleared.

If you wear contact lenses, you should be particularly careful about eye hygiene, especially with cosmetics. Do not wear your contact lenses while you have a stye. ∎

EYE CARE

- Avoid rubbing your eyes.
- Do not touch your eyes when you are gardening – some plants can cause an allergy.
- Wear protective eye goggles when swimming. If you're shortsighted, you can obtain goggles with your prescription.
- Avoid wearing contact lenses overnight.
- Do not touch your eyes when cooking, particularly when handling chillies, ginger or other hot foods.
- Take care of your immune system (pp.26–27 and pp.268–69), which is important to the health of your eyes.

Allergies

The number of people who suffer from allergies is on the increase across the industrialized world. As many as 25 percent of people develop an allergic reaction at some time in their lives.

When allergens enter the body they are met by lymphocytes, which produce immunoglobulin antibodies to the specific allergens. Mast cells cling to the exterior of blood vessels throughout the body. The antibodies attach to these cells, causing them to release histamine, which triggers the symptoms of allergy.

An allergic reaction occurs when the body wrongly identifies a substance as harmful. It reacts as it would to a bacterium, parasite or virus – by sending out antibodies to destroy the invader.

In normal circumstances, this would protect us from the agents that cause disease and help set up immunity to them. But in allergy, the reaction is mistargeted. Rather than protecting the body, the antibodies sensitize it and produce a range of troubling symptoms.

Many experts believe that allergy occurs because modern life compromises the immune system (see pp.26–27). This system instructs individual cells to pursue and destroy intruders. The allergic agent, known as an allergen, triggers the release of histamine (see left), which causes the muscles of the airway to tighten and blood vessels to leak. Prostaglandins are also released, producing pain. The familiar allergic symptoms of inflammation, soreness and itching are the result. The nose, throat, airways, skin and eyes are most often affected.

There is some disagreement as to which immunoglobulins are responsible for allergic reactions. It is widely accepted that immunoglobulin E (known as IgE) is involved. But some experts believe that immunoglobulins A and G (IgA and IgG) are also involved in certain allergies, particularly those to food. Others believe that many allergic reactions are the result of the activity of immune-fighting white blood cells, which are thought to fire toxic chemicals at allergens.

HEREDITY

Whatever the exact process involved, it is known to be, at least in part, genetically programmed, explaining why allergies often run in families. If both parents have allergy problems, an individual has an 80 percent chance of developing them. Where only one parent is allergic, there is a 50 percent chance. And if neither parent suffers, the odds fall to 20 percent.

HOW AN ALLERGY FORMS

1. Lymphocyte recognizes allergen   **2. Lymphocyte makes antibodies**

3. Antibodies attach to mast cell   **4. Mast cell releases histamine**

CAUTION

A common treatment for many allergic reactions is the use of antihistamine drugs, which relieve the symptoms. However, many antihistamines have a sedative effect. This may be inappropriate for daytime use, particularly when driving a car or operating machinery. Check with your doctor. Several of the newer antihistamines do not cause drowsiness, but worries about their side-effect profiles are increasing.

Several individual genes are involved. It is thought that the more of these that have mutations in any one individual, the higher the risk of developing an allergy. If only one or two of the genes carry the mutation, the person needs more exposure to the allergen before symptoms appear.

NOT ENOUGH PRACTICE

Some experts believe that the increase in allergies is due to over-protected immune systems. The eradication of many diseases and the use of immunization in childhood means that our immune systems do not get enough practice. Like muscles that are not exercised, the immune system may be unable to perform properly when needed. Proponents of this theory cite the widely recognized fact that children from small families and firstborns get more allergies and infections than those from large families and later-born children. This may be because the latter are exposed to more infections from an early age.

Other analysts point to affluence as a factor. Central heating and well-insulated homes, for example, encourage the reproduction of the house dust mite, an invisible insect that resides in soft furnishings, where it deposits microscopic droppings that can trigger asthma.

Traffic pollution exacerbates many allergies. The recent history of allergies in Germany suppports this argument. Before reunification, they were much more prevalent in the affluent West. Now that the East has adopted a similar lifestyle, it has as many allergy sufferers as the West.

In principle, any substance can cause an allergy. But some cause allergies more frequently than others do. Outdoors, pollen is the main culprit. It comes from many plants and causes hayfever. Indoors, it is the house dust mite. Other common allergens in the environment are moulds, feathers, nickel, latex, paint and dandruff of furry animals. There is also a whole range of potential food allergens.

SYMPTOMS

Allergic reactions are highly individual. An allergen that causes a set of symptoms in one person can cause different symptoms in another. The same allergen can also affect a different part of the body and to a different extent. The most common symptoms are rhinitis (runny nose), rashes, asthma, urticaria (nettle rash or hives) and eczema.

Some practitioners attribute any physical reaction that routinely occurs when the person is in contact with a particular substance to an allergic response. According to them, symptoms of some ailments, including irritable bowel syndrome and migraine (which can be caused by a food intolerance), would qualify as an allergic response. Because the symptoms of these so-called allergies do not necessarily follow a recognizable pattern, they may be overlooked by

---

ANAPHYLAXIS

Anaphylaxis is a severe allergic reaction in which the body goes into a state of alert minutes after exposure to the allergen. The most common causes are peanuts and other nuts, sesame seeds, shellfish, eggs, wasp and bee stings, latex, paint and penicillin.

On contact with the allergen, the cells release huge quantities of histamine, which causes the blood vessels to suddenly swell. This affects the lungs, throat and mouth, causing breathing difficulties that can be life-threatening. The skin also becomes flushed and urticaria (itchy weals) often appear. Blood vessels leak and can cause a dramatic drop in blood pressure. The person may lose consciousness. This type of shock can be fatal.

Anaphylaxis must be treated immediately with an injection of adrenaline. Steroid injections may be needed. People susceptible to the condition should always carry an injection kit with them.

doctors if they do not involve the classic IgE reaction such as anaphylactic shock (which always involves IgE) or hayfever, asthma and eczema (which generally do).

DIAGNOSIS

The increase in allergies has been met with a proliferation of diagnostic tests, some of which are much more scientific than others. The two that are routinely used by specialists are the skin-prick test and the radioallergosorbent test (RAST).

The skin-prick test involves pricking the skin and placing solutions of suspected allergens on it (see p.128). The RAST is a blood test in which a sample of blood is mixed with the suspected allergens. The IgE antibody response is then measured. The enzyme-linked immunosorbent assay (ELISA), which is becoming more widespread, works along similar lines. Controversial methods include cytotoxic tests such as the antigen, leucocyte cellular antibody test (ALCAT) or food allergen cellular test (FACT), which measure the activity of white blood cells. Vega testing and applied kinesiology (AK) used by complementary practitioners are also disputed by doctors.

FOOD SENSITIVITY

It is estimated that one in three people has a food sensitivity at some time in his life. It is generally accepted that there are two types of food sensitivity. Although the conditions are different, they are often confused because they both involve food.

The most serious type is a food allergy. It is usually severe, resulting in vomiting, rashes, asthma, eczema or anaphylactic shock. It always involves immmuno-globulin E (IgE) and occurs as soon as the allergen is eaten. Even a tiny amount of the food can provoke a serious reaction. This type of allergy appears in childhood

The dust mite (above, magnified 26 times), which lives in carpets, furniture and beds, and pollen (left, magnified 1000 times) are two common allergens. Meticulous house cleaning, such as daily vacuuming, can help eliminate these allergens from the home.

and can be lifelong. Common triggers are peanuts, eggs, sesame seeds, citrus fruit and shellfish. The other type of sensitivity is known as a food intolerance. Symptoms occur when the body does not produce the enzyme necessary to break down certain food chemicals such as lactose, or milk sugar, found in milk. Some nutritional therapists and complementary practitioners suspect that another kind of food intolerance can occur if certain foods are undigested or their breakdown products too easily absorbed.

The most reliable method of tracking down the offending food is by using the elimination, or exclusion, diet. However, this takes time and commitment on the part of the individual and needs to be supervised by a specialist practitioner or qualified nutritionist.

The person is allowed to eat a limited range of foods, which is selected from those that rarely prove allergenic. Some of the foods that fall into this category include lamb, pears, rice, turkey and parsnips. New foods are then gradually reintroduced into the diet to see whether they provoke a reaction. Positively identifying the particular culprit can

To identify true allergens responsible for an allergy, a skin-prick test may be performed. A variety of allergens, including dust, pollen and fungal spores, are placed in contact with the skin. Any skin inflammation near a prick indicates the source of the allergen.

be a slow process because foods can be reintroduced only at three-day intervals, and with each one it can take 72 hours for a reaction to occur. However, these diets have been shown to help even in chronic inflammatory conditions such as rheumatoid arthritis and Crohn's disease.

TREATMENT

It is hardly surprising, for a condition that divides medical opinion as allergy does, that there should be no proven treatment for allergy that is at present accepted across the professional world. The most effective treatment for an allergy is, simply, avoiding the allergen. Anyone who is allergic to eggs, for example, should avoid eating eggs or any dishes containing eggs. If the allergen is pollen, avoidance is not so straightforward, although keeping the car windows closed while driving and closing the bedroom windows at night will provide some protection. However, with certain other allergens, as simple as avoidance may seem, it is not always possible.

Some practitioners put their faith in a method known as desensitization. This is based on a similar principle to that of immunization. If a sufferer is given injections of the suspected allergen, the body is thought to build up an immunity to it. The dosage is gradually increased over the course of the injections. The great disadvantage of this approach is that injections have to be taken all year, they sometimes provoke a severe allergic reaction and they necessitate regular visits to the hospital for them to be given.

Various research groups are now concentrating on developing vaccines to particular allergies such as hayfever. These are intended to reprogramme the immune system to block the biochemical processes that lead to allergic reactions.

SELF-HELP FOR HAYFEVER

There are many steps you can take to avoid pollens:

- Listen to the weather forecast. Do not stay outside for long if the pollen count is above 50, especially if it is dry and windy.

- Rub vaseline inside your nose to trap the pollen and stop it irritating the nose and throat lining.

- Bring in your washing and close bedroom windows before the evening, when pollen grains descend as the air cools.

- Shower and wash your hair after a trip to the country to get rid of any residual pollen grains.

- Keep the car windows closed if travelling in the country.

- Wear wrap-around sunglasses to keep pollen out of your eyes.

- Take holidays by the sea or in mountainous areas where the pollen count is lower.

Allergic reactions to pets can be reduced and possibly eliminated by washing the animal thoroughly. Immersion in water is more effective than washing with a hose, as it removes more of the skin scales that trigger allergy (the fur is not the culprit).

It is important to carefully examine labels on all products to avoid an allergen. Fortunately, growing awareness of allergy is leading to much better labelling of foods such as those containing peanut oil or products made with latex.

Many of the allergies that appear in childhood will disappear with time. Only one-quarter of children who suffer from asthma at the age of seven, for example, will continue to suffer from it as adults.

HAYFEVER

One of the most common allergies is hayfever, affecting up to 20 percent of people. It is known as allergic rhinitis because it affects the mucous membranes of the nose. The condition has little to do with hay: it is a reaction to pollens from trees, grass and weeds. During their pollinating seasons (see box, right), these irritate the membranes, making the nose, throat and eyes itchy; the nose stuffy and runny; and the eyes sore and red.

Because of the nasal symptoms, sufferers often use decongestants, which shrink the nasal membrane. But these give only temporary relief and can make the problem worse, as after the effect of the spray wears off the membrane swells up more than beforehand. They also dry up the protective mucus in the nose. If the sufferer relies on them in the long term, the body may stop responding to them and they will provide no relief at all.

Antihistamine tablets are usually effective, but these act on the whole body. Many sufferers prefer local, targeted anti-inflammatory treatments, such as nose or eye drops, made with antihistamines or steroids that do not cause drowsiness.

Surprisingly, town-dwellers seem to be worse affected than those who live in the country. This may be because pollutants from traffic reinforce the irritant effect of pollens. This may explain why the incidence of hayfever has risen fourfold in as many decades.

The cause of hayfever has now been identified as part of a protein in pollen called profilin. The discovery may lead to a new treatment for the condition. ∎

POLLINATING SEASONS

Pollinating season	Species
Mid winter to early spring	Hazel (Corylus)
Mid winter to mid spring	Alder (Alnus)
Late winter to mid spring	Yew (Taxus) Elm (Ulmus)
Late winter to late spring	Ash (Fraxinus) Willow (Salix)
Early to mid spring	Poplar (Populus)
Early to late spring	Birch (Betula)
Mid spring to early summer	Oak (Quercus) Oil seed rape (Brassica napus) Pine (Pinus) Plane (Platanus)
Mid spring to mid summer	Plantain (Plantago)
Mid spring to late summer	Grass (Gramineae) Nettle (Urtica)
Late spring to mid summer	Dock (Rumex)
Early to late summer	Mugwort (Artemisia)
Mid summer	Lime (Tilia)

Copyright: Pollen Research Unit

CAUTION

Do not, on any account, attempt to dislodge a foreign body by poking a cottonwool bud into your ear. This may only push the foreign body farther in.

Ear problems

Your ears are not just for hearing – they are also important organs of balance. There are a number of possible problems that can occur in an ear, from an infection to a persistent ringing.

The most common ear problem is an earache. The main symptom is pain, which can be sharp and stabbing or dull and throbbing, or a combination of the two. There may be a yellow discharge, which indicates an infection and requires treatment, or your hearing may be muffled because of wax accumulation or fluid in the middle ear. If an earache persists for more than half a day, consult your doctor without delay. Do not attempt to treat it yourself. An earache can be caused by a number of factors:

- middle ear infection (bacterial or viral)
- colds and flu
- blockage of wax
- prolonged exposure to loud noise
- a blocked Eustachian tube due to catarrh and infection

- pressure injury, known as barotrauma, from flying or diving
- tooth or gum infection
- external ear infection, usually a bacterial or allergic problem, causing itching, pain and discharge from the outer ear canal.

INFECTION AND BLOCKAGE

If the earache is caused by an infection, the doctor may send a sample of pus for analysis. She will clean the ear and prescribe drops or tablets of antibiotics or steroids, and you may be given painkillers. If there is a chronic infection, the ear may require cleaning on a regular basis.

If a blockage of wax is causing the problem, your doctor can flush the ear clean by syringing it with warm water. She may soften the wax first, using ear drops. Syringing does present a risk of a perforated ear drum and should only be carried out when it is medically necessary and both patient and doctor have sufficient time for the process.

CHILDREN AND GLUE EAR

Glue ear, in which fluid accumulates in the middle ear, is a common cause of poor hearing in children. The doctor will prescribe decongestant or antihistamine medication to reduce swelling of the Eustachian tube. This allows the build up of fluid to run out of the middle ear, down the Eustachian tube and into the nose and throat.

In severe cases, the child will have to be hospitalized for the ear to be operated on.

TINNITUS

Tinnitus is a persistent ringing, whistling, buzzing or whooshing noise in the ears, or a combination of any of these. It can sound like a television that is not tuned in. The fact that tinnitus continues or recurs makes it hard to bear. Causes include head injuries, prolonged exposure to loud noise, syringing the ear, infection, large doses of aspirin, deafness, Ménière's disease (a disorder of the inner ear, causing severe vertigo) and neck problems. Often there is no obvious cause.

Although 1 in 10 people suffers from tinnitus, it is severe enough to affect work and lifestyle in only 1 in 1000 cases. There is no cure for tinnitus, but 11 percent of cases spontaneously recover and 13 percent improve to some extent. About 8 percent of cases become severe.

ANATOMY OF THE EAR

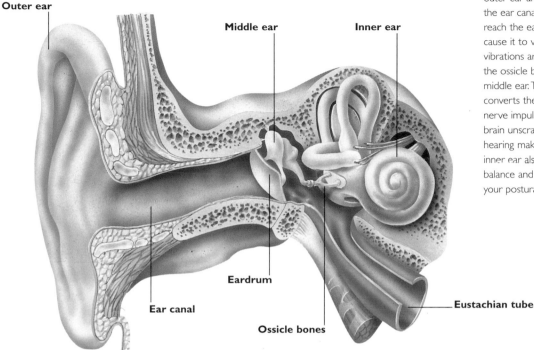

Outer ear

Middle ear

Inner ear

Eardrum

Ear canal

Ossicle bones

Eustachian tube

Sound waves enter the outer ear and travel along the ear canal until they reach the eardrum and cause it to vibrate. The vibrations are amplified by the ossicle bones in the middle ear. The inner ear converts the vibrations into nerve impulses, which the brain unscrambles so that hearing makes sense. The inner ear also controls balance and a sense of your postural position.

Under general anaesthetic, the surgeon will pass a fine needle through the eardrum and remove the fluid with a syringe. Or she may make a small cut in the eardrum and insert a plastic tube (called a grommet, or stopple) into the hole in the eardrum to allow air to enter and dry out the middle ear. The tube is usually left in place for a few months, after which time it is removed and the hole heals spontaneously.

FLYING PROBLEMS

If you usually suffer from earache when you fly, see your doctor before your next flight. She can make sure that there is no low-level infection or blockage of wax, which can be treated with antibiotics or syringing. When you are on board the plane, suck on boiled sweets and try to swallow as often as possible in order to encourage the free passage of air through the Eustachian tube. If an earache persists for more than 24 hours after the flight, you should consult a medical practitioner without delay.

AVOIDING EAR PROBLEMS

If you suffer from repeated outer ear problems, do not share face flannels or towels, and take care if you swim or dive. Scuba divers should make sure to equalize pressure as they dive or surface.

Avoid high noise levels. If you have to work with loud equipment, such as a pneumatic drill, wear ear protection. Prolonged exposure to high noise levels can cause deafness or tinnitus. ■

To remove an insect in an ear, have the person bend his head to one side, with the affected ear upward. Gently pour warm water into the ear to flush out the insect. If this does not succeed, go to the doctor or your nearest hospital accident and emergency department without delay.

Sinusitis

An acutely painful inflammatory condition of the sinuses is known as sinusitis. Some people never suffer from it; others have to endure it each time they contract a cold.

The sinuses provide air cavities in the skull and serve to lighten the head. But bacterial or viral infection, such as a common cold or flu, can cause the mucous membranes that line the sinuses to become inflamed. They may then fill with pus and catarrh. The resulting pain affects the eyes, face and temples and often causes severe headaches. These may be accompanied by fatigue and weakness. A raised temperature is also likely.

Because the infection becomes trapped in the sinuses, it often persists after other cold or flu symptoms have disappeared. The nose becomes increasingly blocked

and produces an infected green discharge. If the passages between the nose and the sinuses also become blocked, the nose will be more congested, but the discharge may stop. At this stage, breathing is possible only through the mouth and sleep is often disturbed. The headache is usually most painful in the morning. Occasionally, sinusitis can occur after dental treatment, when infection spreads from the root of a tooth through the bone into the sinus.

If the infection is bacterial, your doctor will probably prescribe antibiotics to clear it up, before it spreads through the

THE SINUS CAVITIES

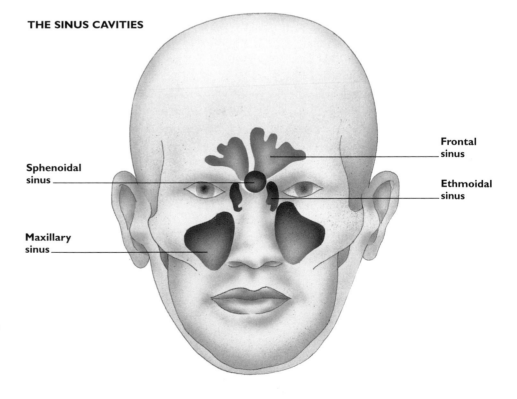

Sphenoidal sinus

Maxillary sinus

Frontal sinus

Ethmoidal sinus

The sinuses are the four cavities in the face that contain air and lie above and below the eyes. The frontal sinuses in the forehead and the maxillary sinuses in the cheekbones are most often affected by blockage and swelling.

mucous membranes of the sinuses into the bones. He may also prescribe a decongestant, either in the form of pills or a nasal spray. Follow the instructions for use precisely because, if used incorrectly, decongestants can do further damage, and if used too often, they can produce a rebound effect, in which the nasal passages become even more congested.

ALLERGIC REACTION

Sinusitis can also be a symptom of an allergy such as hayfever. In this case, the doctor may prescribe antihistamine medications to reduce the swelling and improve breathing. These, too, should be taken with care as the long-term use of antihistamines can dry out the sinuses excessively. This can make the mucus thicker and even more difficult to expel.

MINOR SURGERY

For those suffering from chronic sinusitis in whom home medication is no longer effective, an ear, nose and throat (ENT) surgeon may perform a minor operation to improve the drainage of the sinuses, which reduces the likelihood of sinusitis. The operation involves piercing a bone between the nose and the sinuses in order to make an extra passage. The sinuses are then washed out and the resultant liquid analysed to identify the bacteria so that the most appropriate medication can, when necessary, be prescribed.

PREVENTING RECURRENCE

Once you have had sinusitis, the membranes become more susceptible to later reinfection – so take no chances. If someone you know has a cold or flu, avoid all contact until they recover. Wear a scarf over your nose and mouth when you are in warm overcrowded conditions such as trains and buses.

SELF-HELP MEASURES

- Take aspirin or paracetamol to relieve the pain as necessary.

- Stay at home in a room with a stable temperature and high humidity. Dry, overheated rooms usually make sinusitis worse. Place several bowls of water around the room if you have central heating.

- Blow your nose gently when you have to and throw away the tissue after each use.

- Do not allow the condition to persist for more than three or four days before you visit your doctor.

- Do not smoke. Tobacco smoke and tar prolong the condition and make it much more difficult to treat.

- Take as much exercise as possible. This encourages the rapid elimination of toxins that have become trapped in the sinuses and helps to loosen infected mucus.

Make sure that your own home has a reasonable level of humidity, and when you feel a cold starting, keep the room temperature stable. At this point, avoid any strenuous exercise because it may lead to rapid heating followed by rapid cooling of the body. Look after yourself by eating properly and getting plenty of rest. Some people find it helpful to sleep with two pillows rather than one so that the head is slightly raised.■

Inhaling steam from a basin of hot water with a towel over your head can help to moisten the sinuses and relieve congestion.

CAUTION

Any persistent cough puts strain on the airways and can cause a blood vessel in the airways, lungs, nose or throat to rupture. Coughing up blood is usually related to an infection, but it could be a sign of congestion in the blood vessels of the lungs due to heart failure, a blood clot in the lungs or lung cancer. All require prompt medical attention.

■ Seek medical advice for a cough accompanied by fever for more than three days.

Because there are more than 200 cold viruses, it is difficult to acquire immunity to colds. The colour-enhanced one shown below is magnified 215,000 times.

Colds and coughs

The common cold, often accompanied by a cough, is the most widespread winter infection, affecting 70 percent of people each year. Despite its name, it is not caused by low temperatures or feeling cold.

Colds are caused by viruses that circulate in the air. They are more common in winter because people spend more time indoors close to each other. The symptoms appear two to three days after contact with the virus. Everyone is familiar with them. First comes a need to sniff and discomfort in the back of the throat, followed by mild aches and a general unwell feeling. Then comes the runny nose and congestion, often with a temperature, sore throat and headache.

The first two days are the worst. This is the time when you are most infectious, but you will be producing the live virus for five or more days. While you are infectious, stay away from young babies or other vulnerable people. It is unusual for a cold to last more than 10 days.

RELIEVING COLD SYMPTOMS

There is no single effective treatment for a cold. The most you can do is relieve the worst symptoms with medicines from the chemist and some self-help measures. For aches and pains, take aspirin or paracetamol. Watch the quantity if you are also taking over-the-counter cold remedies, as many already include these drugs. Gargling with water containing a crushed aspirin can help a sore throat.

You can use nasal decongestants (see pp.132–33) for a blocked nose, but do not overuse them because they can stop working. You can try sniffing eucalyptus or olbas oil from drops on a handkerchief. Spicy food can also help clear a blocked nose. Cut down on fatty foods if you have a runny nose: evidence suggests they encourage the formation of mucus.

Take vitamin C supplements daily. Vitamin C has antiviral properties. Even in high doses it is not toxic, though more than 3 g a day can cause loose bowels.

For a sore throat, suck zinc lozenges. They provide some relief and zinc is important to the immune system. Do not smoke, as it makes congestion and coughs worse. You should drink plenty of fluids, because the virus will linger in a dry respiratory tract.

DEALING WITH A COUGH

A cough is a reflex action to clear the airways. It results in a sharp expulsion of air, which causes the often irritating noise. The blockage in the airway can be caused

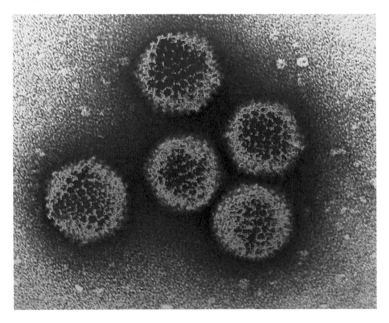

by dust, smoke, gas and food or another foreign body, or by phlegm and mucus associated with a viral infection. Such an infection may also inflame the airways, which makes the problem worse.

There are many types of cough, but they fall into two categories: productive (producing phlegm) or unproductive (dry). Treat a productive cough with an expectorant, which loosens it by stimulating the watery secretions in the lungs. An unproductive cough may require a suppressant, which acts on the coughing reflex in the brain. Simply resisting the urge to cough can help. The mistaken feeling that there is phlegm to bring up leads to unproductive coughing, a sore wind pipe and further irritation. So if there is no apparent reason to cough, try to suppress the urge. If any cough goes on for two weeks or more, you should contact your doctor. ■

CAUTION

Never give aspirin to a child 12 years of age or younger: it has been linked to a dangerous condition known as Reye's syndrome. Treat a fever or aches and pains with paracetamol.

CONDITIONS THAT CAN CAUSE A COUGH

Condition	Symptom	Treatment
Bronchitis	Severe coughing with thick mucus and phlegm; breathlessness on exercise.	Breathing exercises and postural drainage (lying in a position that drains secretions from the lungs into the windpipe, from where you can cough them up).
Bronchiectasis	Chronic, severe cough with thick mucus.	Antibiotics and postural drainage.
Bronchiospasm (Associated with asthma and allergies)	Dry cough that is worse at night.	Bronchodilator or corticosteroid drugs if related to asthma. Avoidance of allergen if caused by allergy.
Pneumonia	Painful, persistent cough, accompanied by breathlessness and raised temperature.	A course of antibiotics.
Tuberculosis (TB)	Persistent cough with shortness of breath, chest pain and, sometimes, bloody phlegm.	A course of antibiotics.
Pneumoconiosis (Lung dust disease)	Cough and shortness of breath.	No treatment; avoid dust that caused it.
Foreign object blocking bronchus	Persistent, sharp cough with mucus.	Removal of the object.
Lung cancer	Persistent mild cough, becoming severe then producing blood-stained phlegm; shortness of breath, chest pain, wheezing.	Surgery and/or radiotherapy and chemotherapy.
Smoker's cough	Recurrent cough producing thick phlegm.	Stop smoking.
Whooping cough	Attacks of violent coughing, ending with strong inhalation and "whoop" sound; may continue up to 3 months.	A course of antibiotics.

SEE ALSO
Herbal medicine 186–191
Aromatherapy 192–195
An immune-boosting diet
268–269

CAUTION

Call your doctor only after a few days if the symptoms are not improving or are worsening. Some doctors prescribe amantidine hydrochloride for people at high risk. It reduces the severity and duration of the illness, but it only acts against the type A virus and has uncomfortable side effects in 10–20 percent of people.

■ At-risk groups, including diabetics and people over 75 years old or with chronic lung disease, heart failure, an immune deficiency or splenectomy, should receive annual flu vaccinations.

Influenza

Every few years influenza, popularly called flu, hits the headlines when an epidemic occurs. This viral infection of the respiratory tract is one of the most infectious diseases and usually occurs in winter outbreaks.

There are three types of flu virus, known as A, B and C. Types A and B are the fickle ones that mutate every year. Even someone who has had flu every season over the previous years is not immune to the new strains that these can produce. Type C, by contrast, produces a milder illness to which sufferers build up immunity, so they can only have it once. The great flu epidemics, where large numbers in a community or region are affected, and pandemics, in which illness crosses national boundaries and spreads worldwide, are usually caused by type A.

SYMPTOMS AND RELIEF

Flu symptoms start to appear about three days after contact with someone carrying the virus. They vary according to the strain, but typically include high fever, shivering and shaking, muscle aches, nausea and vomiting, loss of appetite, a painful chest and fatigue. A type C flu can feel like little more than a strong cold, but A and B take a greater toll on the body.

There is no cure for flu. As with the common cold (see pp.134–35), you can only treat the individual symptoms. Aspirin and paracetamol can help relieve aches and pains and reduce a high temperature. Drinking plenty of fluids helps to replace those lost through sweating. You should also eat well even if you do not have much of an appetite.

Inevitably, drug manufacturers are working on more complete cures. Most hope has been invested in a drug to block the action of the enzyme on the flu virus that enables the virus to spread through the body. Until this is available, the only real weapon is the flu vaccine.

PREVENTIVE MEASURES

You are less likely to catch a viral infection such as flu if you start building up your defences early in the winter. Consume plenty of vitamin C (see pp.246–48), which is a powerful antiviral agent. As well as a daily supplement (see p.249), eat plenty of foods containing the vitamin. Fresh fruit and vegetables, especially kiwis, broccoli, blackcurrants and Brussels sprouts, are rich sources. Those that are red, yellow or orange also contain betacarotene, which aids immune function.

THE VIRUS AND THE VACCINE

Like any other virus, the flu virus has antigens, which the immune system recognizes and attacks. However, the flu virus not only has three different strains, but each season its antigens mutate so that they can outwit the immune system. The flu vaccine works by stimulating the body's production of antibodies to fight these antigens, but without causing the disease. Each year, the World Health Organization (WHO) formulates a new vaccine that contains strains of the virus they predict will be circulating the following winter.

The vaccine is usually 75 percent successful. It takes a few days before it becomes effective, and there may be side effects, which appear 6–12 hours after being vaccinated. The most typical are mild fever and aches, which last up to 48 hours.

You shoulc keep your fluid intake up. Infections find it harder to take hold in the membranes of a well-lubricated respiratory tract. Avoid air-conditioned places as they dry the membranes. Avoid, too, crowded and warm places where viruses readily spread. Long-haul flights, for example, are a fertile breeding ground.

Try to reduce your stress levels. Too much stress lowers your immune system. Rest and relaxation will shorten the bout of flu and make complications less likely. You can also take echinacea, available as tablets or a tincture, which is a herb that increases the number and potency of white blood cells and fights off infection.

INTERNATIONAL SUPERBUGS

Superflu is the popular term for a flu caused by a new virus that spreads quickly because there is no immunity to it. It becomes a pandemic about every 10 years and can cause 10 times as many deaths as in a normal year. Fortunately, prompt modern vaccination programmes usually contain the spread.

It is not certain how the "superbugs" that cause these pandemics emerge. The strongest theory is that they cross from the animal community into humans. Birds and pigs are thought to be prime sources of superbugs. This would explain why the viruses often originate in rural China, where animals and people live closely together; an example is the "chicken flu" in Hong Kong in 1997.

Superflu viruses are usually of the type A variety. The infection starts when parts of the new virus – haemagglutinins (H) and neuraminidases (N) – bind on to a human cell. These are the virus "subtypes" and give the flu its name. ■

CAUTION

Be on the alert for the symptoms of a severe chest infection or pneumonia – a persistent high temperature and cough, rapid heartbeat, fast breathing and shortness of breath when at rest. These all suggest that you should see a doctor urgently.
■ *Never give aspirin to a child 12 years of age or younger: it has been linked to a dangerous condition known as Reye's syndrome. Treat a fever or aches and pains with paracetamol.*

SUPERFLUS AND PANDEMICS

Name	Date	Cause	Impact
Spanish flu	1918	HINI virus. Origin unknown, but may be the United States.	Spread worldwide, infecting more than a billion people and causing 20–30 million deaths over three years. Mainly affected young adults.
Asian flu	1957	H2N2 virus, originating in China.	Quickly spread to Hong Kong and Singapore, then throughout world. Many deaths in later waves, especially in the United States in 1960. Deaths limited by use of antibiotics to fight secondary infections.
Hong Kong flu	1968	H3N2 virus, originating in south-eastern China.	Spread around the globe within a year of appearing in China and remained prevalent for 11 years. High mortality in the United States in the first year.
Swine flu	1976	Originated among military recruits in Fort Dix in the United States.	The United States government instigated an emergency vaccination programme, vaccinating 41 million people in six to eight weeks, which stopped it becoming a pandemic.
Red (Russian) flu	1977	HINI, originating in northern China.	Initial outbreaks concentrated in primary and middle schools. Spread rapidly into southern China and Russia, and spread around world within a year. Mainly affected young people, as older people had obtained some immunity to the HINI virus that was around in the 1950s.

SEE ALSO
Colds and coughs
134–135
Aromatherapy 192–195
Adjusting your diet
264–267

CAUTION

■ *Never touch a cold sore, then your eye. You could develop a serious condition known as corneal ulcer, which can cause blindness.*
■ *Touching genitals after touching a cold sore can cause genital herpes (pp.144–45). Direct contact between cold sores on the lips and genitals can also cause genital herpes.*

Cold sores

Highly infectious small skin blisters, called vesicles, that gather on the skin around the mouth and nose, typically on the lip margins, are known as cold sores. They often occur after a cold, hence their name.

The infection that causes cold sores is the herpes simplex virus. By the age of 25, over 90 percent of people carry the virus. However, people may not be aware that they carry it because they may not have symptoms. Only a minority of people experience recurrent cold sores and few have more than two outbreaks a year. The frequency and duration of cold sores usually diminish with age. Many people believe that the start of a cold sore is their body's way of telling them to slow down, because these viruses typically attack when you are stressed (see pp.76–77), run down or tired.

The symptoms of a cold sore usually start as an itchy tingling feeling in the area that is affected. At this point (and no later), antiviral medicines may prevent an outbreak. The skin reddens and a

RECOGNIZING A COLD SORE

vesicle or cluster of them develops. The surrounding skin may become inflamed, and the vesicles may then feel itchy, tingling or simply numb. Within a few days, the vesicles enlarge and burst. They dry out and form an unsightly crust. The symptoms usually manifest themselves on the face but they can also occur inside the mouth, where the sore will look like a shallow ulcer. The gums may be swollen and deep red in colour and the tongue furred, and the temperature may rise.

When a blister bursts, leaving a small raw area, it is at its most infectious. This is when you are most likely to transmit the virus through skin to skin contact via the mucous membranes, for example, by open-mouthed kissing.

TREATMENT AND PREVENTION
For people who have severe attacks, a doctor can prescribe an antiviral drug that reduces the rate at which the virus multiplies. Pressing a small icepack on to the area may reduce itchiness. Use a fresh, clean pack each time you treat the sore.

Some people find that wind or sunshine or both precipitate an attack. Protective sunblock, available from a chemist or supermarket, can be helpful if this is the cause. If you find that cold sores follow a cold or flu, get plenty of rest in order to help your immune system fight the virus.

Be scrupulously hygienic about face flannels and towels. Make sure that only you use your bathroom items and that you use no one else's during an outbreak. ■

The lips are usually the site of cold sores. A group of vesicles, or tiny blisters. enlarges, bursts and dries out, leaving behind a yellowish crust.

Blisters

SEE ALSO
Stress   76–77

Mouth ulcers

A mouth ulcer is a break or niche in the lining of the mouth or tongue which exposes the underlying tissue. Such ulcers are common, affecting 10 percent of the population at any one time.

Most ulcers look much the same – light yellow or whitish spots inside the mouth or on the tongue – but they vary considerably in cause and severity. The two most common and painful types are aphthous and traumatic ulcers.

Aphthous ulcers, which are normally no more than 2–3 mm ($\frac{1}{16}$–$\frac{1}{8}$ inch) across, usually occur in response to fatigue, stress or illness. Traumatic ulcers, which tend to be larger than aphthous ones, occur after an injury. This may be a broken tooth, excessively hot food or a bite on the inside of the mouth or on the tongue.

Other ulcers are caused by infection such as cold sores (see facing page) if the vesicles in the mouth remain untreated and turn into ulcers. Occasionally, large deep mouth ulcers are malignant.

Sometimes, ulcers on the tongue are a sign of a tumour or a symptom of an underlying disease such as anaemia.

Simple mouth ulcers usually clear up of their own accord within a week or two and do not need treatment. You can obtain from any chemist a soothing ointment or lozenges that numb and protect the exposed tissue in the mouth. These not only relieve the pain but can also help the ulcer to heal more quickly.

PERSISTENT ULCERS

If the ulcer does not go away, you should consult your doctor. She will advise you if there is an obvious cause, as is often the case with traumatic ulcers. You may need to visit a dentist to see if your tooth formation is causing the problem.

If you suffer with recurrent mouth ulcers, your doctor may take swabs or blood samples for analysis to find an underlying cause. You may be referred to your local hospital for a biopsy if you have a large mouth ulcer. Ulcers that are the consequence of herpes simplex viral infection (see facing page) can be treated with the antiviral drug acyclovir.

PREVENTION

Aphthous mouth ulcers are a warning sign that your system is tired or run down. Aim to improve your diet, enjoy as much sleep as you need and take regular exercise in the fresh air. Adjusting your lifestyle should improve your wellbeing and make you less susceptible. ∎

IDENTIFYING A MOUTH ULCER

Ulcerated sores on the inside of the mouth usually last for up to 10 days. You tend to notice them first when you eat spicy food or something acidic, such as a grapefruit.

Ulcerated sore

SEE ALSO
Colds and coughs
                    134–135
Influenza   136–137

CAUTION

Whatever else you may do, do not smoke if you have tonsillitis. Cigarettes can exacerbate the damage to your tonsils, increase the painful inflammation and prolong the illness.

Tonsillitis

An acute infection and inflammation of the tonsils, tonsillitis affects children much more often than adults. The infection can be caused by bacteria or a virus and is highly contagious.

The two tonsils are spongy nodules of lymphatic tissue that guard the entrance to the respiratory and digestive systems. New infections are constantly entering the respiratory tract, and the tonsils are thought to play a valuable part in keeping them away from the lower respiratory tract. As they do so, the tonsils themselves become infected and swollen.

Typical symptoms of tonsillitis are a sore throat, a cough and pain on swallowing. The inflamed tonsils may be covered in tiny white pus-filled spots, the neck glands may be swollen and there may be a raised temperature. Weakness and fatigue are normal, in the same way as with a cold. A high temperature may follow, particularly in children, possibly accompanied by febrile fits.

In adults, treat tonsillitis in much the same way as flu or a bad cold. Stay in bed, take two aspirins every four hours and drink plenty of fluids, especially water. If the tonsillitis persists for more than two to three days, contact your family doctor, who may decide to prescribe antibiotics if he thinks that the infection is bacterial. Adults should refrain from going to work until the inflammation has subsided. Tonsillitis is contagious and easily passed on.

CHILDREN

Children catch tonsillitis more easily than adults because they have not yet built up resistance to many infections. As they gain immunity with age, attacks become less likely. By the age of six or seven most children have developed resistance.

Before antibiotics became widely used, tonsils were often removed in children. Today this is regarded as a last resort and the operation is performed only on children who repeatedly suffer with tonsillitis beyond the age of seven.

A child with symptoms of tonsillitis should be kept away from school and in a warm room, although not necessarily in bed. To reduce a fever, use paracetamol; never give aspirin to a child 12 year of age or younger. He should be given plenty of fluids, especially water. Appetite will be poor but soft, cool foods (scrambled eggs, fruit pureés, even a little ice cream) may be tempting. If the illness shows no sign of abating within a day or two, you should consult your doctor. ∎

If you open your mouth wide and look into a mirror with a light above it, you can clearly see the two tonsils on either side of the back of your throat.

THE TONSILS

Tonsil

Throat

Tongue

SEE ALSO
Chest infections 32–33
Colds and coughs
134–135

CAUTION

If the voice box becomes so inflamed that it is difficult to speak, make sure that you take care not to inflict worse damage. Do not talk and, above all else, do not smoke.

Laryngitis

An infected or inflamed larynx (voice box) is called laryngitis. It usually follows infection by a cold or sore throat, but it can also be caused by straining the voice box, for example, by shouting or smoking. Laryngitis may be accompanied by a general sense of weakness that is similar to what is experienced during a mild flu.

The larynx lies at the back of the throat at the top of the trachea, or windpipe. It has a vertical slit in it, which lies open when you are silent, allowing air to pass through without a sound. On each side of the slit there is a fold of muscle and a mucous membrane. These folds, known as vocal cords, tighten as you speak, making the slit almost close. The voice box is powered by the diaphragm and lungs. Tension and poor breathing can constrict the voice, whereas relaxation can deepen it.

The larynx swells when it is affected by a bacterial or viral infection. This swelling can restrict the flow of air through the vocal cords, just as when you whisper. Once vocal cords are quite swollen, or if the laryngeal muscles are extremely tense, you temporarily lose your voice.

The opening of the larynx is smaller in children, so if the membrane becomes swollen, sometimes it can dangerously impede breathing. This condition is referred to as croup.

Laryngitis is best treated like a mild attack of flu or bad cold. You should stay at home, try not to talk, stop smoking cigarettes and drinking alcohol and eat lightly and often, as well as drink plenty of fluids throughout the day.

PERSISTENT LARYNGITIS

You should consult your doctor if the hoarseness or loss of voice continues for more than a week. The larynx can develop tumours, either benign or malignant, so it is important that any persistent huskiness or change in tone of the voice is properly investigated by your doctor.

If you suffer with persistent attacks of laryngitis, seek your doctor's advice about the possible causes, other than straight-forward and unavoidable infection. Chronic laryngitis is often caused by smoking cigarettes (see pp.20–21) and polluted air, which both continually irritate the mucous membranes. Stress (see pp.76–77) and tension can also cause the condition. You should discuss your lifestyle with your doctor with a view to making any appropriate changes. ∎

When the vocal cords are swollen, air passing over them during speech distorts the sound. The result is a hoarse voice.

THE LARYNX

Pharynx

Vocal cord

Larynx

Trachea (windpipe)

SEE ALSO
Sexually transmitted
diseases   144–145

CAUTION

*Many women are prone
to recurrent vaginal yeast
infections and are familiar
with the symptoms and
treatment. However, if you
have not had vaginal trouble
before or if the problem
is not responding to
treatment, see your doctor.*

The most common form of
yeast infection is candidiasis,
or thrush. It is caused by a
funguslike microbe called
Candida albicans (shown
magnified 2400 times),
which is found naturally in
the mucous membranes of
the mouth, intestinal tract,
vagina and on the skin.

Yeast infections

Fungal yeasts normally live in the human body and, in most instances, cause no problems. However, if a yeast begins to multiply rapidly, you may develop the uncomfortable symptoms of an infection.

There are different types of yeast infections, or thrush, defined by the area affected. By far the most common is vaginal thrush. It is estimated that three in four women worldwide are infected with thrush at some time, and one-third of them have at least one attack a year.

Oral thrush is a type of yeast infection that affects the mouth. It is most common in babies, the elderly and those already weakened by illness. In some cases, it may spread to the oesophagus, making swallowing difficult.

Yet another variation affects the skin, nails and mucous membranes of the body. Thrush can occur in the moist folds of

skin, and babies may develop skin thrush along with nappy rash.

In rare cases, the yeast can spread throughout the body, causing systemic thrush. This occurs in people who have severely weakened immune systems such as those suffering from leukaemia or AIDS or taking potent anticancer drugs.

CAUSES OF THRUSH

Candida albicans, the most common type of fungal yeast, is normally found in the mouth and vagina, but it is kept in check by harmless bacteria that are also present. It is when these bacteria fail in their task that the yeast grows uncontrolled and thrush develops. There are a number of factors that can affect the delicate balance between bacteria and yeast. For example, illness or stress may lower the body's natural defences and lead to a range of infections, which include thrush.

Medications such as antibiotics, steroids and other immunosuppressant drugs can make you more vulnerable to thrush. The drugs may destroy not only the bacteria causing the illness but also the beneficial bacteria that control fungal growth.

Diabetes can increase the risk of thrush because of the high blood sugar levels associated with the disease. Yeast feeds on sugar, so this promotes fungal growth. In addition, the hormonal changes that occur during pregnancy can lead to more sugar in the vaginal tissues and encourage fungal growth. It is suspected that some oral contraceptive pills may have the same effect. Anyone prone to thrush should cut down on her sugar intake – and alcohol, which is sugar in another form.

Because yeast grows more readily in a warm, moist environment, clothes that increase sweating around the groin area can cause thrush. Heavily scented bubble bath or oil, vaginal deodorants or douches may irritate the groin area and alter the natural acidity of the vagina, which may allow thrush to thrive unchecked.

SYMPTOMS

Vaginal thrush can cause a white discharge that resembles cottage cheese, itching and soreness around the vagina and vulva, a burning sensation when urinating and pain on intercourse. Men can catch it from an infected partner. Symptoms include irritation, redness, burning or itching under the foreskin or on the tip of the penis, a thick discharge under the foreskin, a slight discharge from the urethra and discomfort when urinating.

Oral thrush causes creamy, whitish or yellow raised patches inside the cheeks and throat. If the skin is affected, you may notice red, itchy skin patches and redness and swelling around the nails. Systemic (widespread blood-borne) thrush may result in fever, headache, weakness and severe symptoms such as endocarditis (inflammation of the heart valves) or blood poisoning.

DIAGNOSIS AND TREATMENT

Symptoms of a vaginal yeast infection are similar to those of other vaginal infections so a proper diagnosis is necessary. This will involve an internal examination by a doctor and a laboratory analysis of any discharge.

Once thrush is confirmed, treatment is provided with antifungal medication. This comes in many forms, including creams,

---

PREVENTING VAGINAL THRUSH

Understanding the factors that may lead to thrush can help you prevent an attack.

- To keep the groin area dry, wear cotton instead of nylon panties, stockings instead of tights and loose skirts or baggy trousers on warm days.

- When the weather is hot, have cool baths or showers rather than soaking in a hot tub.

- Do not use perfumed soaps, bubble baths or bath additives, which may inflame the vaginal area.

- Eat live (also called bioactive) yoghurt regularly, as it contains bacteria that may block the growth of thrush in the vagina.

- After using the toilet, always wipe from front to back to prevent any *candida* from the bowel entering the vagina.

- If you have diabetes, maintain strict control of your blood sugar levels.

- Avoid excessive alcohol and reduce sugar intake.

- Use a vaginal lubricant, if necessary, during intercourse – damage to the vaginal tissues can increase the risk of thrush.

---

pessaries, lotions, lozenges, drops and tablets. In most cases, the treatment works rapidly and eradicates the excess thrush within a few days to a week. However, some forms of thrush that affect large areas of the skin or the nails are more resistant to treatment. They may take weeks or even months to clear.

OTHER INFECTIONS

There are other vaginal infections that cause similar symptoms to thrush but require different treatment. One is trichomoniasis, which causes a fishy, ammonia-smelling discharge. Bacterial vaginosis is another vaginal infection often mistaken for thrush. Symptoms include an off-white discharge and soreness around the genitals. Treatment for both conditions is a course of antibiotics. ∎

CAUTION

It is important to have a sexually transmitted disease treated as soon as you become aware of it. If left untreated in a woman, it can cause pelvic inflammatory disease (PID). The bacteria that cause the initial disease travel up the pelvic cavity into the Fallopian tubes. Infertility may occur if the tubes are damaged. This process can develop over many years, without any symptoms.

Sexually transmitted diseases

Anyone can catch a sexually transmitted disease if they have unprotected sex with someone who is infected. Some of these conditions can have serious consequences if not correctly diagnosed and swiftly treated.

Sexually transmitted diseases, often called venereal diseases or STDs, are a problem throughout the world. There are about 25 different types of infection and the prevalence of these diseases has changed over time. Gonorrhoea and syphilis, once widespread, can now be contained with antibiotics.

In the developed countries, the most common diseases in this category are now chlamydia, nonspecific urethritis, genital herpes and genital warts. The incidence of all these rose sharply in the 1960s and '70s, when women started to use the oral contraceptive pill and stopped using barrier contraception.

Chlamydia and genital herpes became even more prevalent in the '80s and '90s. Chlamydia is responsible for many cases of infertility and some countries have introduced routine screening. Unlike the older types of venereal disease, it causes few or no early symptoms and is often undiagnosed.

Most sexually transmitted diseases are caused by bacteria or other microbes, such as viruses, that are transmitted by the infected partner during sex. Yet some infections in this category, such as hepatitis B and HIV, are transmitted not only sexually but can also be passed on through a blood transfusion, infected needles or from mother to baby.

DIAGNOSIS AND TREATMENT

If you suspect you have a sexually transmitted disease, act promptly to have it diagnosed. In many cases, you can visit a sexual health clinic and consult a specialist in genitourinary medicine. As well as a physical examination, you may have blood and urine tests performed. Swabs of any discharge will be sent to a laboratory for a diagnosis.

For most common diseases, antibiotics can clear up the infection. Others, such as genital herpes, have no cure but can be kept under control. You will be asked to notify your sexual partner of the infection so that he can also be examined and treated. In most cases, you will also be advised to avoid sexual contact until the infection has completely cleared. ∎

HOW TO HAVE SAFER SEX

Apart from celibacy, there is no guaranteed way to avoid becoming infected with a sexually transmitted disease. However, you can limit your risk of contracting one by practising a few safety precautions when having sex.

- Be selective in your choice of sexual partner and limit the number you have.

- Use condoms for all penetrative sex.

- Wash carefully before and after the sexual act.

- If having oral or anal sex, wash in between acts.

HOW TO IDENTIFY AND TREAT SEXUALLY TRANSMITTED DISEASES

Infection	Symptoms	Treatment	Complications
Chlamydia Protozoal infection	***In women:*** slightly increased vaginal discharge; need to urinate more frequently; lower abdominal pain; pain during intercourse; failure to conceive. ***In men:*** discharge from penis; pain or burning when urinating.	Antibiotic tablets	***In women:*** infertility. If pregnant, ectopic pregnancy or premature labour. Infection can pass to baby, causing eye or lung infection. ***In men:*** inflammation of testicles, causing infertility. ***In both:*** Reiter's syndrome (inflamed eyes and joints; rash on feet and genitals).
Nonspecific urethritis Infection, often chlamydia; may be due to an allergy or excessive alcohol.	Pain or burning when passing urine; white or cloudy discharge from tip of penis; frequent urination.	Antibiotic tablets	Rarely serious complications, but may cause inflammation of the testicles or Reiter's syndrome (see Chlamydia).
Genital warts Human papilloma virus or HPV.	Contagious, small, pink-white fleshy lumps around genital area, singly or in groups; may itch but usually painless.	Podophyllin liquid painted on warts or liquid nitrogen to freeze them. Warts disappear, but recur in half of sufferers.	Some types of HPV linked to increased risk of cervical cancer. May require more frequent cervical smears.
Pubic lice "Crabs"; parasitic insects transmitted sexually and by close contact or towels.	Itching; black powder in underwear from lice droppings; brown eggs or lice on pubic or other hair.	Insecticide shampoos and lotions. Wash clothing and bedding in hot water to avoid reinfection.	None
Genital herpes Herpes simplex virus	Itching or tingling in genital or anal area; painful, small, fluid-filled blisters in genital area; flulike fever, backache, headache or swollen glands.	Antiviral medication can reduce symptoms and help prevent recurrence if taken in early stages of infection.	Small risk of miscarriage if in early pregnancy. If passed on to baby in labour, may cause brain damage or blindness. Caesarean delivery advised.
Trichomoniasis *Trichomonas vaginalis* (protozoan)	***In women:*** fishy, watery vaginal discharge; itchy, swollen vulva. ***In men:*** stinging after urinating; urethral discharge.	Antibiotics	None
Syphilis *Treponema pallidum* (a spirochaete, or spiral-shaped bacterium).	Open sore on penis, vagina, cervix, rectum or throat; skin rash, fever, headache, bone pain, fatigue, appetite loss.	Penicillin or other antibiotics effective at all stages. In late stages, organ damage may be irreversible.	If untreated, fatal heart disorders, brain damage, paralysis, damage to skin and bones. Can pass to foetus.
Gonorrhoea *Neisseria gonorrhoeae*	***In men:*** white discharge from penis; pain on urination; irritation of anus; inflamed testicles and prostate gland. ***In women:*** similar symptoms but less marked.	Antibiotics	Gonoccocal arthritis, with crippling pain and swelling, and fatal septicaemia. ***In women:*** may affect fertility. Can be passed on in childbirth and blind baby.

SEE ALSO
Yeast infections   142–143
Aromatherapy   192–195
Hydrotherapy   236–237

Urinary tract infections

Any part of the urinary tract – which is made up of the kidneys, ureters, bladder and urethra – can become infected if large numbers of bacteria enter the urethra and spread through the system.

The most common cause of urinary tract infections (UTIs) in the lower part of the tract is the *Escherichia coli (E. coli)* bacterium, which is commonly found in the gastrointestinal tract. If *E. coli* bacteria enter the urethra, they can cause urethritis, an infection of the urethra; and if they travel to the bladder, the result can be cystitis, an inflammation of the bladder.

The unmistakable key symptom of a lower urinary tract infection is a painful burning or stinging sensation during urination. You may also have an urge to urinate frequently, even though only small

amounts come out. The urine often appears cloudy, contains pus or blood or has a strongly pungent smell. The area just above the pubic bone may also feel particularly tender.

WHO IS AT RISK?

Women are much more susceptible to urinary tract infections than men because their urethral opening is closer to the anus. While a man's bladder is about 15 cm (6 in) from his urethra, a woman's is only about 2.5 cm (1 in) away, so the bacteria have much less distance to travel, making transmission that much easier.

A number of factors can trigger infection. Poor hygiene, putting off urination, sexual intercourse, childbirth and gynaecological surgery can all easily introduce bacteria into the urethral area. Hormonal changes during pregnancy and menopause also increase the risk.

Pregnant women are especially prone to cystitis because the developing foetus presses on the bladder, preventing it from completely emptying. Even certain forms of contraception, such as spermicidal foams and jellies, diaphragms and condoms are linked to irritation of the urethra or difficulty emptying the bladder.

SEEING THE DOCTOR

Mild urinary tract infections often disappear without treatment. However, anyone who has symptoms which last more than 24 hours, who develops fever or chills, has lower back pain, vaginal or

The urinary tract processes urine. The kidneys make it by filtering and removing waste products from the blood. This waste fluid passes down the ureters and into the bladder, where it is stored until there is enough liquid to trigger micturition – the passing of urine. The bladder contracts and urine is released from the body through the urethra.

THE FEMALE URINARY TRACT

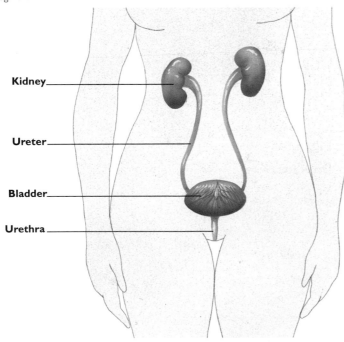

Kidney

Ureter

Bladder

Urethra

penile discharge or bloody urine should see a doctor. Any of these could be a sign of a kidney infection.

You should also see your doctor if you have a medical history of diabetes, high blood pressure, kidney disease or if you are or might be pregnant. Preventive action can preempt complications from untreated bladder infections.

Diagnosing a urinary tract infection is not complicated. Most doctors will take a urine sample and, using a dipstick, check it for blood or pus – a concentration of white blood cells signifying infection. If the urine test is positive, the sample will usually be sent to a laboratory to determine the exact nature of the bacterium responsible for the infection.

TREATING THE INFECTION

If the infection appears straightforward, your doctor will probably prescribe an antibiotic without waiting for the results of the urine culture. Previously, courses of antibiotics of up to two weeks were given, but recent studies have found that simple urinary tract infections can be effectively cleared with shorter courses of antibiotics, ranging from one to five days. Although the treatment usually provides quick relief from symptoms, it is important to complete the entire course prescribed. If you stop taking the medication before your doctor's recommendation, the original bacterial infection may not be completely eradicated, and you are likely to have a relapse.

Some women are prone to recurrent infections and will need further testing to see if there is a physical abnormality in the urinary tract that predisposes them to infection. This may involve cystoscopy (looking at the bladder using an endoscope), an ultrasound scan to thoroughly study the kidneys and bladder

or an intravenous pyelogram (IVP), a procedure in which a dye is injected into the veins before an X-ray of the bladder and kidneys is taken.

COMPLICATIONS

Lower urinary tract infections are rarely serious. However, if left untreated they may spread up to the kidneys and inflame them, a condition called pyelonephritis. Untreated attacks may eventually cause permanent damage to the kidney.

Acute pyelonephritis is more common in women and most likely to occur during pregnancy. Symptoms include a high fever, chills, back pain, nausea, vomiting, a burning sensation during urination and a need to urinate frequently. Any woman with these symptoms should see her doctor immediately for diagnosis and antibiotic treatment. ∎

PREVENTING CYSTITIS

Some women find that they are prone to recurrent attacks of cystitis. Rather than resorting to regular courses of antibiotics, which may in turn trigger thrush, the following self-help tips can prevent the infection developing in the first place.

- Drink plenty of fluids throughout the day. Liquid helps to dilute the urine.

- Empty your bladder regularly, which helps prevent stagnation.

- Avoid bubble baths, vaginal deodorants or douches, which may irritate the area around the urethra.

- Drink cranberry juice, which is thought to help prevent bacteria from sticking to the lining of the bladder.

- Urinate before and after intercourse to flush out any bacteria that may be near the urethral opening.

- Always wipe yourself from front to back after a bowel movement. This avoids spreading bacteria from the intestinal tract into the urethra.

- Change sanitary towels or tampons regularly.

Hepatitis

The term "hepatitis" refers to inflammation of the liver, which is most commonly caused by viruses. Viral hepatitis is a potentially serious disease and there are several recognized viruses that transmit the illness.

An illness due to hepatitis can take two forms: acute (short term) and chronic (long term). Acute hepatitis is usually caused by one of the viruses, but taking certain medications, including an overdosage of paracetamol, or exposure to chemicals such as dry-cleaning agents can also cause it.

The hepatitis viruses have an acute phase, but only infection with the B, C and D strains involve a chronic phase. Chronic hepatitis can also be caused by heavy alcohol consumption and an auto-immune disorder, in which the body's own defence system attacks the liver.

Chronic hepatitis may be persistent or active. In chronic persistent hepatitis, the virus is present in the liver but does not seem to be damaging it – this is the least serious type of chronic hepatitis and there is usually little risk of complications. Chronic active hepatitis causes inflammation and progressive destruction of cells in the liver and can eventually lead to cirrhosis and liver cancer.

COMMON TYPES OF VIRUS

Hepatitis A is one of the most common infections in the world. About 40 percent of the population of western Europe get this infection, although not everyone becomes ill from it. It is transmitted by faecal contamination. The virus multiplies in the liver and produces viral particles, which are excreted in faeces. Infection results from close contact with infected individuals or contaminated water, hands, cooking utensils or food – particularly fresh fruit and salads, ice and shellfish. Infection with hepatitis A does not progress to chronic illness. During the infection, antibodies develop, providing lifelong immunity.

More than one-third of the world's population is infected with hepatitis B. It may cause chronic liver damage, including liver cancer. Between one and two million people die each year from the infection, which is passed on through contact with contaminated blood. Male homosexuals and intravenous drug abusers are at high risk of infection. People with the disease are carriers and can pass it on to others through certain body fluids, particularly blood.

The hepatitis D strain affects only those already infected by hepatitis B. This form is common in Italy, the Mediterranean region, eastern Europe and South

---

ABOUT THE LIVER

The liver is the body's chemical factory. It regulates the level of amino acids in the blood and is responsible for producing several proteins, including albumin, which helps control the exchange of water between tissues and blood, and coagulation factors, which enable blood to clot when a blood vessel wall is damaged. It also stores glucose in the form of glycogen, which it converts back into glucose when more energy is needed.

The liver helps to eliminate drugs and poisonous substances from the blood. About three-quarters of the liver's cells can be destroyed before it can no longer function.

America. A proportion of sufferers go on to develop chronic liver disease.

Hepatitis C is more common than the B strain. About 1 in 100 people is a carrier of hepatitis C, which can be detected in donated blood by screening. (Before screening was available, donated blood was one route of transmission.) The virus is usually transmitted by syringes shared by intravenous drug abusers and improperly sterilized needles used by tattoo artists, yet it is not known how one-third of the cases are transmitted. At least 80 percent of sufferers are carriers of the virus and a large proportion develop chronic liver disease.

Hepatitis E is found in southeast Asia, India, Africa and Mexico. Infection follows contact with contaminated water.

SYMPTOMS

In hepatitis A, symptoms appear two to six weeks after contact with the virus. They typically include fever, nausea, vomiting, lack of appetite, diarrhoea and abdominal pain and may last for a week or more before jaundice develops. The skin and whites of the eyes turn yellow, because the inflamed liver cannot remove the pigment bilirubin from the blood.

The jaundice phase can last for weeks or several months. In severe cases, coma and death can result.

The symptoms of the other forms of hepatitis are similar and can range from a mild flulike syndrome and weakness to vomiting and jaundice. However, some people experience no symptoms. Because there may be no symptoms or they may be attributed to flu, chronic forms of the disease may not be diagnosed.

TREATMENT

Sufferers of acute hepatitis are advised to stay in bed, eat a nourishing diet and avoid alcohol for six months after recovery from the disease, which usually takes a few weeks. Alcohol damages the liver and can prolong the illness or cause a relapse.

Vaccines are available for the A and B strains. People at high risk of exposure to the virus, such as healthcare workers and travellers to the developing world, should be vaccinated. A convenient double vaccine containing A and B is available. Immunization against hepatitis B also protects against the D strain, which can co-exist only with hepatitis B. Babies of mothers who are hepatitis B carriers can be treated at birth to prevent infection. ∎

PROTECTION AND PREVENTION		
Virus	How it spreads	Protection methods
Hepatitis A and E	Faecal contamination of water and food; contact with infected person's faeces.	Scrupulous hygiene; vaccination against hepatitis A for long-term protection or immunoglobulins (antibodies) for the short term.
Hepatitis B and D	Contact with infected blood and blood products.	Avoid unprotected sex; avoid penetration of skin with contaminated items such as needles; vaccinate against hepatitis B.
Hepatitis C	Contact with infected blood and blood products.	Avoid penetrating the skin with contaminated objects, including needles.

HIV

The human immunodeficiency virus, or HIV, attacks the body's T-cell lymphocytes (a type of white blood cell), which normally trigger the actions of the immune system. The immune system is the body's defence against disease and, when it is damaged, it cannot fight off certain infections. The result is acquired immunodeficiency syndrome, or AIDS.

Magnified 86,000 times, the HIV virus is shown budding from an infected T-cell lymphocyte. Once free (below, far left), the virus infects other T-cell lympho-cytes, weakening the body's immune response.

When HIV attacks T-cell lympho-cytes, it alters the codes within them: instead of fighting against the virus, they make more HIV. As the HIV spreads to more T-cells, the number of healthy cells decreases, making it increasingly difficult for the body to recover from any illness. Eventually, there are not enough T-cells to protect the body from opportunistic infections (ones that can only attack if the immune system is weak)

and the person has AIDS. Some people experience a flulike illness when first infected, but many people are infected for years without realizing it, until the HIV develops into AIDS.

WHO CATCHES AIDS?

The HIV virus is contained in blood, saliva and seminal and vaginal fluids. Anyone whose blood, semen or vaginal fluids interchange with those of someone who is HIV-positive risks being infected. This can occur during sexual intercourse (both vaginal or anal) a blood transfusion, use of an infected needle or syringe or between mother and baby during childbirth or breast-feeding. However, it seems that the virus cannot be passed on by the exchange of saliva, for example, in open-mouthed kissing.

The virus is extremely infectious. It exists in over 140 countries and, worldwide, there are 8,500 new infections every day. HIV is not a homosexual disease. Unprotected sex with any infected person, homosexual or heterosexual, is a risk. The number of cases among heterosexuals has grown steadily, and women are more vulnerable than men. An HIV-negative woman is four times more likely to contract the virus from an HIV-positive man than the other way round.

HIV PREVENTION

Both sexes can reduce their risk of virus transmission, particularly by practising safe sex (see Caution, right).
- Intravenous drug abusers should use only new, disposable syringes; never share a needle or syringe or use an old one.
- If you are HIV-positive and pregnant, discuss the proposed method of giving birth and the issue of breast-feeding with your hospital consultant.
- Make sure that your dentist and dental hygienist wear fresh rubber gloves.
- Make sure any form of skin piercing is carried out with disposable needles.
- Any cuts or open wounds on an HIV-infected person should be covered.

TREATMENT

There is as yet no cure for AIDs, but some treatments and lifestyle changes can alleviate symptoms, treat secondary infections or slow the spread of the virus.

Drugs are often given in combination. The type and amount given depend on the individual, the stage of the disease and the secondary infections involved.

A healthy lifestyle can alleviate the burden on the immune system. This entails a healthy diet with lots of fruit and vegetables and no junk food, alcohol, nicotine, caffeine or illegal drugs. Gentle exercise in the fresh air also helps.

In some people, complementary therapies appear to have a beneficial effect on general wellbeing and may help to boost the immune system. Professional counselling with a doctor or through one of the national support groups can help psychologically. ■

CAUTION

Because it takes up to three months for the virus to be detectable by current tests, safe sex (using a condom, p.169) is essential until both partners are certain that neither has had intercourse with anyone else for at least three months before testing HIV negative. Women can protect themselves (and their partner) with the use of the female condom. Especially strong condoms are available for use in anal sex.

TESTING FOR HIV

If you suspect that you could be HIV-positive, it is wise to have a test, especially if you are planning to become pregnant or to become involved in a new sexual relationship. If you are infected with HIV, you will have produced antibodies to it – the HIV test looks for these antibodies. It must be carried out at least three months after the last time you could have been infected; this is the amount of time it can take for the antibodies to register. The test involves taking a sample of blood, which is sent to a laboratory for analysis.

Information about the availability of tests in your area can be obtained from national support and advice organizations. Tests are routinely offered at sexual health clinics. You can also obtain the test through your family doctor. If you do, the result may be noted in your medical records.

A trained counsellor will advise you in detail of the implications of having the test done and what the results mean. Only if you are psychologically prepared to accept the result, whatever it may be, should you go ahead. A positive result can be devastating news, even if you are expecting it. It does, however, enable you to seek medical advice and treatment and to change your lifestyle at the earliest opportunity. Despite a positive result, many people have lived in relatively good health for more than 10 years before the onset of AIDS.

SEE ALSO
Adjusting your diet
264–267

Cancer

Despite decades of research and advances in treatment, cancer affects one in three people, a quarter of whom die of it. Although cancer is widely regarded as a disease of modern times, it is not new – however, it does affect far more people than in previous centuries. One-quarter of all people in the industrialized world now develop some form of the disease.

The more than 200 forms of cancer all follow a similar pattern of development. A cancer occurs when cell growth goes out of control. This happens when a cell is affected by carcinogens – for example, from cigarettes, the sun or radioactivity – and its DNA mutates. DNA is the genetic material that tells each cell how to behave. When the DNA is transformed, it cannot pass on the correct information. The cell misbehaves: the most obvious manifestation is in accelerated cell division. The mutant cells are unable to perform the function for which they were designed, and they produce harmful substances and can learn to move and set up new growths.

Cells contain many safeguards against mutations occurring, so multiple, consecutive changes are necessary to produce a cancerous cell. This is why cancers are common in old age or when the exposure to carcinogens is repeated, as in smoking or sunbathing. Mutation is caused by a random chain of events, with individual cells in different parts of the body transforming in their own way. This is one reason why treatment is difficult.

THE GROWTH OF A TUMOUR

Cancer cells usually reproduce themselves every 24 hours, each time passing their abnormality on to their offspring. After three weeks there may be millions of new

All cells need nutrients and oxygen, supplied by blood (below left). Cancer cells, which ignore the normal messages telling them to stop multiplying, require more blood than other cells. They release tumour angiogenesis factor (TAF), a substance that triggers the growth of secondary blood vessels near the site (below, centre). The extra supply of nutrients allows the cancer cells to grow even more rapidly (below, right), destroying healthy tissue and eventually seeding to other parts of the body.

HOW A CANCER CELL GROWS

Blood vessel   **Normal cell**

TAF   **Cancer cell**

Blood vessel drawn toward tumour

cancer cells. Once cells grow in an uncontrolled way they form a tumour, which gradually enlarges, spreading into healthy tissue. It was because of this that the ancient Greeks named the disease *cancer,* or crab.

Tumour cells can form a benign or malignant growth. If benign, it may grow in size and press on surrounding tissues, but cannot invade them or cause new growths in other parts of the body.

A malignant growth will continue to grow and can spread from the original tissue to others. When cells from a malignant tumour break free, they are carried onward – usually in the lymph system or bloodstream – to other tissues or organs, where they continue to reproduce. A secondary growth is known as a metastasis. There may be just one or many metastases and they can occur in parts of the body unrelated to and distant from the original, primary tumour.

If any tumour develops in a vital organ, such as the liver or lungs, it will interfere with its essential functions. Similarly, a tumour that presses on a main artery can reduce blood supply to vital organs. In both of these cases, life-threatening complications can result.

WHO DEVELOPS CANCER?

Cancer is in large part a disease of aging. More than 70 percent of cancer sufferers are over 60 years old. However, cancer can affect people at any stage in their lives. Leukaemia, for example, is more prevalent in children, and testicular cancer mainly affects men from 19 to 44 years of age.

A susceptibility to cancer can be inherited. It is now known, for example, that two genes, called BRCA1 and BRCA2, are linked to breast cancer. By 70 years of age, 85 percent of women with a mutated BRCA1 gene have breast

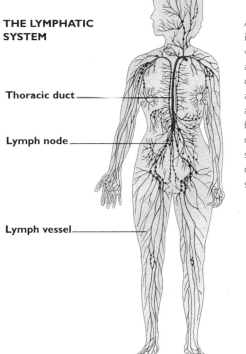

THE LYMPHATIC SYSTEM

Thoracic duct

Lymph node

Lymph vessel

A crucial part of the body's immune system, lymphatic vessels and ducts provide an alternative to blood circulation in carrying fluids around the body. However, as well as transporting beneficial antibodies to fight off infections, the lymphatic system can be a route for cancer cells to quickly spread through the body.

THE WARNING SIGNS

Cancer has a variety of symptoms, and their nature and severity depend on how established the cancer is, in which organ or tissues the tumour is and its secondary effects on other parts of the body. There are 11 possible symptoms that should always be taken seriously. Usually, they are not related to a cancerous growth, but you must always tell your doctor if you experience:

- rapid, unexplained weight loss
- severe recurrent headaches
- persistent hoarseness, sore throat or difficulty swallowing
- persistent, unexplained abdominal pain or indigestion
- a lump or thickening of tissue anywhere in the body
- a change in bowel or bladder habits
- unusual bleeding or discharge
- blood in your urine or phlegm
- a scab, sore or ulcer that fails to heal
- a mole that changes colour or size, bleeds or itches
- vaginal bleeding after sex, between periods or after menopause

CAUTION

The best method for detecting cervical cancer early is screening. It is important to attend all sessions you are called for, as it may be three to five years between breast or cervical screenings.

cancer. Similarly, a light smoker carrying a gene known as CYP1A1 has seven times the risk of developing lung cancer as one without the gene. However, behaviour can also affect the risk of developing cancer. Nine out of 10 people with lung cancer, for example, are smokers, and most skin cancer sufferers are fair-skinned people who spent too much time in the sun.

It has been estimated that more than 90 percent of cancers stem from an interaction between genes and the environment. In most cases, even if you carry a gene that predisposes you to a form of cancer, you can reduce your risk by adopting a certain lifestyle.

DIAGNOSIS AND TESTS

Any cancer is more easily treated if caught in the early stages, so early diagnosis is important. This is not easy because symptoms usually do not develop until millions of cancer cells have reproduced or until the primary tumour is the size of

a small grape. Growths deep in the body are undetectable except by special kinds of medical examination. The exceptions are cancers of the breast (see p.157), testicles (see p.158) and skin (see p.158), which you can feel or see yourself. Most cancers are found when a person develops symptoms and visits the family doctor.

If the doctor suspects that a cancer may be present, he can arrange for various tests to confirm the diagnosis. There are four types of test. In cytology, cells from the suspect area are removed for examination. This test can reveal abnormal cells, which are shed by the affected area. The cervical smear test is the most common example.

The doctor may perform a biopsy by removing a sample of tissue from the suspect area. The sample is studied for microscopic changes in its structure in a procedure known as a histology. The doctor may take a blood sample for examination, which can detect changes or abnormality in its components. An X-ray can help to detect the increased density of a tumour, which shows up as a lighter area in bone or lung tissue.

Other newer imaging techniques can be used instead of or in conjunction with a conventional X-ray. Computerized X-rays (known as computerized tomography, or CT scanning), ultrasound and magnetic resonance imaging (MRI) can all produce images of suspect tissue to aid diagnosis. Radio-isotope scans, in which low doses of radioactivity are injected, can be used to view certain cancers, such as those of the thyroid and bone.

TREATMENT

Once the diagnosis of cancer has been confirmed, the best ways to tackle it can be discussed. There is no single cure for cancer and it is up to the specialists to whom you are referred to decide on the

Radiotherapy is a method of destroying cancerous cells with radiation. This linear particle accelerator delivers high-voltage X-rays that penetrate the skin and reach the target area.

best form of treatment. Cancer can be treated in four ways: through surgery, radiotherapy, chemotherapy or biological therapy – or with a combination of two or more of them.

Surgery can eliminate about 40 percent of malignant tumours. If the tumour has attacked an organ, "radical surgery" is often recommended. This procedure involves removing not just the diseased organ, but also its surrounding lymph nodes. It reduces the chances of a malignant tumour spreading to other parts of the body through the lymphatic system. Radiotherapy or chemotherapy are sometimes used before surgery to shrink a tumour and destroy cancer cells, which may be metastasizing.

Radiotherapy works by killing cancer cells with radiation. This treatment works best on well-nourished cancer cells, which are those on the outside of the tumour. The treatment is usually given in several doses, allowing the inner cells to be exposed in stages.

Treatment with anticancer drugs is known as chemotherapy. The drugs are cytotoxic chemicals that attack fast-dividing cells, and they can effectively destroy the cancerous cells. However, they cannot discriminate between these and other fast-dividing cells in the body that are not cancerous, including those in the bone marrow, intestinal lining, hair follicles and reproductive organs. Consequently, chemotherapy produces many unwanted side effects.

RECENT DEVELOPMENTS

Biological therapy is the newest type of treatment. It aims, through the use of substances such as manufactured antibodies and interferons, to alter the body's response to cancerous cells. It can sometimes be used to carry radioactive isotopes to the affected areas. However, it is still experimental and rarely used.

Scientists have discovered that the self-destruct mechanism for a cancer tumour is located on the outside of the cells. This may open the way for a new generation of drugs that could make cancerous cells self-destruct while leaving the normal ones untouched.

Apart from new drug treatments, the good news about cancer is that in many cases it is preventable. Up to 60 percent of cancers may be avoided by making changes in lifestyle such as stopping smoking and improving your diet.

STOPPING SMOKING

Smoking is the single greatest preventable cause of cancer, and it is not only the lungs that are damaged by smoking (see pp.20–21). It is estimated that smoking is responsible for a third of all cancer deaths.

CAUTION

It is particularly important to give up smoking if you have or are planning to have children. Children are more sensitive than adults to passive smoking. Smoking can increase a baby's risk of developing leukaemia.

RECEIVING THE BEST TREATMENT

Cancer is a serious disease which requires you to put yourself in the hands of specialists. You can help to maximize your chances of recovery by avoiding delay in investigation and treatment.

- If your family doctor believes you need diagnostic tests, you should see a hospital specialist within two weeks.

- Your specialist will order diagnostic tests. Ideally, they should be performed within two weeks and the results offered within the subsequent two weeks. Test results should be given by the specialist in person and in private.

- Treatment is best in the hands of a multidisciplinary hospital team – one in which radiotherapists, oncologists, surgeons and cancer care nurses work together.

- Make sure you are given all the possible treatment options and a basis on which to make a confident judgment of them.

- Ask your specialist or family doctor about pain-relief and supportive care.

CAUTION

Consumption of a low-fibre diet has been linked to an increased risk of bowel and stomach cancers. Most experts now recommend wholemeal bread and high-fibre cereals, with several servings of vegetables and fruit a day. Cancers of the colon, breast, skin and lung are all much less common in southern Europe, where people eat three times as much fresh fruit and vegetables as those in northern Europe.

The answer to those who smoke is theoretically simple: stop. The benefits are soon felt. Eight hours after giving up, blood oxygen levels rise to normal; in 48 hours, the sense of taste and smell recover as the last traces of nicotine leave the body; and 72 hours afterward the lungs are capable of holding more air.

In practice, it is difficult to break the habit because nicotine is an extremely addictive chemical. If you need convincing that it is worth the struggle, bear in mind that within five years of giving up smoking, your risk of cancer falls to half that of a smoker – and there is also a huge financial benefit.

ADJUSTING YOUR DIET

An estimated 35–40 percent of cancers could be prevented by changes in diet. Stomach cancer, for example, was much more common before the invention of the refrigerator, when foods were preserved by curing and salting. Today, it is still more common in countries whose cuisines feature a lot of these foods.

Try to cut down your meat intake, particularly if it goes hand in hand with poor eating habits. Big meat eaters tend to eat more fat. Increased fat consumption, besides leading to an overweight problem, increases the risk of certain cancers such as that of the uterus. Hearty meat consumers also tend to eat fewer fresh fruit and vegetables. That means less fibre and fewer antioxidants, both of which protect against many cancers.

A good intake of natural fibre (see p.253) decreases the risks of bowel cancer and breast cancer. In women, high fibre intake decreases the amount of circulating oestrogen, a hormone that is linked to breast cancer. Fibre also helps the food to pass through the gut more quickly, decreasing the risk of bowel cancer.

Fruit and vegetables are rich in antioxidants – vitamins C and E and betacarotene (see pp.242–43). These mop up harmful substances in the blood called free radicals, which are associated with cancer. You should eat at least 400 g (14 oz) and, ideally, 800 g (1 lb 12 oz) of fresh fruit and vegetables each day. Within two months of raising your intake, the level of antioxidants in your blood will be significantly higher.

In particular, women are advised to eat fruit and vegetables that are high in phyto-oestrogens such as soya, yams and rhubarb. These are believed to block the oestrogen receptors in the blood, which may reduce the risk of breast cancer. Vitamin D, which is available from dairy foods, fish and sunlight, has also been associated with a lower risk of breast cancer.

Fish oils (see pp.250–51) are thought to protect against many cancers by reducing the level of prostaglandins – inflammatory agents that may help tumours grow – in the blood. Other fats should be restricted. Transfatty acids, such as those found in margarine and biscuits, are thought to increase the risk of breast cancer and prostate cancer by acting on the sex hormones oestrogen and testosterone.

SUN EXPOSURE

Skin cancer is much more common than it used to be. The popularity of holidays in hot countries, the appeal of tanned skin and the availability of sun beds have all encouraged people to expose their skin to damaging UVA and UVB rays (see p.119). Anyone can develop skin cancer from sun exposure, but fair-skinned people are more vulnerable, because their skin contains less of a pigment called eumelanin, which protects from burning. The best advice is to stay out of the sun.

EXAMINING YOUR BREASTS

One in 12 women in the industrialized world develops breast cancer. Doing a monthly breast self examination can detect the cancer early, giving you a better chance of recovery. You should carry out an examination four days after the end of your period, when your breasts are least swollen or lumpy. Look and feel for any changes. Regular examination will help you become familiar with your breasts, making it easier to detect a change.

1 With your arms by your sides, look at your breasts in the mirror, noting their shape, size and position, first from the front and then from the side. Look for any swelling, change in size or colour, puckering or dimpling of the skin or increased prominence of the veins. Don't worry if your breasts are different sizes – this is normal.

2 With your hands on your head, look at each of your breasts from the side and front for any changes. Note and become familiar with their outlines.

3 Repeat your observations with your hands pressed on your hips, then with your arms raised in the air.

4 Squeeze each nipple in turn to see if there is a discharge. You should also inspect the nipples for any changes in skin colour or texture, inversion or change in direction.

5 Lie with a pillow under your shoulders and head, with the arm on the side of the breast you are examining behind your head. Using the flat parts of your middle fingers, firmly press the breast all over, working from the nipple and spiralling outward.

6 After you have palpated the whole breast, feel from the breast to the armpit and along the collarbone for any unusual lumps, lumpy areas or thickening of tissue. Then repeat steps 5 and 6 on the other side.

CAUTION

Ninety percent of changes are benign, but always contact your doctor if you find a lump or suspect that there might be a problem.

CAUTION

The fairer your skin, the more you need to shield it from the sun. Sun creams provide a barrier, but they must protect against both UVA and UVB rays. Make sure the sun protection factor (SPF) is strong enough for your skin type. The SPF number indicates how much longer you will take to burn if using the cream. For example, if you usually burn after an hour in the sun, when you are covered with an SPF15 cream it will take 15 hours.

THE BENEFITS OF EXERCISE

Keeping fit (see pp.10–11) seems to reduce the risk of cancer by influencing weight and metabolism, which affect hormone production. Inactive people are more likely to get colon and breast cancer. Women who gain a lot of weight (more than 20 kg/42 lb) between their late teens and mid-50s increase their risk of breast cancer by 40 percent.

Exercise also reduces the risk of heart disease, so it makes sense to take it up. At least half an hour three times a week is recommended. If you cannot go to a gym or take up a vigorous sport, leave the car at home and do some brisk walking. Any activity that generates sustained warmth and heavier breathing is helpful.

TESTICLE EXAMINATION

As rates of testicular cancer in men are rising, testicle examination is more important than ever. It is the most common cancer in men 20–35 years old. However, 90 percent of testicle cancers are curable if caught in the early stages.

Examine your testicles regularly, preferably in a warm shower or bath. Hold each testicle in your hands to become familiar with its size and weight. One may be larger than the other, or may hang lower, both of which are normal.

Roll each testicle between your thumb and finger. It should feel smooth, apart from the soft, tender tube toward the back, which is the epididymis that carries and stores sperm. You should see your doctor if you feel a hard lump on the front or side of a testicle or if there is any swelling or enlargement, an increase in firmness, an unusual difference between the two testicles or any discomfort or pain. Also report any heavy or dragging feeling or dull ache in the groin.

CHANGES IN YOUR SKIN

Skin cancer has become much more common over the past 40 years and is usually ranked as the second most common cancer. However, because it is underdiagnosed, it is probably the most common cancer.

There are three common types of skin cancer: basal cell carcinoma, which occurs mostly on the face and neck and is relatively slow to spread, and squamous cell carcinoma and malignant melanoma, both of which are common on areas exposed to the sun. They are all easily preventable by protecting yourself from the sun (see box, left). Be aware of the condition of your skin, particularly if you are fair-skinned, and visit the doctor immediately if you notice any of the following signs:
- the growth of a new mole or enlargement of an existing one
- a change to mixed brown or black colourings on a mole
- an irregular outline to a mole
- itching, inflammation, bleeding or crusting of a mole
- a failure of the skin to heal
- persistent ulcers on the skin. ■

SUN SENSE AND SAFETY

- Stay out of the midday sun (11:00am–3:00pm).
- Cover up with loose cotton clothing and a wide-brimmed hat.
- Put sunscreen on exposed skin and reapply it regularly.
- Never allow the skin of babies or young children to be exposed to the sun – their sensitive skin burns more easily. The younger you are when sunburnt, the greater the chances of developing cancer in later life.
- Do not use sun beds if you have fair skin, a lot of freckles or moles or a history of sunburn. No one should use them more than 20 times a year.

GUIDE TO THE SIX MOST COMMON CANCERS

Site of cancer	Symptoms	Who it affects	Treatment	Survival (5 years after diagnosis)
Lung	Persistent cough and breathlessness; chest pain; coughing up of blood-stained phlegm; malaise, lethargy and weight loss.	Mostly all smokers. Twice as many men as women, but women who smoke the same amount as men have a three times greater risk.	Radiotherapy. Surgery is appropriate in 20 percent of cases – chemotherapy may be used beforehand.	Less than 10 percent.
Breast	Lump or pain in a breast or armpit; eczema on or discharge from a nipple; wrinkling of the skin around a nipple.	One in 12 women, mostly over 50 years old – unless they carry the breast cancer gene, in which case they may develop it earlier.	Removal of tumour if small, whole breast (mastectomy) if large. Removal of lymph nodes if cells spread. Chemotherapy to shrink tumour. Drugs to block production of oestrogen or its action on breast.	About 60 percent.
Skin	Changes in moles; persistent skin ulcers; shiny patches on skin; any skin injury that does not heal within 2 weeks.	Fair-skinned people who sunbathe and those who have a tendency to freckle heavily; outdoor workers.	Surgery in early stages, later combined with chemo-, radio- or biological therapy. For non-malignant melanomas, cryo surgery (freezing).	More than 90 percent if caught early, but declining sharply with time.
Bowel	Blood in stools; constipation; diarrhoea; flatulence, with pain; constant sense of fullness in the bowel.	Mainly in people over 60 years of age, but 5 percent of people are under 40 years old (there is usually an inherited factor).	Removal of a section of the bowel; chemo-therapy if cancer is in an advanced stage.	About 35 percent recover. Up to half of bowel cancers diagnosed too late because patients delay seeing doctor.
Prostate	Difficulty urinating; frequent urination at night; passing blood in urine; feeling of incomplete emptying.	Mainly in men over 70 years of age.	Surgery; radiotherapy if small. Drugs that inhibit testosterone sometimes used before radiotherapy.	About 45 percent of men who receive treatment recover.
Bladder	Blood in urine; pain during urination; urgent or frequent need to urinate.	Smokers and men up to three times greater risk; chemical, leather and textile workers, mechanics, printers, painters and hair-dressers are at risk.	Removal of tumour if small with cytoscope; removal of bladder if large or several tumours; radio- and chemotherapy.	About 60 percent of those treated recover.

SEE ALSO
Cancer   152–159

Prostate problems

The prostate gland is partly responsible for producing semen – the fluid that the sperm travel in during ejaculation – and for making secretions to moisten the lining of the urethra. Prostate disorders affect half of all men over 50 years old. The most common problems are prostatitis, benign prostatic hyperplasia and prostate cancer.

At birth, the prostate gland in a boy is the size of a pea. It grows bigger during puberty and, by adulthood, the gland is the size of a chestnut, weighing an average of 20 g (¾ oz). The gland enlarges once more after a man reaches 50 years of age, which is when a prostatic problem can develop. It is rare for one to occur in men under 30 years old.

PROSTATITIS

An umbrella term covering several disorders that involve the prostate gland, prostatitis occurs when the prostate becomes inflamed. This often happens when bacteria spread from the intestines to the gland via the urethra. Prostatitis is common, particularly in men between 30 and 50 years of age. It is estimated that as many as one in three men suffers from prostatitis at some time in his life.

The main symptoms of prostatitis are frequent urination and pain on doing so; swelling of the testes; pain in the lower back, prostate, genitals or rectum; a watery discharge from the penis; pain on ejaculation; blood in the semen and premature ejaculation.

A doctor may perform a rectal examination to determine if the gland is tender and enlarged. Tests of the urine and urethral secretions can identify the type of infection. Prostatitis is treated with antibiotics. However, it can take a while to clear up, and it may return.

Drinking plenty of water can help prevent infection of the prostate. This may seem perverse advice, given that the chief symptom of an enlarged prostate is frequent urination. However, a high fluid intake helps to reduce the possibility of any residual urine in the bladder causing infection.

ANATOMY OF THE PROSTATE

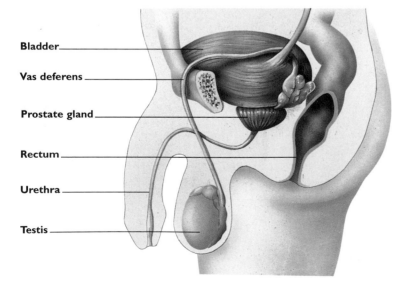

Bladder

Vas deferens

Prostate gland

Rectum

Urethra

Testis

The prostate gland is an organ situated in front of the rectum and immediately below the bladder; it surrounds the urethra – the outlet for urine – as this tube exits the bladder. The positioning of the gland makes it possible for a doctor to judge its size during a rectal examination.

ENLARGED PROSTATE

Benign prostatic hyperplasia (BPH), or hypertrophy, is an enlarged prostate gland. Because the prostate gland encircles the urethra, when it enlarges it increases pressure on the bladder. This produces the sensation of wanting to urinate frequently. However, the ability to urinate is impaired by the pressure exerted from the gland.

At least 1 in 3 men over 50 years of age experiences one or more of the symptoms of an enlarged prostate (see box, right), but only 6 out of 10 sufferers visit their doctor. Diagnosis can be confirmed by a rectal examination and an ultrasound test. An enlarged prostate can be treated with drugs or surgery.

CANCER OF THE PROSTATE

After lung cancer, prostate cancer is the second most common fatal type in men; worldwide, it accounts for 149,000 deaths every year. Prostate cancer usually occurs in men over 55 years of age, although it can affect younger males. Evidence of cancer can be found in 10–30 percent of men between 50 to 60 years old. The figure rises to 50–70 percent in men between 70 and 80 years of age.

In many cases, prostate cancer is a silent disease: the sufferer does not know that he has it. However, because it usually occurs at a late age, a man with the disease is not likely to die of it – most men will die from some other disorder, such as a stroke or heart disease, before prostate cancer has a chance to be fatal.

The symptoms of prostate cancer are similar to those of a benign prostate enlargement. If you have difficulty in starting the flow of urine and a weak sluggish urinary stream, you suffer from dribbling or incontinence, or score high in the box on the right, you should have a professional diagnosis.

A blood test can be used to detect the early signs of prostate cancer, making treatment more effective. The test measures the level of prostate specific antigen (PSA, a protein), which, if raised, can indicate the presence of cancerous cells. Other diagnostic tests, such as ultrasound, can confirm the diagnosis.

Cancer of the prostate in younger men is treated by the surgical removal of the prostate gland or by radiotherapy. In older men it may be left untreated. ∎

INTERNATIONAL PROSTATE SYMPTOMS SCORE

This is a system devised by the World Health Organization (WHO), which enables an individual and his doctor to judge the severity of his prostatic enlargement and whether or how urgently he needs treatment.

To each question, score 0 points if the answer is not at all; 1 if it is less than once in 5; 2 if less than half the time; 3 if about half the time; 4 if more than half the time and 5 if almost always. Over the past month, how often have you:

- Had the sensation of not completely emptying your bladder after urinating?
- Needed to urinate again within two hours of previously urinating?
- Stopped and started again several times when urinating?
- Found it difficult to postpone urinating?
- Had to push or strain to start urinating?
- Had to get up in the night to urinate?

How did you score?

0–8: Your symptoms are nonexistent or mild. You may not need treatment but if you develop any symptoms, these will be closely monitored by your doctor.

9–17: Your symptoms are moderate. Your doctor may prescribe a drug treatment, provided that your rectal examination and blood tests are normal.

17 and above: Your symptoms are severe. Your doctor will probably refer you to a specialist for further tests and treatment.

CAUTION

Hormonal treatments for premenstrual syndrome have side effects. In fact, the progestogen in the oral contraceptive pill can lower the level of natural progesterone in the body, potentially making symptoms worse.

Premenstrual syndrome

More than two-thirds of women are affected by premenstrual syndrome (PMS) at some time in their lives, and one-third of these suffer from it throughout their reproductive years. Although premenstrual syndrome can occur at any time between puberty and menopause, it is most common in women over 30 years of age.

The cause of premenstrual syndrome is not clear. It is thought to be a result of hormonal fluctuations that are a normal, integral part of the menstrual cycle. There also may be a cumulative effect of hormonal changes over the long term. This is why women who have been pregnant often suffer most.

Many medical conditions are known to get worse just before a period. In medical terms, these are often unrelated conditions, ranging from asthma and migraine to skin rashes and conjunctivitis.

Common symptoms of premenstrual syndrome are fatigue, bloating, back pain, headaches, breast tenderness and aching joints. Many women also experience psychological symptoms such as mood swings, depression and anxiety.

LOW BLOOD SUGAR

One symptom of premenstrual syndrome is low blood sugar. For some reason, women seem to use their blood sugar more quickly in the premenstrual stage of their cycle. Blood sugar levels usually stay up for five hours after a meal, but this can drop to three hours before a period. Low blood sugar can result in tiredness, poor concentration and sugar cravings.

According to one school of thought, low blood sugar may also be responsible for some of the psychological symptoms. When the blood sugar level is low, the body releases the hormone adrenaline. This triggers the liver into releasing glycogen, which is converted to sugar and released into the blood. However, the surge in adrenaline could lead to feelings of aggression and anxiety. An alternative theory is that the symptoms are caused by a lack of serotonin in the brain. Small amounts of serotonin can be derived from tryptophan, which the body metabolizes from carbohydrates.

The simple answer is to eat frequent small meals or snacks that are rich in

LIFESTYLE AND DIETARY SELF HELP

- Eat often and include plenty of unrefined carbohydrates in your diet such as brown rice, wholemeal pasta, baked potatoes, wholemeal bread and breakfast cereals.

- Cut down on smoking or give it up. Cigarettes disrupt blood sugar levels.

- Decrease your salt intake, which encourages water retention.

- Eat plenty of fruit and vegetables and wholegrain cereals to prevent constipation.

- If you are on the contraceptive pill, come off it for a few months to see if symptoms improve.

- Time your important work appointments and social dates outside your premenstrual week.

- Take regular exercise, which encourages the production of natural opiates and can improve some symptoms.

complex carbohydrates or protein, which the body breaks down into sugar. These are preferable to sugary snacks, which provide the body with a sudden but short-lived supply of blood sugar. Energy requirements seem to rise premenstrually, so you should not put on weight.

DIAGNOSIS

Because individual sufferers display different symptoms and because there is no diagnostic test for the condition, it is often overlooked by doctors. Timing is the key to diagnosis. If symptoms start before your period and abate when bleeding becomes heaviest, it is likely that you are suffering from premenstrual syndrome. The premenstrual stage may start anywhere from only a few days before your period to as much as two weeks beforehand, when you ovulate.

The best way to assess your condition is to keep a menstrual chart. You should note the date and nature of the main symptoms you experience over two or three months. Then look back to see if their is an obvious cyclical monthly pattern. Only with such documentation can your doctor make a confident diagnosis of premenstrual syndrome.

TREATMENT

For the 90 percent of sufferers whose symptoms are mild to moderate, no drug treatment is necessary. Most can handle their symptoms by making lifestyle and diet changes and taking natural vitamin supplements. Severe sufferers may need medication. Antidepressants known as selective serotonin reuptake inhibitors (SSRIs), such as Prozac, can work.

Hormone treatment is sometimes prescribed but does not help everyone. The aim is to balance the fluctuations in hormonal levels. Progesterone therapy is the most established. It involves a regular dose of progesterone, given by injection or suppository. Some specialists use oestrogen given continuously by patch or implant. Another approach is to suppress oestrogen and progesterone production with drugs known as gonadotrophin-releasing hormone analogues. The contraceptive pill may also be prescribed. ∎

SUPPLEMENTS FOR REDUCING PREMENSTRUAL SYMPTOMS		
Symptoms	**Cause**	**Treatment**
Fatigue; poor concentration; sugar craving	Low blood sugar or lack of serotonin.	Regularly consume starchy food; magnesium supplements may help.
Bloating; mental sluggishness	Water retention.	Reduce salt intake; in some cases, take vitamin B_6 in food or as supplements.
Tender breasts	Inflammation of tissues caused by prostaglandin hormones.	Take evening primrose oil, which can reduce sensitivity to hormones; reduce or stop coffee intake.
Nervous tension	Hormonal changes affect transmission of messages from the brain.	Try relaxation exercises (pp.14–15); vitamin B_6 helps in some cases.
Migraine and menstrual pain	Unknown	Extra calcium and vitamin D may help.

Menstrual problems

The term menstruation refers to the shedding of the endometrium, the lining of the uterus. It occurs as a result of a complex chain of hormonal interactions. This delicate process is often painful and easily disrupted, so most women will consult their doctor about a menstrual problem at some point in their lives.

Today, the average age at which the first menstruation occurs – called the menarche – is about 12½ years. Women start their periods younger than their ancestors did: 100 years ago the average age was 16½ years. Menstruation will continue until you reach the menopause, usually at about 50 years old – except during pregnancy (see pp.172–77).

THE NORMAL CYCLE
Although the average menstrual cycle is 28 days – from the first day of bleeding to the first day of the following period – the normal range can be anywhere from 21 to 38 days. The length of each period in which there is a loss of blood is usually from three to seven days. Although it may seem as if you are losing a lot of blood, most women only lose about 60 ml (4–6 tbsp) of menstrual fluid.

The menstrual pattern may change over your lifetime, and it often takes a few years for your cycle to settle down when you first start having periods. They may become erratic again when nearing the menopause, and women over 35 years of age often notice shortened cycles and increased or decreased blood loss.

WHEN TO SEE YOUR DOCTOR
Many factors, such as stress, travel or illness, can affect your cycle, making your period start early or late. If a problem continues for more than a few cycles, see your doctor. Always see your doctor if:
■ You notice bleeding between periods or after sexual intercourse.
■ Severe pain or heavy bleeding stops you participating in normal activities.
■ You start bleeding at any time after you have reached the menopause. ■

At the midpoint of the menstrual cycle an ovary releases an egg into the Fallopian tube. If the egg is not fertilized by a sperm, the uterus sheds the spongy layer of endometrium that lined the uterus to support a pregnancy.

THE FEMALE REPRODUCTIVE SYSTEM

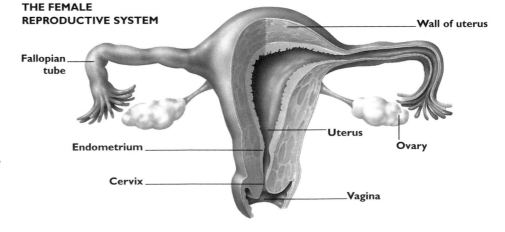

Fallopian tube

Wall of uterus

Uterus

Ovary

Endometrium

Cervix

Vagina

COPING WITH MENSTRUAL DISORDERS

Problems and symptoms	Causes	Treatment
Painful periods (*Dysmenorrhoea*) Pain and abdominal cramping, ranging from mild to disabling. Severe pain may be combined with constipation or diarrhoea, nausea or vomiting.	Mild cramping is probably caused by an imbalance in the production of prostaglandins – natural chemicals that help close off blood vessels and make the muscles of the uterus contract during the release of the endometrium. Severe pain or periods that suddenly hurt may be because of endometriosis, an ovarian cyst, a pelvic infection, fibroid tumours or insertion of an intrauterine device (IUD).	Relieve cramping and mild pain with painkillers such as aspirin or ibuprofen. Some medications are available that are designed specifically for period pain. A hot water bottle on the abdomen, a warm bath or exercise may all help. More severe pain can be treated with a prescription antiprostaglandin medication, nonsteroidal anti-inflammatory drugs (NSAIDs) or hormone treatment.
Heavy periods (*Menorrhagia*) Excessive blood loss, passing of blood clots, flooding or prolonged bleeding (lasting more than 7 days).	Hormonal imbalance, stopping the oral contraceptive pill (it decreases blood loss), an intrauterine device (IUD), an early miscarriage, fibroid tumours, approach of menopause, polyps (noncancerous growths of the cervix or endometrium), endometriosis or pelvic infection.	If there is no underlying cause, antiprostaglandins or nonsteroidal anti-inflammatory drugs (NSAIDs) are prescribed. Severely heavy periods in women who do not plan to have children may be treated with endometrial ablation, which removes the lining of the uterus, or a hysterectomy. Dilatation and curettage (D and C), in which the uterus lining is scraped, is used for diagnosis.
Infrequent periods (*Oligomenorrhoea*) Periods more than 6 weeks apart.	More common at the beginning and end of reproductive years. If you have recently been pregnant, it may take 6 months – more if you breastfeed – for a regular cycle to resume. Other causes are stress; weight loss or gain; excessive dieting or anorexia nervosa; chronic illness such as diabetes or thyroid disorders; polycystic ovaries; or taking antidepressants.	Any underlying condition should be investigated and treated. Otherwise, no treatment is necessary although you may have difficulty conceiving. In this case, hormone treatment may be given to stimulate ovulation.
Irregular periods Inconsistent menstrual cycles, which may combine short, long and normal intervals.	More common when first menstruating or nearing the menopause. They may also be related to stress, anxiety, excessive dieting, eating disorders or, more rarely, liver, kidney or thyroid disease.	No treatment is necessary unless there is an underlying disorder or you have difficulty conceiving.
Absent periods (*Amenorrhoea*) Known as primary amenorrhoea if a women has not begun to menstruate by the time she is 18 years of age; referred to as secondary amenorrhoea when periods stop in a woman who has previously menstruated.	Usual cause is late puberty for no reason or from poor nutrition, an endocrine disorder, an underactive thyroid or Turner's syndrome, when one of the female sex chromosomes is missing. Secondary amenorrhoea may be caused by starting or stopping the contraceptive pill, a hormonal imbalance, excessive dieting or weight loss. More rarely, it is because of an endocrine disorder, an ovarian cyst or polycystic ovary syndrome.	Once any underlying condition is investigated and treated, no further treatment is necessary. Hormone treatment can stimulate ovulation.

SEE ALSO
Menstrual problems
164–165

Endometriosis

Occurring in women between 25 to 40 years of age, endometriosis is a condition in which cells similar to the endometrium cells that line the inside of the uterus become established elsewhere in the body.

One school of thought is that when the endometrium surface layers are shed as a period, some of the cells may travel through the Fallopian tubes into the pelvic cavity. Like cells inside the uterus, endometrial deposits respond to changes in hormones and bleed when a woman has her period. They are usually trapped inside the pelvic area and become sticky and spread. As the deposits spread, they can join organs to each other or to the peritoneum. These areas of tissue are called adhesions. They can also form cysts, swellings that fill with blood.

SYMPTOMS AND DIAGNOSIS

Endometriosis can produce severe pain during the period. It may also create pain at the time of ovulation, during bowel

movements and during sexual intercourse. Conversely, there may be no symptoms.

It is important that you see your doctor as soon as you suspect you may have endometriosis – it worsens considerably with time. One possible result of this condition is infertility, which occurs if the passages of the eggs from the ovaries to the Fallopian tubes become blocked. This happens in 30–40 percent of women with endometriosis. Diagnosis may be made only when a couple cannot conceive.

Endometriosis is diagnosed by laparoscopy, in which a tube with a tiny camera at one end is inserted into the pelvic area just below the navel. If the condition is confirmed, it can be treated with drug therapy or surgery.

TREATING ENDOMETRIOSIS

Drugs can be used to stop the production of certain hormones, allowing the endometrial deposits to dissolve. Or they can be removed surgically, often by laparoscopy. If the deposits have spread widely, some of the reproductive organs may also have to be removed. Such drastic treatment will depend on other factors, including age and whether or not the woman has plans to conceive.

While the condition is mild, lifestyle changes may alleviate the symptoms and simple treatments can prevent them from worsening. There is no method of preventing this disorder, although taking the contraceptive pill and pregnancy can protect against endometriosis. ∎

The cells of endometriosis can develop anywhere in the pelvic area – on the ovaries, the Fallopian tubes, bladder, uterus, bowel or peritoneum (the lining of the abdominal cavity). In some cases, they have been found in other parts of the body.

SITES OF ENDOMETRIOSIS

Endometrial deposits

Ovary

Uterus

Bowel

Peritoneum

Fallopian tube

Bladder

Endometrial deposits

SEE ALSO
Menstrual problems
164–165

Fibroid tumours

Varying in size from a pea to a grapefruit, fibroids are tumours made up of bundles of muscle fibres and connective tissue. They are nearly always benign – only in rare cases do they become cancerous.

Normally, progesterone counteracts the sensitivity of the uterus to oestrogen. But high levels of oestrogen, which can occur during the reproductive years, can trigger the growth of fibroids. Levels can rise from being overweight or by taking certain contraceptive pills or hormone replacement therapy (HRT).

SYMPTOMS

There may be no symptoms at all, even when the fibroids are large. However, a proportion of women suffer from heavy menstrual bleeding (including flooding), long periods or clots in their menstrual blood. Heavy bleeding can cause anaemia, which produces exhaustion, breathlessness and depression. Other symptoms include severe cramps, incontinence, constipation, cystitis and infertility.

LOCATION OF FIBROIDS

Fibroids are common – at least 20 percent of women over 30 years of age have them. There are three types: ones that grow inside the wall of the uterus, those that protrude from the uterus into its cavity and those that grow outside the uterus, sometimes attached by a stalk.

Uterus

Fibroid tumour

Uterine wall

TREATMENT

How the condition is treated depends on the size and position of the fibroids, the severity of symptoms and whether the woman wants children. If the fibroids do not cause problems, they can remain untreated. Ask for a second opinion if you are unsure of what to do.

There are three options: transcervical resection of the endometrium (TCRE), drug therapy and surgery. In the transcervical resection, the cells of the lining of the uterus are shaved with a wire loop. Only fibroids that protrude into the uterine cavity can be removed with this option. The second one, drug therapy, reduces the oestrogen levels and shrinks the size of the fibroids.

The two main types of surgery are myomectomy (the removal of only the fibroids) and hysterectomy (the removal of the uterus). A third type, bilateral uterine arterial embolization (which reduces blood supply to the fibroid), is also available. Myomectomy is appealing for women who have not had children, but it has a higher rate of complications than hysterectomy and there is a chance of the fibroids regrowing. The surgeon may also discover that a hysterectomy is necessary once he starts the procedure. However, there is a 50 percent chance of successful pregnancy after myomectomy, whereas after hysterectomy there is none.

It is hard to prevent fibroids, but losing weight if you are overweight and stopping contraceptive pills or HRT may help. ∎

SEE ALSO
Endometriosis   166
Fibroid tumours   167

Ovarian cysts

Cysts are fluid-filled swellings that can occur in or on the ovaries (as well as on other parts of the body). They are nearly always benign and may disappear without treatment.

An ovarian cyst may grow inside the ovary or on the outside, and it may be attached by a stem (which is sometimes called a pedicle). Cysts form because of an abnormal growth of a fluid-producing tissue in which there is no way for the fluid to escape. Ovarian cysts occur more often in smokers than in nonsmokers.

SYMPTOMS

There are often no symptoms at all. However, when they do exist, they can include a swollen abdomen, increased pressure on the bladder or bowels (causing more frequent visits to the lavatory), painful sexual intercourse, irregular periods and periods with heavier or lighter bleeding than usual. If a cyst becomes twisted, it will cause acute abdominal pain, nausea and fever. There is a slight risk that this will lead to peritonitis.

DIAGNOSIS AND TREATMENT

Some types of cyst may disappear without treatment, and the contraceptive pill may improve the chances of this occurring. Other cysts require surgery by laparoscopic fenestration or by laparotomy. Your doctor will confirm diagnosis from a complete physical and pelvic examination. She may decide to give you an ultrasound scan to produce a detailed image of the pelvic organs or use laparoscopy, in which the abdominal cavity is viewed while you are under general anaesthetic.

SURGERY OPTIONS

Laparoscopic fenestration (similar to laparoscopy, in which a tube with a viewing device is inserted into a small incision) allows the cyst to be removed by draining its contents. Laparotomy requires a larger incision, which allows the removal of all of the tumour or cyst. Some ovarian tumours are cancerous, in which case the affected ovary or ovaries and the Fallopian tubes may also be removed.

The type of surgery you will need will depend on your age and whether or not you are planning to have children. One factor to consider is the possible removal of some or all of the reproductive organs to avoid any risk of cancer. ∎

POLYCYSTIC OVARIES

Polycystic means "many cysts" and refers to immature follicles (fluid-filled cavities), which each contain an egg. A polycystic ovary has at least 10 cysts just below the surface, which cause the ovary to become enlarged. The covering of the ovary thickens, which increases difficulty in ovulating or prevents it.

It is a common condition, affecting 20 percent of women. Symptoms include irregular, scanty or absent periods, infertility, miscarriage, hair growth on the face, chest, abdomen, arms and legs, acne, weight gain, pelvic discomfort and depression.

Because hormones are responsible for all of these symptoms, drug treatments are designed to change hormone levels. Because treatment may be different for each symptom and what is helpful for one woman may not work for another, it is important to decide which of the symptoms is the most troubling. If you are planning to become pregnant in the future, this, too, will influence the choice of treatment.

Contraction

Used to avoid an unwanted pregnancy, contraception can work in three ways: by halting the woman's production of eggs, by preventing sperm meeting the egg or by stopping a fertilized egg implanting in the womb.

SEE ALSO

Sexually transmitted
diseases   144–145
HIV   150–151

CAUTION

Contraceptive efficiency is usually lowest in the first year of use, when a couple is growing used to the method. If you realize you have used a contraceptive incorrectly, or that you have forgotten it, you may want emergency postcoital contraception. You have a choice of two methods. The "morning-after pill" has to be taken within 72 hours after sex, usually in two doses, or an IUD can be inserted up to five days after sex.

To avoid pregnancy, contraception is needed during sexual intercourse throughout a woman's reproductive years, from the menarche (onset of periods) to the menopause. There are times when she is unlikely to become pregnant, such as during her period or when she is fully breast-feeding, but it is still possible.

Although reliable and convenient forms of contraception are available, there is as yet no perfect contraceptive. Each method has its advantages and disadvantages. The needs of the individual couple vary, too, according to how often they have sex, how carefully the method is used, whether they have completed their family and the age of the woman. Every couple should consider which method to choose in the light of their circumstances. You can discuss these with your family doctor or a family planning counsellor.

There are five principal types of contraception. Barrier methods include the condom, diaphragm, cervical cap and sponge. Hormonal methods are provided in the oral contraceptive pill, implants or injections. Intrauterine devices or systems (IUDs and IUSs), sterilization and natural family planning are further options. Withdrawal (*coitus interruptus*), in which the male partner withdraws his penis before ejaculating, is still used. However, it is not a reliable method because sperm can escape before ejaculation.

METHODS FOR WOMEN

Most forms of contraception are used by the woman, so she is usually the one to visit the health practitioner. Some methods, such as the diaphragm, cervical cap and intrauterine device, need to be fitted by a trained doctor or nurse.

The woman will be examined to make sure she is given the right size cap or diaphragm for her body and instructed on how to insert it herself before sex. In the case of an intrauterine device, once fitted it can be left in place for five years, but should be checked each year. Losing or gaining a large amount of weight or having a baby can affect the efficacy of any internal device. In such circumstances the doctor should re-examine you and, perhaps, fit a new one in place.

A permanent choice is sterilization, in which the Fallopian tubes are cut or sealed to prevent sperm from reaching the egg. This method may be preferred by a woman who has decided not to have any children in the future.

HOW TO PUT ON A CONDOM

When the penis is fully erect, take the condom in your hand. Find the teat at the tip of the condom and squeeze it to expel any air. Keeping hold of the teat, roll the condom all the way down the penis. If the condom does not reach the base of the penis, it is probably inside out, so start again with a new one.

Never use a condom twice. Once the man has ejaculated, he must withdraw his penis while holding the base of the condom to prevent any sperm escaping. Dispose of condoms in the bin, not down the toilet.

OPTIONS FOR MEN

The only current contraceptive options for men are the condom (see box, p.169) and vasectomy (male sterilization). Vasectomy, an irreversible procedure, involves severing the vas deferens – the tube that carries sperm. Ejaculation will be normal, but without any sperm.

Male hormonal methods are in development and may be available soon. Among those that have been successfully trialled are a weekly testosterone injection and a daily progesterone pill. These are seen as suitable only for couples in a stable and trusting relationship.

NATURAL FAMILY PLANNING

Anxiety about side effects and long-term drawbacks of hormonal contraceptives have led to a surge of interest in natural methods of family planning. These aim to identify the days of the menstrual cycle

GUIDE TO CONTRACEPTIVE CHOICES

Method of contraception	How it works	Efficiency
Oral contraceptive pill Pill taken orally every day.	Oestrogen and progestogen combined prevent ovulation. Progestogen-only pill thickens cervical mucus to stop sperm reaching uterus and thins the uterus lining, making egg implantation difficult.	One of the most efficient methods, at over 99 percent.
Intrauterine device (IUD) or system (IUS) IUD inserted into the vagina and changed every 3 to 5 years.	Prevents sperm from meeting the egg or fertilized egg from implanting. IUS releases progestogen, which thickens the cervical mucus to stop sperm reaching the uterus and thins the lining of the womb to make egg implantation difficult.	An efficient method at 98–99 percent.
Condom Rubber sheath put over erect penis or, with female condom, inserted in vagina.	Collects sperm and prevents it entering the vagina.	If used properly, 98 percent for male condom; 95 percent for female.
Diaphragm or cervical cap Dome-shaped protective rubber device inserted into the vagina before sex.	Prevents sperm reaching the cervix and travelling into the uterus.	Between 92 to 96 percent when used with spermicide.
Hormonal treatments Injection of hormones or hormone-releasing implant inserted under skin.	Injection releases progestogen into bloodstream to prevent ovulation. Implant prevents fertilization of egg.	One of the most efficient methods, at over 99 percent.
Natural methods Timing intercourse to occur when woman is not fertile.	Record of menstrual cycle kept, along with system to monitor changes in hormone levels (using cervical mucus, body temperature, urine or saliva).	Between 95 to 98 percent, depending on the method used, but totally dependent on proper method and disciplined use.
Sterilization and vasectomy Cutting of Fallopian tubes that carry egg or vas deferens that carry sperm.	Sperm or egg not able to travel to achieve fertilization.	Over 99 percent efficiency rate.

when fertilization can occur, so that a couple can avoid sex at that time or use a barrier contraceptive.

Formerly, couples who did not want to use contraception merely estimated when ovulation would occur, around the middle of the cycle. Called the "rhythm method", it was a hit-and-miss affair and many women became pregnant. Various techniques have now been developed that enable couples to pinpoint the days around ovulation with much greater accuracy. During this time there is a change in the woman's body temperature, cervical mucus, saliva and the hormones excreted in the urine, and all of this can be monitored. You will gain the most reliable results if you monitor more than one of these changes. Various kits are available to help a woman do this, but it is best to learn from an experienced natural family planning teacher. ▪

GUIDE TO CONTRACEPTIVE CHOICES continued

Benefits	Side effects or risks	Who should avoid
Easy to use. Does not interfere with sexual intercourse. Can ease period problems and premenstrual syndrome. Protects against cancers of the ovary and womb and some pelvic infections.	Weight gain; loss of libido; breast tenderness; headaches; and mood changes.	Not suitable for smokers over 35 years of age or breast-feeding women.
Effective as soon as inserted. Intrauterine device stays in place for 5 years; intrauterine system, 3 years. Intrauterine system also lightens and shortens period and can reduce period pain.	Longer, heavier periods with intrauterine device. Slight bleeding between periods for the first few months with intrauterine system. Increased risk of pelvic infections.	Those with heavy periods or who have had an ectopic pregnancy or a pelvic infection. With the intrauterine system, also avoid if you have had cancer of the womb or ovary or arterial disease.
Protects against sexually transmitted diseases, including HIV.	May slip off or split if used improperly.	
Can be put in any time before sex (but if over 3 hours, more spermicide needed). May protect against sexually transmitted diseases and cervical cancer.	May trigger cystitis (pp.146–47). The rubber or spermicide can cause irritation in some people.	
Long-lasting: injection 2–3 months and implant 3–5 years. Fertility returns as soon as implant is removed.	May cause irregular periods or weight gain. Up to a year for fertility to return after stopping injection.	Those with a risk of breast or ovarian cancer; with implant, if you have heart disease or had an ectopic pregnancy.
Nonintrusive method with no side effects. Can also be used to achieve pregnancy when desired.	Risk of pregnancy rises markedly if not used carefully.	
Permanent and works immediately in case of woman; takes a few months for all sperm to disappear in men.	Rarely, tubes can rejoin.	

CAUTION

If you smoke, it is important that you stop before having children. The effect on the foetus during pregnancy is serious. Smoking can stunt the growth of the baby in the womb, which can have severe health repercussions into adult life, such as an increased risk of developing heart disease.

Pregnancy

The beginning of a pregnancy occurs when a female egg is fertilized by a male sperm. If a couple has regular unprotected sex, a healthy woman has a 25 percent chance of conceiving in an average month.

A missed period is the first indication of pregnancy for most women, but there are other signs, including nausea, tender breasts, a change in taste for food or drink, a metallic taste in the mouth, a need to urinate more frequently, tiredness, increased vaginal discharge and emotional swings. To confirm your pregnancy, your doctor or gynaecologist can take a test or you can do a home pregnancy test. All tests detect the presence in urine of the pregnancy hormone human chorionic gonadotrophin (HCG). Tests work from the week after your period was due.

Once you have a positive result, you can calculate when the baby is due by counting 280 days, or 40 weeks, from the first day of your last period. Even if you do not see a doctor to confirm your pregnancy, you need to visit her to arrange your antenatal care and find out about any antenatal tests you may need.

Conception and early foetal growth are complex events, so pregnancy can go wrong, even if you do everything by the book. About 20 percent of pregnancies end in a miscarriage, usually in the first 13 weeks. Most of these are caused by

THE DEVELOPING EGG

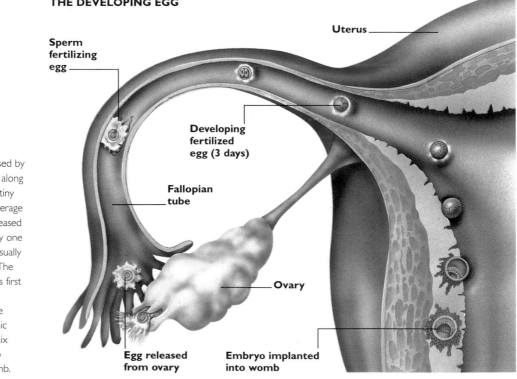

Sperm fertilizing egg

Uterus

Developing fertilized egg (3 days)

Fallopian tube

Ovary

Egg released from ovary

Embryo implanted into womb

When an egg is released by the ovary, it is carried along the Fallopian tube by tiny hairlike cilia. Of the average 400 million sperm released during ejaculation, only one can fertilize the egg, usually in the Fallopian tube. The fertilized egg makes its first cell division in about 36 hours, signalling the beginning of embryonic development. About six days later, the embryo implants into the womb.

random developmental mistakes; however, the woman usually goes on to conceive again and carry a healthy baby to term.

FIRST TRIMESTER

Doctors divide pregnancy into three periods of 13 weeks, called trimesters. By six weeks after conception, the uterus will have grown to the size of a small peach and the embryo inside will have a head, trunk, limb buds and a rudimentary spinal cord and brain.

The hormonal changes and energy used to produce all these physical changes may make you feel tired, vulnerable, weak and nauseous. Look after yourself, as poor nutrition, lack of sleep and the increased expenditure of energy as the baby grows all make fatigue more pronounced. By eight weeks your breasts will be heavier and more tender. Your gums will soften by 10 weeks, requiring you to pay extra attention to your dental hygiene.

With critical developments occurring from the earliest weeks of pregnancy, it is vital that you take steps to protect the foetus and provide it with the nutrition it needs. This means avoiding cigarettes and any nonessential pharmaceuticals, cutting down on alcohol, limiting stress and having a healthy diet.

SECOND TRIMESTER

By 12 to 13 weeks, your waistline will start to disappear. You should begin to feel better, as morning sickness passes and fatigue is not so intense. However, other minor problems may start.

The baby's development is complete by the 16th week, and from then on it grows in size rather than complexity. From around 7.5 cm (3 in) long at the beginning of the second trimester, the foetus grows to about 35 cm (13 in) at the end. Not only will you be protruding

WHY PREGNANCY MAY NOT HAPPEN

For successful fertilization to occur, a healthy egg must be penetrated by a healthy sperm. But a woman does not always release an egg every month or produce healthy ones, especially late in her reproductive years. Similarly, a man may ejaculate sperm that are not fully healthy, particularly if he smokes or drinks heavily. Because fertilization is a hit-and-miss affair, couples are usually advised to persevere for a year at trying to conceive before seeking help. However, a doctor will often agree to a shorter wait for a woman who has reached her mid-30s.

Common obstacles to conception include sexually transmitted diseases in either partner, ovulatory failure or infrequency and blocked Fallopian tubes in the woman and a low sperm count in the man. The doctor can carry out various tests. For the woman, these include a blood test to check hormone levels, an X-ray or laparoscopy to see if the Fallopian tubes are open or if there are any uterine growths and a post-coital mucus test to check the condition of the vaginal mucus. The man will be asked for a sperm sample to see if he is making enough active sperm of the correct shape. Treatment may include ovarian-stimulating drugs, tubal surgery or hormones to increase sperm production.

perceptibly around the middle, but your heart and lungs will be working 50 percent harder than usual, which may make you sweat more. The rapid growth of the baby will make you urinate more often, as the baby presses on the bladder, and you will need to eat little and often, as your stomach capacity will be reduced.

From about the 18th week, the baby's movements become noticeable – especially when you are resting. The combination of increased metabolism, night sweating, the need to urinate and the baby kicking may cause insomnia. To help combat sleeplessness, wear light night clothes and do not drink too much before bedtime. Be sure to wear loose, comfortable clothes during the day, too, and get properly measured for new bras as your breasts enlarge and ribcage expands.

The "rehearsal" contractions, known as Braxton Hicks, that go on throughout pregnancy become marked toward the end of the second trimester. Your midwife or doctor will now be able to pick up the baby's heartbeat with a monitoring aid.

THIRD TRIMESTER

As your abdomen protrudes more, it is important to adopt a good posture to prevent or minimize backache. To combat

---

MORNING SICKNESS

So-called morning sickness can occur at any time of day, but it rarely lasts beyond the first trimester. It is caused by the sudden surge in hormones that occurs in pregnancy, especially of human chorionic gonadotrophin (HCG) and prolactin. Morning sickness makes some women merely a little nauseous, but others vomit persistently. It is unwise to take any drugs during pregnancy, especially in the early weeks, so try the following measures to help ease the symptoms:

■ Eat little and often.

■ Eat something while still in bed in the morning to prevent dizziness when you get up.

■ When nausea strikes, try eating dried fruit or plain biscuits and drinking ginger tea (prepared from a piece of root ginger). Ginger is an anti-emetic.

■ Keep up your fluid intake. If you suffer from trapped wind related to nausea, drink effervescent water – the bubbles can help the gas escape from the gut.

■ Cut down on tea and coffee, which aggravate nausea and vomiting (and interfere with the absorption of essential iron).

■ Have some fresh air before eating. Walking will help you work up an appetite.

■ Make sure you have an adequate intake of chromium (found in brown rice, cheese, wholegrains and meat), because this helps keep the blood sugar level up.

■ Make up your calorie intake on the days you feel better. Energy needs increase in pregnancy by up to 400 calories a day.

---

fatigue, rest when you can, eat a balanced diet and sleep as much as you need.

By the 32nd week, the baby is usually in the head-down position until the birth. If it is your first baby, it should descend into the pelvic cavity by the 36th week. This may ease any breathing or digestive problems you have experienced.

WEIGHT GAIN

The amount of weight put on varies with individuals and with each pregnancy. The average is 11 kg (25 lb), but there is a large margin on either side within the acceptable limit. You will not gain weight at the same pace throughout pregnancy. It is slow in the first trimester, gradually increasing to a peak between the 24th and 32nd weeks, then tailing off at the end. The extra weight is from a combination of the uterus, placenta and fluids, larger breasts, increased blood volume, fat laid down for breast-feeding – and the baby.

Only in exceptional circumstances are women advised to diet in pregnancy, and then it should only be done under the strict supervision of a doctor or qualified nutritionist. If you know you are putting on weight too quickly, exercise is a much better way to keep it in check.

The combination of dry, thin skin and your rapid growth may also produce stretch marks, but these should gradually fade after the birth.

EXERCISE IN PREGNANCY

If you are used to taking regular exercise, there is no need to change your routine during pregnancy. Indeed, women who go into childbirth fit often have easier labours and recover more quickly afterward. However, not all kinds of exercise are appropriate. Well-paced aerobic activities such as brisk walking, cycling and swimming are ideal. Avoid

ESSENTIAL NUTRIENTS DURING PREGNANCY

Nutrient	Why you need it	When you need it	How much to take	Sources
Protein	For the building of new body tissues.	Throughout pregnancy.	Fifty percent more than normal levels.	Meat, fish and dairy products.
Fibre	Helps prevent constipation.	Throughout pregnancy, particularly at the end.	Some in all meals.	Fruit, vegetables, pulses and wholegrain cereals.
Folic acid	Supplies nucleic acids needed by rapidly dividing cells of the embryo. Can prevent neural tube defects such as spina bifida.	Most important before conception and in the first trimester, but also necessary in the other trimesters.	300 mcg a day: equivalent to 300 g (10½ oz) of peanuts or 350 g (12 oz) of spinach. In first 12 weeks, also take a 400 mcg supplement.	Spinach, lamb's liver, peanuts, green leafy vegetables and walnuts.
Zinc	Vital for cell replication; for growth of mother and baby; and for nerve and brain development.	Throughout pregnancy.	20 mg a day: equivalent to 350 g (12 oz) of red meat or 400 g (14 oz) of brazil nuts.	Red meat, brazil nuts, almonds, wholemeal flour and oats.
Iron	For increased haemoglobin, as blood volume rises. The baby needs to build up a reserve, because breast milk contains little iron.	Throughout pregnancy, but especially in the second and third trimesters, when blood volume will increase the most.	15 mg a day: equivalent to 300 g (10½ oz) of fortified breakfast cereal, 400 g (14 oz) of lentils or 500 g (1 lb 2 oz) of soya beans.	Breakfast cereals, soya, lentils, shellfish, egg yolks, red meat, dried apricots, kidneys and molasses.
Calcium	Formation of baby's teeth and bones; regulates mother's blood pressure.	Throughout pregnancy.	Twice as much as normal levels.	Especially dairy foods; also in leafy green vegetables, pulses and nuts.
Vitamin C	Helps body to absorb iron and strengthens mother's and baby's resistance to infection.	Throughout pregnancy.	500mg a day.	Fresh fruit and vegetables, especially citrus fruit, kiwis and peppers.
Vitamin D	Helps the body absorb and use calcium.	Throughout pregnancy.	10 mcg a day: equivalent to 150 g (5½ oz) of margarine or 200 g (7 oz) of cereal.	Oily fish, margarine, eggs (especially yolk), fortified breakfast cereals and sunlight.
Magnesium	Essential to bone growth. Helps the body to use calcium and essential fatty acids.	Throughout pregnancy, especially in the last trimester.	500 mg a day: equivalent to 200 g (7 oz) of almonds or 400 g (14 oz) of wholemeal flour.	Green leafy vegetables, pulses, nuts and seeds and wholemeal flour.
Essential fatty acids (EFAs)	Assist the brain and nerve development of the baby.	Throughout pregnancy, but particularly in the early weeks.	Some in each meal (oil must be eaten cold to preserve EFAs).	Oily fish, seeds, nuts and cold-pressed sunflower, soya or rapeseed oil.

sports that require sudden bursts of energy, particularly in the later stages.

Any weight-bearing exercise should be done at a moderate level, as your joints will be more vulnerable to dislocation. They have to bear the extra weight at a time when hormonal changes make the ligaments looser. This is why swimming or aquarobics are ideal forms of exercise, especially toward the end.

Yoga is beneficial in the later stages. As well as keeping you supple and toned, it can help you relax and breathe properly. In the last trimester, it is a good idea to attend an antenatal exercise class. They teach appropriate routines that can be used to minimize pain in labour.

PLANNING FOR DELIVERY

Most women give birth in hospital, but a growing number are opting for home deliveries. Studies show that these are as safe as hospital for women who are not at high risk. Those that are include women who have had previous birth complications, a Caesarean section or are at the end of their reproductive years.

Have everything prepared two weeks before your due date. The date is only an estimate and the baby could arrive earlier or later. Among the practical items to prepare are breast pads, sanitary towels, baby clothes and nappies. If you are going to hospital, also pack underwear and nightwear. Make arrangements with your partner so that you can contact him at short notice when labour starts.

SIGNS THE BIRTH IS DUE

Labour usually starts between the 39th and 41st week. Among the signs that labour will soon start are a "show" of the gelatinous, blood-tinged mucus that has plugged the cervix during pregnancy, the rupture and leakage of the amniotic sac and a dull backache.

There are three stages of labour: the dilatation of the cervix, the descent of the baby down the birth canal and the delivery of the placenta (see pp.310–11). ■

As the foetus grows, it presses down on the bladder and up against the diaphragm. The ribcage splays out and organs such as the bowel and stomach are squashed. At the end of the third trimester, the baby usually swivels round, ready to be born head first.

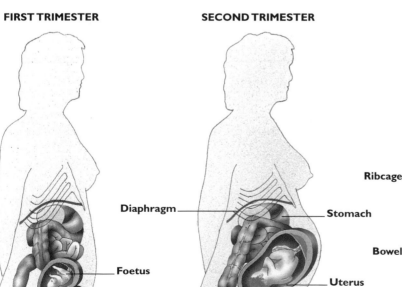

FIRST TRIMESTER

SECOND TRIMESTER

THIRD TRIMESTER

Diaphragm

Foetus

Bladder

Stomach

Uterus

Ribcage

Bowel

COMMON COMPLAINTS DURING PREGNANCY

Condition	When it occurs	Causes	How to treat it
Backache	Can occur in the early months, however, it is usually at its worst in the last 4 to 8 weeks.	Bad posture; sometimes excess weight gain. In later pregnancy, relaxation of the ligaments and muscles supporting the joints makes it worse.	Keep shoulders back but relaxed, chest and ribcage raised, back straight, bottom tucked in and knees relaxed. Rest lying on your back with legs supported on a chair.
Leg cramps	Middle to late pregnancy.	Probably muscle tension, but possibly a shortage of calcium.	Massage vigorously and flex legs and feet repeatedly. Increase your calcium intake.
Indigestion	Middle to late pregnancy.	Growing baby pressing on the stomach; relaxation of muscles at top of stomach.	Eat little and often rather than one or two main meals. Avoid heavy, fatty, spicy food.
Bleeding gums	Throughout pregnancy.	Hormonal changes cause softening of the gums and an increased blood supply.	Brush teeth gently but thoroughly after meals. Floss after brushing.
Frequent urination	Beginning and end of pregnancy.	In early stages, hormonal changes; later, growing uterus pressing on bladder.	Ensure bladder is fully emptied when urinating. Reduce caffeine intake.
Cystitis	Throughout pregnancy in susceptible women.	Muscle wall around bladder relaxes, predisposing it to infection.	Drink plenty of water. If it does not clear up, ask doctor if she can prescribe antibiotics that will not affect baby. If untreated, can cause kidney infection.
Thrush	Throughout pregnancy in susceptible women.	Unknown, but may be hormonal changes.	Antifungal pessaries or cream; eat yoghurt with "live" cultures.
Varicose veins	Middle to late pregnancy.	Baby's head pressing down on pelvic veins, causing blood to pool in legs, where veins can balloon.	Avoid putting on too much weight and standing for long periods. Sleep with your feet raised. Exercise to improve circulation in legs.
Nasal congestion	Throughout pregnancy.	Increase in supply of blood to small vessels in nose; softening and thickening of membranes in nose.	None – but blow nose gently to prevent bleeds.
Constipation and piles	Throughout pregnancy.	Progesterone relaxes smooth muscles and slows down intestines.	Drink lots of water or juice; eat plenty of fresh fruit and vegetables and whole-grain cereals.

SEE ALSO
Herbal medicine 186–191
Aromatherapy   192–195
Homeopathy   196–201

Menopause

The term menopause literally means "the end of periods", and this is what most women see as its defining factor. In fact, the menopause is a gradual process that begins several years before menstruation ceases.

As women approach their early 40s, the ovaries that produce oestrogen start to decline. As the oestrogen level falls, fewer healthy eggs are produced and fertility drops. This period is called the perimenopause. The process speeds up in the late 40s and is often accompanied by increasingly irregular and abnormally heavy or light periods. It culminates in the termination of periods, typically around the age of 50.

The decline in oestrogen production results in a host of symptoms. The most common one is hot flushes and related night sweats, which affect 70 percent of Western women. These produce sudden increases in body temperature, often accompanied by red flushes of the skin that are as uncomfortable as they are embarrassing. Hot flushes are caused by changes in the hypothalamus, the part of the brain that controls temperature and sleep. These same changes can also result in headaches, dizziness and insomnia. Although these symptoms usually last two to five years, they can last much longer.

Over the longer term, the reduction of oestrogen affects the genitourinary tract and causes two distressing symptoms. The sphincter muscles surrounding the urethra lose their tone, resulting in incontinence, and the vagina becomes shorter, drier and less elastic, often making sex painful.

Oestrogen deficiency also has long-term implications for health. As it declines, the level of bad cholesterol in the blood rises and women begin to store fat around their middle. These factors increase a woman's risk of heart disease fourfold – at this stage, she is as susceptible as a man. Without oestrogen, the loss of the mineral calcium is also accelerated. A woman's bones can lose up to five percent of their mass in a year (see box, facing page).

Although not all women will experience the obvious symptoms, most will know they are menopausal. If you are uncertain, your doctor can give you a blood test. This measures the level of follicle stimulating hormone (FSH), which rises in menopausal women. Women with a family history of osteoporosis or heart disease should discuss with their doctor hormone replacement therapy (HRT), which can reduce their risks of developing these conditions.

Reaching the menopause does not mean that you have to slow down or curtail your activities. Many women enjoy full, active lives.

REPLACING THE OESTROGEN

Up to one-third of menopausal women use hormone replacement therapy (HRT). This replaces the lost oestrogen, which eliminates the symptoms and decreases the risks of osteoporosis and heart disease. It is particularly important for the one percent of women who experience a premature menopause and face more years without the protection oestrogen offers.

The oestrogen can be given in various forms. The most popular one is the pill; however, some women prefer patches, which remain attached to the skin for up to a week, or implants, which last six months. Another option is a gel that is rubbed into the skin. Women who are concerned about genitourinary symptoms may choose the vaginal ring, which releases hormones locally.

Hormone replacement therapy can cause side effects and does carry some risks. By raising the level of oestrogen, it slightly increases the risk of cancers of the womb and breast. A combination form of oestrogen and progesterone limits the risk of womb cancer. Women with a history of breast or endometrial cancer should not use the therapy.

Oestrogen can cause fluid retention, nausea, breast tenderness and vaginal discharge. Progestogen may cause headaches, abdominal cramps, fibroid tumours, acne, tiredness and dizziness. The risk of developing a blood clot in the legs increases threefold for women on hormone replacement therapy but the risk is still small. These women also develop thicker breast tissue, making it more difficult to detect cancer.

OTHER TREATMENTS

A new class of drugs called selective oestrogen receptor modulators (SERMs), which protect against heart disease and bone loss but do not increase the risk of hormone-related cancers, may be a better alternative for some women. Women who do not want to rely on synthetic hormones could consider consulting a qualified practitioner of homeopathy or herbal medicine. Plant medicines containing naturally occurring oestrogens (called phyto-oestrogens), herbs known as adaptogens and homeopathic remedies such as *Sepia* and *Pulsatilla* may help. ∎

OSTEOPOROSIS

After your mid-30s, your bones gradually start to lose calcium. The drop in oestrogen after the menopause accelerates this process, so that by the age of 70, one-third of women have osteoporosis, or brittle bones. However, few know it, as osteoporosis is a silent disease. The first symptom is often a bone fracture. In the industrialized countries, it is estimated that every three minutes someone has an osteoporotic fracture. One-quarter of all old people who fracture their hips die as a result.

Because bone cannot be rebuilt once it has lost mass, there is no cure for osteoporosis – prevention is the only solution. The following measures can help:

- Stop smoking.

- Eat plenty of calcium-rich foods: cheese, yoghurt, tinned fish with their bones, milk and dark green leafy vegetables.

- Do regular weight-bearing exercise such as walking, running and lifting weights.

- Cut down on tea, coffee and alcohol.

- Get plenty of sunlight because it provides vitamin D, which the body needs to absorb calcium.

- Consider hormone replacement therapy. If taken continuously from the start of the menopause, the therapy reduces the risk of osteoporosis by preventing bone loss.

These measures are important for women at high risk of osteoporosis. This includes women who began menopause early on, who have had one or both ovaries removed, who have taken corticosteroid drugs for a long time, suffered eating disorders or been on a low-calcium diet and those who do little exercise.

SEE ALSO
Vaccinations   120–121

CAUTION

■ *Pregnant women who have not had measles should avoid all contact with affected children. The foetus may die in some cases of maternal measles.*

■ *Never give aspirin to a child 12 years of age or younger: it has been linked to a dangerous condition known as Reye's syndrome. For fevers and aches and pains, use paracetamol.*

Measles

A highly contagious viral disease, measles spreads throughout the body, causing a fever and characteristic rash. It is usually contracted in childhood, but it is considerably more serious if picked up as an adult.

The symptoms of measles typically appear one to two weeks after being in contact with the virus. They include fatigue, malaise, fever, runny nose, sore watery eyes, dry throat, a cough, croup and diarrhoea. They may be accompanied by febrile convulsions, although these are rarely serious.

After three or four days, a crop of tiny white spots on a reddened base will appear on the inside of the cheeks. The child may develop a headache and high temperature, normally 37.7–38.9°C (100–102°F). Some children will have swollen lymph glands or become sensitive to light. A brownish pink rash may then appear on the head or neck, then spread down the trunk. Sometimes the spots spread so much that they appear to merge and produce large red blotches. By the sixth day, the rash will begin to fade. A child's symptoms usually disappear after 10 days, although an adult may take up to four weeks to recover.

TREATMENT

The fever is treated with bedrest, plenty of fluids and paracetamol. Antibiotics will not treat the measles, but the doctor may prescribe them for any secondary bacterial infection. If the child complains of light sensitivity, keep him in a darkened room.

Measles and rubella (see box, left) can be prevented by vaccination. An attack of measles usually confers lifelong immunity.

COMPLICATIONS

A case of measles can have complications: these include chest and ear infections, conjunctivitis, diarrhoea, vomiting, abdominal pain and, rarely, pneumonia. Although viral pneumonia is not a great cause for concern, a bacterial type is serious, requiring immediate treatment with antibiotics.

About 1 in 1000 children develops encephalitis, a potentially life-threatening inflammation of brain cells. He will have a headache, a fear of bright lights, become drowsy and sometimes lose consciousness. This requires urgent medical attention. ■

WHAT IS RUBELLA?

Also known as German measles, rubella is a viral infection that normally causes only a mild illness in children. It is more serious in adults, particularly in pregnant women, because it can cause serious defects to a baby in the womb, including deafness, heart disease, eye disorders and cerebral palsy. As an attack of rubella usually confers lifelong immunity, it is important for girls to have the disease or be immunized before they become adults.

Symptoms typically appear two to three weeks after contact with the virus. The first sign is a rash that takes the form of small pink spots, but they do not run together as they do in measles. The spots appear first on the forehead and face, then spread to the trunk and limbs. Sufferers often develop a sore throat and mild conjunctivitis. There may also be a slight temperature and swollen lymph nodes at the back of the neck. By the fourth or fifth day, all the symptoms will disappear. Symptoms are more severe in older children and adults and may include headache and a higher fever. Treatment and prevention are the same as for measles.

SEE ALSO
Vaccinations 120–121
Meningitis 183

CAUTION

■ *If the fever exceeds 38.5°C (101°F), call the doctor. If it exceeds 40°C (104°F), immediately call for emergency services.*
■ *Never give aspirin to a child 12 years of age or younger: it has been linked to a dangerous condition known as Reye's syndrome. For fevers and aches and pains, you can use paracetamol if necessary.*

Mumps

This viral illness is usually caught during childhood. Although it is mild in young children, after puberty it may have serious complications. One attack of mumps usually confers lifelong immunity.

The symptoms of mumps first appear from two to three weeks after contact with the virus that causes it. The virus is spread by air-borne droplets, and an affected person can spread the virus from a week before symptoms develop to two weeks afterward.

The most recognizable symptom is the inflammation of one or both of the parotid glands, a pair of glands that produce saliva. The glands become swollen and painful, and the child may have trouble opening her mouth, chewing or swallowing. A fever and headache may develop, although the temperature will drop after two or three days. The swelling will probably subside within a week or 10 days. If the gland is swollen on only one side of the face, the second side may

then swell just as the first one subsides. However, many children experience no symptoms or are only slightly unwell and uncomfortable around the glands.

Treatment consists of painkillers, lots of fluids and plenty of bedrest. If the salivary glands are particularly painful, the doctor may prescribe an anti-inflammatory medicine to reduce pain and swelling. Vaccinations are available that prevent development of the disease.

COMPLICATIONS

One-quarter of teenage and adult males who catch mumps develop orchitis, a painful inflammation of one or both testes. It usually lasts about two to four days, after which time the affected testis may be smaller than it was before. If both testes are affected, orchitis can lead to infertility, although this is rare. Cases of severe orchitis can be treated with cortico-steroid drugs to reduce inflammation and with powerful painkillers.

Occasionally, mumps can develop into meningitis, but it is not usually serious. Among other rare complications are pancreatitis (abdominal pain and vomiting) and meningoencephalitis, deafness, facial palsy, arthritis, rheumatic fever and thrombocytopenia (a blood disorder that is characterized by a lack of platelets in the blood).

If a post-pubertal male shows signs of having mumps, an immunoglobulin injection may be beneficial in preventing the development of orchitis. ■

Cheeks swollen like those of a hamster are the most obvious symptom of mumps. The swelling occurs in the parotid glands, which are located along the curve of the jaw below the ears.

CAUTION

Never give aspirin to a child 12 years of age or younger: it has been linked to a dangerous condition known as Reye's syndrome. For fevers, aches and pains, you can give paracetamol.

Chickenpox

An infectious disease, chickenpox is caused by the varicella-zoster virus, a member of the herpes group. It is not usually dangerous and rarely causes complications in children. An attack usually confers lifelong immunity.

The virus spreads from one person to another in airborne droplets. The initial symptoms, including malaise, mild fever, headache and nausea, start two to three weeks after contact with the virus.

A rash of small, dark red itchy spots appears on the torso and spreads to the legs, arms, head and face. After a few days, the spots burst or dry out, then crust over and form scabs. The spots disappear after about 12 days, and they rarely leave scars. The child will be contagious from the day before the rash appears until it disappears.

Rest is usually all that is needed for a complete recovery. If a secondary infection arises from scratching the spots, your doctor may prescribe an antibiotic. If the child cannot resist scratching, you should keep his nails short to limit the damage. By 10 years of age, most children have had chickenpox.

SHINGLES

During an attack of chickenpox, the virus finds its way into the root of a nerve in the spinal cord and lies dormant. It can be reactivated as shingles, especially in elderly people or in those whose immune systems are compromised by disease or stress.

A shingles attack can produce intense, stabbing pain in the affected nerve, with goups of blisters forming on the skin over it. The pain can persist for several weeks after the rash has cleared. Calamine lotion can soothe the itching and the antiviral drug acyclovir can limit the severity of the attack and the pain. ∎

Chickenpox is itchy and uncomfortable but rarely serious. Keep the child at home, out of contact with others who have not yet had the disease.

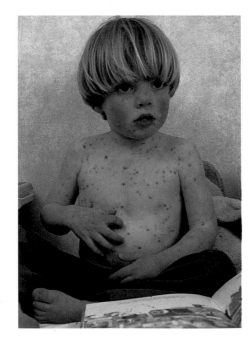

TREATING A FEVER

Treating a fever is the same for a child or adult. Keep the ill person in a warm, well-ventilated room. If the person is sweating, wipe his face and neck with a lukewarm wet flannel or sponge and change his bedclothes and bedlinen often. Lower a temperature with paracetamol, following the stated dosage. When the temperature starts to drop, stop the medication.

Call a doctor immediately if a baby less than six months has an armpit (axillary) temperature over 38.3°C (101°F) or rectal temperature over 39.7°C (103.5°F) or an older child or adult has a temperature over 40°C (104°F).

SEE ALSO

Vaccinations   120–121

CAUTION

Bacterial meningitis is a medical emergency that requires urgent hospital treatment with large doses of intravenous antibiotic drugs. If the patient is not treated immediately, the chance of recovery is slim.

Meningitis can cause cerebrospinal fluid to accumulate in the brain, a condition which is known as hydrocephalus. In some cases, there may be brain damage, which can cause blindness or deafness. The younger the child, the greater the risk of complications. Elderly people are also at risk of brain damage or death.

Meningitis

A viral or bacterial infection can cause meningitis, an inflammation of the meninges, or the thin layers of membrane that cover the brain and spinal cord. Bacterial meningitis is rarer and more serious.

Meningococcal meningitis is the most common form of bacterial meningitis and often occurs in winter epidemics. Haemophilus influenzae b (Hib) meningitis is the bacterial form that occurs mostly in children 6–15 months old. About 60 children in 100,000 will contract Hib. Up to 6 percent of these die, while a further 14 percent have long-term problems such as deafness, learning difficulties and cerebral palsy.

SYMPTOMS

The main symptoms of bacterial meningitis are a raised temperature, severe headache, a stiff neck, red or purple spots that do not fade under pressure (see box, below), nausea and vomiting and photophobia (an intolerance of bright light). The symptoms of viral meningitis are much milder; in fact, they are often mistaken for influenza.

In meningococcal meningitis, the symptoms can develop within a few hours. The sufferer may feel an intense throbbing pain in the back of the head and begin to shiver and vomit violently. There may be a temperature of 38.9°C (102°F) or higher, convulsions and delirium. An infected person often holds the neck rigid because any stretching of the inflamed membranes can cause painful spasms. She may feel drowsy and eventually lose consciousness. A red skin rash may develop anywhere on the body. In young children, the fontanelle (the soft spot on top of a baby's head) can become swollen and taut instead of being slightly sunken as normal. This is from increased pressure of the cerebrospinal fluid.

TREATMENT AND PREVENTION

Meningitis is diagnosed by a lumbar puncture, a procedure in which a small sample of the fluid that surrounds the brain and the spinal cord is withdrawn. In cases of viral meningitis, the treatment is bedrest in a darkened room, plenty of fluids and painkillers. It usually clears in a week or two, with no after effects. Bacterial meningitis requires emergency medical treatment in a hospital, where intravenous antibiotics will be given.

Immunization against Hib meningitis is now routinely given to children. Certain strains of bacterial meningitis can be immunized against to control an epidemic during an outbreak; however, these vaccines are short lived. Antibiotic drugs given to those who have come into contact with someone with meningitis are thought to be a more effective form of preventive treatment. ∎

TESTING FOR MENINGITIS

- To test for meningococcal meningitis, press the side of a glass tumbler firmly against the rash. If it does not fade and lose colour under the pressure, contact your doctor immediately.

- Neck stiffness can occur in all sorts of meningitis. Ask the person to bring one knee up to her chest. If this causes neck pain, meningitis should be considered.

Chapter 2

COMPLEMENTARY THERAPIES

INTEREST IN COMPLEMENTARY THERAPIES HAS soared along with people's growing concern for a healthy lifestyle and as they search for ways of promoting health. The therapies range from the medicinal, such as homeopathy and herbal medicine, to the physical such as massage and manipulation. Many of the therapies, including acupuncture and ayurveda, have arisen in the East and been adapted for Westerners. The same could be said for the movement- and posture-based tai chi ch'uan and yoga.

As varied as the therapies and their origins are, they have much in common. They all claim to treat the individual as a whole person to galvanize the body's own defences. Although expressed in different ways, complementary therapies often include the idea of a "life force", whose availability and proper distribution ensures vitality. Most complementary practitioners would agree that health and contentment depend on achieving a harmonious development of our physical, mental, emotional and spiritual natures.∎

SEE ALSO
Homeopathy   196–201

Herbal medicine

Healing with herbs is the oldest therapy in the world and remains the medicine on which many countries, including China and India, largely rely. Herbalists in the Western tradition combine the examination methods of conventional medicine with a "mind and body" approach to diagnosis and treatment. The results can be remarkable.

Marigold (*Calendula officinalis*), which is easy to grow in the garden and has an attractive flower, plays an important part in the herbalist's armoury. Infusions of the flower are used to bathe minor burns and scalds, as well as for acne and skin inflammations.

The underlying aim of all herbal medicine is to restore the body to a state in which it is better able to heal itself. The right herbs can promote health by correcting imbalances within the body. In this "holistic" approach, the aim is not simply to relieve your complaint, but also to improve your overall health and vitality by encouraging your body to work as efficiently as possible.

A herbal practitioner will usually do more than prescribe herbs for an illness. As part of the treatment he will also make recommendations about changing your diet and lifestyle and reducing the amount of stress in your life. The goal is to prevent, as well as to treat, illness.

Herbal medicine has been in use since prehistoric times and is known to have flourished in ancient Egypt, Greece and Rome. It has enjoyed a renaissance in the West in the last century. In controlled laboratory experiments, scientists have documented how a number of herbs traditionally used by herbalists have important medicinal properties. The herbs in question include garlic for combating heart disease and St John's wort (*Hypericum perforatum*), which is used to treat depression.

With such scientific reassurance, there has been increasing interest in herbal medicine among the pharmaceutical manufacturers In fact, they have been scrutinizing "phytochemicals" – the hundreds of thousands of substances contained within the plant world – in their quest to find new drugs.

HOW DOES IT WORK?

The approach to healing with herbal medicine is different in many ways from that of conventional medicine. It aims to work with the body, to gently nudge it into balance rather than attempting to actively tip the scales. For example, in the case of a fever, conventional doctors advise taking drugs such as aspirin or paracetamol to suppress the temperature. However, herbalists take the view that a fever can sometimes be helpful, not harmful – it is one of the body's natural defence mechanisms. Many harmful bacteria and viruses are known to be compromised and even killed by a higher than normal body temperature. The herbal medicine approach is to encourage a cleansing sweat so that the fever is not suppressed. At the same time, the fever is treated to prevent it from becoming dangerously high.

Similarly, in the case of food poisoning, vomiting and diarrhoea are considered by herbalists to be effective protective mechanisms. They allow the body to quickly rid itself of any harmful organisms in the digestive tract. Unlike conventional medicine, which would recommend drugs to halt diarrhoea and vomiting, herbal medicine aims to control these symptoms by recommending medicines that inhibit absorption from the digestive tract. The object is to make it more difficult for any harmful agent to enter and circulate throughout the bloodstream. As in conventional medicine, the patient would be encouraged to drink plenty of liquids to prevent dehydration; however, the diarrhoea or vomiting would not be completely suppressed.

BENEFITS OF WHOLE HERBS

The orthodox medical approach is to identify and isolate the "active ingredient" within a plant, then to artificially synthesize it for formulation into a drug. However, herbalists believe that it is important to prescribe the whole herb: the balance of substances within a whole herb or a mixture of whole herbs works as a combination to heal – in other words,

---

HERBS AND MODERN MEDICINE

Many of the most powerful and best-known drugs that are employed in modern medicine were originally derived from plants, which are often still used in herbal medicine.

Aspirin It contains a synthesized form of salicylic acid, which has remarkable pain-relieving, anti-inflammatory and fever-lowering properties. The chemical was first discovered in its natural form in willow (*Salix alba*). It is also found in many other medicinal herbs such as meadowsweet (*Filipendula ulmaria*) and the quaking aspen (*Populus tremuloides*).

Digoxin A component of the foxglove (*Digitalis lanata* and *Digitalis purpurea*), digoxin is widely prescribed to help regulate the heartbeat and to improve a failing heart.

Morphine This narcotic drug, strictly used for severe pain relief, is extracted from the poppy (*Papaver somniferum*).

Quinine This medicine has been used to combat malaria for centuries. Quinine is found in the bark of cinchona trees.

Contraceptive pill It was the steroidlike substances found in the wild yam (*Dioscorea villosa*) that led to the development of the first oral contraceptive pill.

Vincristine and vinblastine These two important and widely used anticancer drugs are derived from the Madagascar periwinkle (*Vinca rosea*).

CAUTION

Herbs are powerful substances, and some can be poisonous when taken in large doses. It is best to take them under the supervision of a qualified herbalist. If you are taking any conventional medicine, consult your doctor, too.

that the sum of the parts is greater than the whole. The belief is that the components of a herb will balance one another – one part can modify the potentially harmful effects caused by another part.

A herbalist would argue that, in much the same way as vitamins, minerals and other nutritional supplements can never replace whole foods, an isolated active ingredient is a crude and poor substitute for the gentler healing power of the complete herb. What is more, the whole herb is safer because the dose it delivers of any one active ingredient will be much lower than if the ingredient were isolated and formulated into a drug.

NATURAL BALANCE

One case in favour of using a herb in its entirety is that of salicylic acid, which is the active ingredient found in aspirin. If you take regular doses of aspirin, you run a risk of side effects, such as stomach upsets and gastric bleeding. However, if you take meadowsweet (*Filipendula ulmaria*), a herb that contains a form of salicylic acid, you will still receive some pain relief, but there are other substances in the plant that have an antacid effect,

which counters the side effects of salicylic acid. So, unlike aspirin, which is not recommended for people suffering from a peptic ulcer, meadowsweet is, in fact, a recommended treatment for ulcers and stomach pains.

Another important advantage in prescribing whole herbs is that in nature no two plants of one variety have an identical chemical make-up. It should, therefore, be more difficult for infectious agents such as bacteria and viruses to develop resistance to herbal remedies and for people to develop allergies to them; these are problems that can occur in conventional medicine.

WHAT CAN IT TREAT?

Each herb has different healing properties, which is why the skill of the professional herbalist is important. There is no one herbal cure for any particular condition, and each patient is treated individually. For example, two patients suffering from recurring chest infections are unlikely to be prescribed the same medicines.

Herbs can be valuable for treating many conditions. Hormonal gynaecological conditions, for example, such as those associated with premenstrual syndrome (PMS) and the menopause, respond particularly well. Nervous stress, anxiety and depression, as well as health problems that are aggravated by these factors, often also react favourably.

Herbal medicine can help strengthen the immune system in people who suffer from recurrent bouts of infection, and the herbs are usually successful in treating gastrointestinal disorders. Herbs are also good for many joint problems, such as osteoarthritis, and can improve poor circulation to the hands and feet.

Skin conditions sometimes respond more variably. Treating a condition such

---

IS IT SAFE?

Most herbs used by herbalists are totally safe and can be regarded in much the same way as tonics or food supplements. Some, such as camomile and dandelion, have been used for thousands of years for their therapeutic properties, while others, such as ginger, cayenne and garlic, are routinely used as foods.

However, it is wrong to assume that just because something is "natural", it is automatically harmless. Some herbs used by herbalists, such as *Lobelia inflata* and *Ephedra sinica*, are extremely powerful and, like any drug, they can have side effects if not used correctly. Improperly used, a few herbs can be toxic.

HERBAL FIRST AID

Doses given are for adults. Halve the dose for children six years of age and over. Do not give to children under six years old.

Problem	Herb	How to administer it
Acne and skin infections	Marigold flowers (*Calendula officinalis*)	Make an infusion (p.190) and drink three times daily.
	Tea tree oil (*Melaleuca alternifolia*)	Mix ½ teaspoon of the oil in a cup of warm water and sponge over the affected area.
Anxiety or agitation	Lemon balm (*Melissa officinalis*)	Brew an infusion (p.190) and drink up to six cups daily.
Colds and influenza	Elderflower (*Sambucus nigra*) Peppermint (*Mentha piperita*) Yarrow (*Achillea millefolium*)	Mix equal quantities of the three herbs and make an infusion (p.190). This mixture stimulates sweating to help reduce fever, and it tones the mucous membranes, reducing catarrh. Drink up to three cups daily.
Coughs	Thyme (*Thymus spp.*)	Take up to three teaspoons of thyme syrup (p.190) daily.
Earache	Onion (*Allium cepa*)	Grate a teaspoon of raw onion, lay the person down and place the grated mixture in the hollow just below and behind the ear. Leave in place for 10 minutes.
Hayfever	German camomile (*Chamomilla recutita*) Elderflower (*Sambucus nigra*) Eyebright (*Euphrasia spp.*)	Mix the three herbs in equal quantities, make a double-strength infusion (p.190) and pour in a bowl. Inhale the steam from under a towel tented over the bowl. Also drink up to three cups daily. Start drinking the infusion 2–3 weeks before hayfever usually develops.
Headaches and migraine	Feverfew (*Tanacetum parthenium*)	Grow a pot of feverfew on your windowsill. Two to three fresh leaves eaten daily help prevent headaches and migraines. *Caution:* do not take feverfew if you are pregnant or on anticoagulant therapy (blood-thinning drugs), and do not give to children.
Indigestion	German camomile (*Chamomilla recutita*)	Make an infusion of either herb (p.190) and drink up to six cups daily.
	Lemon balm (*Melissa officinalis*)	
Sore throat	Sage (*Salvia officinalis*)	Brew an infusion (p.190), allow it to cool a little and add a teaspoonful of vinegar and honey. Gargle up to five times daily.
Wind and bloating	Peppermint (*Mentha piperita*)	Brew an infusion (p.190) of either herb and drink up to three cups of it daily after meals.
	Fennel (*Foeniculum vulgare*), crushed seeds	

as acne, for example, could involve prescribing a combination of herbs that improve the elimination of body wastes by stimulating the liver, kidneys and lymphatic system. This treatment may work on its own, but if the patient has noticed that the condition deteriorated during periods of stress, herbs to induce relaxation might be included in the prescription.

Herbal medicines cannot be used for treating mechanical problems such as broken bones, dislocations, and prolapsed vertebral discs. They can, however, be used to encourage the healing process of damaged tissues associated with conditions of this kind.

THE FIRST VISIT

The initial consultation with a herbalist, sometimes called a phytotherapist, may take an hour or so. He needs time to build up a complete picture of you and all your problems – not just those for which you have sought his help – before he can recommend an effective course of treatment for you. Subsequent consultations usually take half an hour.

The herbal therapist places great importance on taking a thorough case history of every new patient. This includes taking your full medical history, along with details of your current ailment and how long you have been suffering from it. He will ask you questions, too, about

BREWING A HERBAL INFUSION

For each cup, place one teaspoon of the dried herb or two teaspoons of the fresh, chopped herb in a teapot. Pour on freshly boiled water. Cover the pot with a lid and leave to infuse for 10–15 minutes before straining the infusion into a cup. Drink it as it is or sweeten with honey.

MAKING A HERBAL SYRUP

Put four teaspoons of dried herbs or eight teaspoons of fresh herbs in a jug. Pour in about 500 ml (16 fl oz) of boiled water. Cover and leave for 10–15 minutes. Strain into a saucepan. Add 500 g (1 lb) of unrefined sugar or honey. Heat gently, stirring until the mixture is syrupy. Cool and pour into a sterilized dark glass bottle and seal with a cork.

your diet, what, if any, exercise you take and how well you sleep. He will probably ask you about your general lifestyle, which should enable him to pinpoint any stressful areas in your life, as well as noting your prevailing state of mind.

The herbalist may give you a thorough physical examination, using exactly the same techniques to do this as your family doctor would use. For example, he will take your blood pressure with a sphygmo-manometer (the familiar blood pressure cuff), and he will use a stethoscope to listen to your heart and lungs. The herbalist may also perform simple urine tests if he considers these to be necessary. Finally, he will be ready to prescribe the appropriate treatment.

Because of the way in which herbs work, improvements tend to be gradual, particularly if the ailment has been a long-standing one. Herbal medicines work more slowly than some conventional medicines because they are much less concentrated. As a rough guide, you can expect to be treated for about one month for each year that you have suffered from your current problem.

TAKING A HERBAL MEDICINE

Herbal medicines can be dispensed in a number of different ways. In liquid form, they can be given as a tincture, where the herb has been extracted in alcohol and water to preserve it; as an infusion brewed from dried herbs; and as a decoction in which herbs containing tough material, such as roots and bark, are boiled before the liquid they were cooked in is strained and drunk. Herbal tablets, pessaries, suppositories, creams and ointments may also be prescribed, either blended or as single herbs.

The flavour of some herbal medicines can be unpleasant. However, herbalists believe that the taste of herbs can have a therapeutic effect in itself. Many herbs, such as yellow gentian (*Gentiana lutea*), have a bitter taste. The bitterness induces a reflex action in the gastrointestinal tract, stimulating the release of digestive juices. This property makes bitter herbs valuable digestive tonics – something acknowledged for centuries in the custom of adding bitter herbs to traditional aperitifs.

You can add a little honey to help disguise the taste. Children, of course, may make a fuss when it comes to taking herbal medicines that taste unpleasant, but it is usually possible to mix the medicine with something more palatable, such as a little milk or fruit juice, to get them to take it. ∎

THE CHINESE APPROACH

The roots of traditional Chinese medicine, which relies greatly on herbs, can be traced back to 200 BC, to an ancient text known as the *Yellow Emperor's Classic of Internal Medicine*. It records the belief that everything in the universe has a mixture of yin and yang qualities, which is still adhered to by today's practitioners of traditional Chinese medicine.

Yin and yang are complementary opposites similar to, for example, day and night, hot and cold, wet and dry. Illness is seen as evidence of an imbalance between yin and yang. For instance, a fever denotes too much yang, while feeling cold and shivery indicates too much yin.

Chinese practitioners look for evidence of disharmony. To make a diagnosis, they take careful readings of the pulse and pay close attention to the appearance of the tongue, which is considered to be a good indicator of health. Over the centuries, many effective herbal recipes have been developed. Chinese herbalists use them as a basis of prescription, fine-tuned for an individual by the addition of other herbs. One of the best known is the Four Things Soup for treating female hormonal imbalances.

Medicines are usually given as decoctions of dried herbs, roots and bark. The ingredients are boiled for 20 minutes or so before the medicinal components can be extracted and drunk.

Aromatherapy

Aromatic substances have been used in bathing and religious rituals for thousands of years in Europe and throughout Asia, but it was not until the 20th century that the therapeutic use of essential oils, often combined with massage techniques, began to evolve into what has now become familiar to us as aromatherapy.

A relatively new discipline, aromatherapy was first developed in France in the 1920s. It was at that time that the French cosmetic chemist René-Maurice Gattefossé made the accidental discovery that the essential oil of lavender was wonderfully soothing and healing for minor burns. This sparked off a quest to explore the possible therapeutic applications of other essential oils, which are the basic tools of aromatherapy.

WHAT ARE ESSENTIAL OILS?

Essential oils are highly fragrant essences that are found in the flowers, leaves, roots, grasses, peels, seeds, resin and barks of plants. These oils are produced from hundreds of different chemicals extracted by a distillation process (which is too complex and hazardous to attempt to undertake at home) that creates a pale runny liquid of a consistency that is more like water than oil. Because essential oils

A field of lavender in bloom is more than a beautiful sight in the countryside. It also yields a powerful pale yellow essential oil that has a unique combination of soothing, relaxing, painkilling, antiseptic, antibacterial, antirheumatic and anti-depressant qualities.

are highly volatile, they can evaporate quickly; store them in sealed containers.

Most essential oils are expensive because the oil comprises, on average, only 1.5 percent of the prepared raw material from which it is derived. Certain oils, such as those of rose, jasmine and melissa, for example, are exceptionally expensive because the raw material yields an even smaller percentage of essential oil than the average. For instance, it has been estimated that it takes about 40,000 jasmine flowers to make just 5 g (⅛ oz) of jasmine oil.

THE POWER OF SMELL

Aromatherapy works primarily through the sense of smell. The human nose is a remarkably sensitive organ. It is, in fact, only through smelling food, rather than tasting it, that you are able to fully appreciate its flavour.

Your sense of smell is also closely linked with your mood, memory and emotions. Smells are perceived via the olfactory nerve, which has strong links with the limbic system of the brain, where emotions such as pleasure and sexual feelings are generated. The fragrance of the oils may affect this area of the brain.

HEALING PROPERTIES

This therapy is a valuable method for dealing with stress. It is excellent, too, for treating ailments that are known to be made worse by stress, such as pre-menstrual syndrome, anxiety, irritable bowel syndrome, hypertension, migraines and eczema. It is recognized for its ability to lift the spirits, and it can also be used to ease pain and tension caused by tight or overworked muscles.

In addition to the therapeutic effect of their fragrance, essential oils have other healing properties. Some oils such as

camomile are anti-inflammatory, while others such as geranium stimulate the circulation, and others still such as tea tree help fight infections.

A UNIQUE THERAPY

Nonmedical aromatherapists tend to prefer massage as the most effective way of transporting essential oils into the body. This is because the fragrant oils have been shown to penetrate through the skin and enter the bloodstream, where they are transported around the body to give further benefits.

With a few exceptions, such as lavender and tea tree, most essential oils should not be applied undiluted to the skin. A neat dose would often be too strong and could cause local irritation, as well as being an expensive waste. Just a few drops are needed and should be added to a light vegetable carrier oil, such as sweet almond, peach or apricot kernel, grape seed, olive, sunflower or safflower seed or soya oil. A standard mixture is 25 drops of essential oil to 50 ml (2 fl oz) of carrier oil. If your skin is sensitive, you should halve the quantity of essential oil.

YOUR FIRST CONSULTATION

At your initial consultation, the aroma-therapist will probably take a detailed medical history and ask you questions about your general health, your lifestyle and any specific health problems you may have. Finding out about your mood, diet, exercise regime, the stress in your life, how well you sleep and whether you drink alcohol or smoke can help build up a picture of you as an individual.

Aromatherapists are not trained to make medical diagnoses. For this purpose, they will rely on the clinical opinion of your doctor or a practitioner such as a medical herbalist or an osteopath.

Essential oils should be kept in tightly sealed containers in a cool, dark place. Make sure that they are stored out of children's reach.

The quality of essential oils can be extremely variable. Because they are often expensive, some manufacturers mix them with cheaper chemical extracts or dilute them to reduce their selling cost. Be wary of essential oils that are inexpensive. The rarer and purer the oil, the more expensive it will be.

CAUTION

Do not use any essential oils on small children, during pregnancy or if you are on medication without first informing your doctor and seeking the advice of a qualified aromatherapist. Although medical aroma-therapists (especially in mainland Europe) prescribe oils to be taken orally, you should never swallow an essential oil unadvisedly. If you do so accidentally, eat bread, drink plenty of milk, and seek professional help right away.

With all the information necessary compiled, the aromatherapist will select the most suitable oils for you, which may be used singly or in blends. Some aromatherapists also use other techniques – such as swinging a pendulum over both the oil and you – to help them make their initial choice of oil.

The aromatherapist may then ask you to smell several of the selected oils. This is because reactions to different smells are an individual matter. For example, some people adore an essential oil such as patchouli, while others have an intense dislike of it.

Using a burner is a pleasant way of dispersing the aroma of an essential oil. A few drops of the oil are placed on top of water in the well of the burner. The candle below provides the heat source to vaporize it. These are not suitable for use around children.

THE BENEFITS OF MASSAGE

In most practices, you will be given a full body massage, which usually takes about an hour, but can last longer. The specific type of massage performed will depend on what the aromatherapist judges will benefit you the most. Some massages are invigorating and energizing, while others aim to be relaxing and calming. A massage may be so relaxing that it can eventually send you off to sleep.

On a physical level, massage stimulates the circulation and the lymphatic system, relieving muscle tension, pain and inflammation. The aromatherapist may draw on various massage techniques, such as acupressure, to devise a massage that suits you best.

Manipulation through massage may make you aware of previously unidentified areas of muscle tension or tenderness, which are often located around the neck and shoulders. Treatment sessions are usually arranged on a weekly basis to begin with and then may eventually be reduced to once a month or so.

Aromatherapy can be utilized to complement other therapies. The one exception to this may be homeopathy, where the aroma of certain essential oils could interfere with the effect of the homeopathic medication.

OTHER WAYS OF USING OILS

As well as massage, there are several other ways of using essential oils, many of which are ideal for self help. A few drops of oil can be put in a warm bath; they can be inhaled, either through a steam inhaler or by sprinkling a few drops on a tissue and inhaling deeply; they can be applied locally in the form of a hot or cold compress to soothe aches, sprains or swelling; or a few drops can be sprinkled on to cottonwool and dabbed directly on to the affected area.

HOW TO STORE THE OILS

Because essential oils evaporate easily and are damaged by light and heat, they are dispensed in tiny dark bottles. They can usually be preserved for at least a year. The citrus oils produced from lemon, lime, orange and grapefruit peel tend to deteriorate more rapidly than others and usually last for only up to six months. ▪

USING ESSENTIAL OILS SAFELY

- ▪ You can test for sensitivity to a blended massage oil by putting a drop on your inner elbow, covering it with a sticking plaster and leaving it in place for 24 hours. Peel the plaster off and, if there is no sign of irritation, the oil should be safe to use.

- ▪ Essential oils that are more likely to irritate the skin include rosemary, verbena, lemongrass and fennel.

- ▪ Those that should be reserved for only professional use are origanum, thyme, sage (not clary sage), wintergreen, savory, cinnamon and clove.

- ▪ Citrus oils such as bergamot, orange, lemon, grapefruit and lime, as well as verbena, react to sunlight; do not apply one of these oils before sunbathing.

ESSENTIAL OILS FOR HOME USE

Name	Problems treated
Camomile, German (*Chamomilla recutita*)	***Massage:*** for menstrual cramps, insomnia, anxiety, stress, indigestion. ***In the bath:*** for stress, anxiety, insomnia. ***Application:*** for acne, eczema, cuts and abrasions.
Clary sage (*Salvia sclarea*)	***Massage:*** for depression, period pains, premenstrual syndrome, general debility. ***In the bath:*** for depression, irritability, premenstrual syndrome, tension. ***Inhalation:*** for sore throats. ***Application:*** for inflamed skin.
Geranium (*Pelargonium* 'Graveolens')	***Massage:*** for depression, colds, diarrhoea, stress, indigestion. ***In the bath:*** for menopausal symptoms, skin inflammation, stretch marks. ***Inhalation:*** for colds and flu. ***Application:*** for minor skin problems.
Grapefruit (*Citrus paradisi*)	***Massage:*** for kidney and liver problems, depression, ***In the bath:*** for depression.
Lavender* (*Lavandula officinalis*)	***Massage:*** for muscle aches, stress, depression, insomnia. ***In the bath:*** for stress, insomnia. ***Inhalation:*** for catarrh, colds and flu. ***Application:*** for burns, bites, stings, acne.
Melissa (*Melissa officinalis;* lemon balm)	***Massage:*** for viral and bacterial infections. ***In the bath:*** for indigestion. ***Application:*** for chapped and sensitive skin.
Patchouli (*Pogostemon cablin*)	***Massage:*** for stress, cellulite, diarrhoea, fluid retention. ***In the bath:*** for eczema, over-excitement. ***Application:*** for chapped skin, hair care.
Peppermint (*Mentha piperita*)	***In the bath:*** for skin inflammation, eczema, acne, dandruff, menstrual problems, headaches. ***Inhalation:*** for colds, flu, asthma, bronchitis.
Petitgrain (*Citrus aurantium*)	***Massage:*** for nausea, indigestion, flatulence. ***In the bath:*** for insomnia, depression, mental fatigue, irritability. ***Inhalation:*** for colds and flu. ***Application:*** for acne and greasy hair.
Rosemary (*Rosmarinus officinalis*)	***Massage:*** for muscular aches and pains, rheumatism, hair loss, dandruff. ***In the bath:*** for menstrual cramps and fluid retention. ***Application:*** for sprains, headaches, indigestion.
Sandalwood (*Santalum album*)	***Massage:*** for anxiety, tension, depression. ***In the bath:*** for cystitis and urinary infections. ***Inhalation:*** for catarrh, throat infections, dry skin. ***Application:*** for eczema, sunburn, nettle rash.
Tea tree* (*Melaleuca alternifolia*)	***Application:*** for cuts, stings, cold sores, acne, verrucas, warts, athlete's foot, rashes from chicken pox and shingles. ***Inhalation:*** for colds and flu.
Ylang ylang (*Cananga odorata*)	***Massage:*** for depression, anxiety, tension. ***In the bath:*** for depression, insomnia. ***Application:*** for acne, bites and stings.

*These oils can be applied neat in small amounts.

SEE ALSO
Herbal medicine 186–191

Homeopathy

Although homeopathy has been practised for about 200 years, its fundamental underlying principle that "like cures like" would have been familiar to the ancient Greeks and, in particular, to Hippocrates, the so-called father of medicine who practised in the fifth century BC, and to Paracelsus, a great 15th-century European physician.

If you had been seriously ill in the late 18th century, you would have had good reason to dread a visit from the doctor. Medical treatments in those days were often harsh and could sometimes, unwittingly, be life-threatening in themselves. Purging, blood letting and the dispensing of drugs that could lead to addiction were all among the medical establishment's stock in trade.

After becoming disillusioned with this aggressive form of medicine, the German physician and chemist Samuel Hahnemann (1755–1843) decided to find a different way to treat his patients.

A KINDER WAY TO HEAL

Hahnemann looked back to the ancient wisdom of the Greeks and discovered pointers to the more gentle approach that he was looking for. He refined and formulated what he called the Law of Similars, establishing the principles for the therapy of homeopathy.

"Homeopathy" is a combination of two Greek words: *homeo,* meaning the same or similar, and *pathos,* meaning hardship or suffering. Together, homeopathy means "similar suffering". The fundamental homeopathic principle that "like cures like" refers to Hahnemann's observation that if a substance triggers symptoms similar to those from which a patient is suffering, then a small dose of that same

Hahnemann's new ideas on medicine were inspired by the discovery that a herbal remedy for malaria, cinchona tree bark, produced malarialike symptoms when taken by a healthy person. He concluded that symptoms indicate the body's way of fighting illness.

substance will actually encourage the patient's body to fight and overcome the disease in question.

LIKE CURES LIKE

If you were to cut up an onion, the fumes that it would release might give you a runny nose, streaming, stinging eyes and a sore throat. So it follows that the homeopathic remedy based on onion, known as *Allium cepa,* is prescribed to treat patients suffering from a cold with the same type of symptoms. Similarly, the poisonous hedgerow plant, deadly nightshade, or

CAUTION

A wide variety of low potency homeopathic medicines are available over the counter. These can be useful for first aid and for treating many minor acute illnesses. However, although homeopathy is a safe form of therapy, a professional homeopath should monitor the treatment of any long-term condition – self treatment is not advisable for chronic and recurring conditions.

Belladonna, provokes a high fever, a throbbing headache, heart palpitations, hot dry skin and a bright red face. Given in its ultra-diluted homeopathic form, however, it is used to treat patients who are feverish and have an acute sore throat or a throbbing headache.

Homeopathic remedies are tested on people and not on animals. Groups of volunteers, under supervision, take a safe dose of a substance prepared as a homeopathic remedy repeatedly until they produce a range of symptoms. These symptoms are carefully recorded.

MAKING A REMEDY

The natural substances that are used in homeopathic remedies are derived from plants, minerals, metals, insects and recognized poisons, which have been used medicinally for generations. The remedies are manufactured by first making an alcoholic extract of the raw material, which is known as a "mother tincture". This is done by steeping the raw material in alcohol for several weeks and then straining off the resulting liquid.

A series of dilutions are then made of the mother tincture. Besides diluting the raw material, each successive dilution, or potency, is "succussed", which entails shaking it vigorously to "potentiate" or activate the treatment. The remedy is rendered useless without succussion.

The mother tincture can be used as it is or diluted as an external remedy, or it can be impregnated into lactose (milk sugar) tablets, granules or powder. Lactose tablets are the most common way of taking a homeopathic remedy, but if you are lactose intolerant or have a milk allergy, it can be administered as a diluted tincture. For babies and children, the granules or powder are usually the easiest way of taking a remedy.

THE POTENCY

Because so many remedies are derived from poisons, Hahnemann realized that he had to dilute them. To his surprise, he discovered that, providing the dilutions were succussed with each dilution, their action became stronger and more specific.

Homeopathic remedies are prescribed in different strengths, or "potencies". The lower potencies are shorter lasting and less powerful in their effects. High potency remedies should be prescribed only by experienced, qualified homeopaths.

To make a "1c potency", one part of the mother tincture is diluted with 99 parts of an alcohol and water mixture. If one part of the 1c potency is then diluted in another 99 parts alcohol and water, this produces a 2c potency. A 6c potency, which has been processed another four times, is recommended for self-treatment.

Remedies also come in x potencies. In this case, a 1x potency indicates that the mother tincture has been diluted by only one part to nine of alcohol and water, and a 6x means this process has been repeated five more times. The x potencies are not as diluted as the c potencies and, therefore, not as strong.

The mother tincture is progressively diluted many times over, with a vigorous shaking after each dilution, which "potentiates" the mixture, or increases its therapeutic powers by transferring energy to it. Insoluble substances are ground up with lactose and progressively mixed with more lactose, which is eventually dissolved in alcohol. Alcohol is used to make the potentiated remedies.

Some highly poisonous substances form the basis of certain homeopathic remedies. However, they are totally safe administered in homeopathic doses as they have been diluted to such a degree that not even a chemical trace of the original substance remains. Some of the remedies derived from poisonous substances are shown, right.

EXPLAINING THE UNEXPLAINED

According to homeopaths, the more diluted a remedy, the more powerful its potential effect. This is perhaps the most contentious aspect of homeopathy. Sceptics argue that it is absurd to suggest that homeopathic remedies can work when they are so diluted. But one theory suggests that homeopathy owes its success not so much to chemistry as to physics and, in particular, to electromagnetism.

The process of dilution and succussion may imprint the characteristic energy pattern of the original substance on to the liquid in which it is diluted. This can be likened to the transmission of television signals, where an original image is converted into an electromagnetic energy pattern or signal, which is then broadcast to a receiver in your home, where it is unscrambled again to form the television picture.

So it may be that a homeopathic remedy acts as a signal that energizes or stimulates the body's self-healing, thus mobilizing the defence systems and working simultaneously on the mental, emotional and physical levels of the body.

WHAT HOMEOPATHY CAN TREAT

Homeopaths claim all kinds of health complaints are suitable for homeopathic treatment. These include mental health disorders such as depression, chronic conditions such as arthritis and post-viral fatigue syndrome and acute illnesses that come on suddenly such as ear infections.

Unfortunately, there is little research to confirm these claims. Homeopathy should not be regarded as a cure-all. Homeopaths themselves are the first to acknowledge that mechanical complaints such as broken bones, a life-threatening heart attack, severe asthma or epilepsy, as

POISONS USED IN HOMEOPATHY

Substance		Description
Aconite		Made from the deadly *Aconitum napellus* (monk's hood or wolf's bane), *Aconite* can help treat heart and respiratory problems, as well as anxiety, arthritis, fevers, middle-ear infections, eye inflammations and other problems.
Belladonna		This is made from the poisonous plant *Atropa belladonna* (deadly nightshade). Some of the conditions it is used to treat include cold- and flu-related symptoms, gallstones, toothache, varicose veins, arthritis, painful periods and measles.
Spanish fly		The beetle known as Spanish fly, which contains a powerful irritant and poison, forms the basis of *Cantharsis*. It is used for urinary problems, such as bladder infections, as well as for burns and blisters.
Arsenopyrite		The main source of arsenic, this is used in the making of *Arsenicum album*. Among the conditions it is suitable for treating are hayfever, skin problems, anxiety disorders and some cold-related symptoms.

well as many other serious conditions, all require the expertise of a practitioner of conventional medicine.

THE FIRST CONSULTATION

Homeopaths take a holistic view and treat the individual as a whole rather than just their symptoms. As one 16th-century physician put it: "Those who merely study and treat the effects of disease are like those who imagine they can drive away the winter by brushing the snow from the door. It is not snow that causes winter, but winter that causes snow."

Before deciding on the appropriate treatment, the homeopath aims to consider every aspect of the person's wellbeing, and treat them simultaneously on physical, emotional and mental levels. The first consultation usually takes between one and two hours, during which you will be questioned in considerable detail not only about your complaint but also about your lifestyle, your attitudes and preferences, any stresses and strains to which you are subject, your emotional state of health and your personality.

The aim of the homeopath is to build up a complete overview of you within the context of your way of life. You may find some of the questions that she asks you rather strange. For example, you may be asked whether you are frightened of thunder or the dark, and how you react to heat or cold. On the face of it, these questions may seem to have very little to do with your complaint, but to the homeopath they contribute to the overall picture of your mental and physical reactions and constitution.

A homeopath views symptoms as evidence of the body's efforts to heal itself, and they will give her clues as to which remedy is likely to suit the patient. This is why it is perfectly acceptable for two

Homeopathic remedies have been available since the late 18th century. This 19th-century wooden case is one example of how the bottles containing the remedies were stored. Compact cases, complete with miniature books, were also available for travelling.

patients who are apparently suffering from the same complaint to be treated with different remedies. A detailed record of your symptoms and the way in which they affect you will be kept during the course of your treatment.

HOW TO TAKE REMEDIES

A homeopathic remedy is prescribed with the intention to use the minimum dose necessary to stimulate the body's natural healing powers. There are no side effects because there is no chemical build up to accumulate in the body, so it is impossible to take an overdose of these medicines. However, homeopaths maintain that because remedies can stimulate the body's reactive forces so powerfully, symptoms sometimes get worse before they improve.

The remedy should be taken in as pure a form as possible: avoid strong aromatic foods or aromas, including coffee and peppermint, which can interfere with the treatment. Avoid handling it by tipping it straight into the mouth, using the cap of the container in which it was dispensed.

Homeopathic remedies are often available in tablet form. The person taking the tablet should dispense it from the container without touching it. Do not eat, drink or clean your teeth for 15 minutes before or after taking a remedy.

If you have been ill for a long time, you may need repeated doses of a remedy to stimulate its recuperative powers, whereas a healthy person may respond quickly to a single high potency remedy. Prescribing remedies effectively requires considerable training and skill, which is why self-medication can be hit and miss.

Homeopathic remedies are absolutely safe to use during pregnancy and can be administered even to the youngest of infants. In fact, they are particularly good for children because the tablets are virtually flavourless and children rarely object to them.

YOUR BODY'S RESPONSE

Although some people report feeling much better and energized almost directly after taking a remedy, generally the effects are more subtle and slower. The original symptoms may become temporarily worse, or previous symptoms may even return for a short time. Nevertheless, any of these reactions is considered to be a good sign and indicates that the process of self healing has begun.

The body has remarkable powers to heal itself. Take, for example, common

conditions such as coughs and colds. Without any treatment at all, a generally healthy person will recover in his own time as the body overcomes the infection. Following a healthy diet and taking plenty of rest can help, too. But with chronic illnesses, such as migraine or depression, the body's vitality may be too depleted to do this without assistance. This is where homeopathic remedies are said to trigger the process of recovery.

The homeopathic approach is to nip a disease in the bud by correcting small imbalances that arise before they can develop into more serious symptoms denoting a particular disease. As a result, homeopaths claim that people who are successfully treated will generally find that their overall state of health has improved. They are better able to resist infection and often develop a greater sense of stability.

HOMEOPATHY VS VACCINES

Controversially, some homeopaths will recommend the use of remedies as alternatives to vaccines because they claim they work according to vaguely similar principles. However, there is no scientific evidence to back this belief. Vaccines introduce a small amount of a particular weakened or dead virus or bacterium into the body in order to stimulate the body's immune response against that disease and develop an immunity to it.

Although homeopathic remedies also boost the immune system response, they differ from vaccines in that the remedies are extremely diluted and no disease material is introduced into the body. Another fundamental difference is that a homeopathic prescription is specific to a particular patient and stimulates the immune system in order to strengthen it against all illness. ∎

TREATMENT TIPS

- For chronic or serious problems, consult a professional homeopath. However, treatments for minor ailments and simple first aid can be given at home.

- If the remedy you are taking for a minor problem works, stop it and recommence only when symptoms return.

- Don't worry if you think you've chosen the wrong remedy – there will be no side effects. Try the next most likely remedy.

- Ailments that are unsuitable for exclusively homeopathic treatment include mechanical problems such as dislocations, back problems and severe physical injury.

HOMEOPATHIC SELF HELP

Ointments, tinctures and remedies can be obtained from pharmacies and health-food stores. Remedies in the 6c potency are recommended for home use. Always consult your medical practitioner if the symptoms are severe, persistent or unexplained.

Complaint		Remedy	What to do
Bruising		Arnica	Apply ointment to any bruise as long as the skin is unbroken and take *Arnica* tablets for shock and injury.
Colds		Aconite	Take in the early stages, especially when there has been exposure to cold weather and when symptoms are worse in a stuffy atmosphere.
		Allium cepa	Take for a runny nose with copious, watery mucus and when the nostrils or lips are red and raw.
		Pulsatilla	Recommended for the thick-headed stage of a cold.
Coughs		Arsenicum album	Suitable for a cough that becomes worse on lying down.
		Bryonia	Take when the chest is sore from coughing and worse at night.
		Chamomilla	Suggested for a dry, tickling, tight cough with a raw throat.
Crushed fingers or toes		Hypericum tincture	Apply neat to soothe and ease pain when children trap fingers in doors or drawers.
Cuts and grazes		Hamamelis	Apply in ointment form, or blend with mother tinctures of *Calendula* and *Hypericum* – mix 10 drops of each tincture with warm, previously boiled water and use to clean the abrasion gently.
Headaches		Belladonna	Take when there is a throbbing type of pain.
		Pulsatilla	Recommended for headaches brought on by too much work.
Indigestion		Pulsatilla	Suitable when discomfort has been caused by indulging in rich food.
		Nux vomica	Take when there is also wind and colic.
Strains and sprains		Ruta	Ointment or tablets ease sprained or strained joints and ligaments. Use alternately with *Arnica* ointment when there is bruising and the skin is unbroken.

Reflexology

According to reflexologists, the health and condition of the body can be read from the hands and feet. By massaging certain reflex points on these extremities, therapists believe that it is possible to improve the health of every organ and body system and, therefore, to encourage the body to work more efficiently.

Like the Eastern therapies of acupressure, acupuncture and shiatsu, reflexology works on the theory that health depends on the flow of energy within the body. In the eastern therapies, energy flows through channels, or meridians. In reflexology, 10 channels, known as zones, are thought to terminate in the feet and hands.

Wallpaintings discovered in Egypt show that a form of foot massage was practised there some 4,000 years ago. However, reflexology as we know it today owes its existence to the American ear, nose and throat specialist Dr William Fitzgerald. In 1917, he developed the concept that parts of the body are intimately linked together in zones and that it is possible to anaesthetize one part of the body simply by applying pressure to another. Dr Fitzgerald's ideas were further refined in the 1930s by another American, physiotherapist Eunice Ingham, who decided that the various zones could best be accessed through the feet. She then went on to invent the familiar reflexology maps of the feet (see p.204).

THE ZONES AND REFLEXES

Reflexologists have defined 10 energy zones dividing the body into longitudinal sections, beginning at the head and terminating at a finger or toe. They believe that any medical condition that upsets the energy flow through a zone of the body will interfere with the healthy functioning of other parts of the body that are located in the same zone.

Two principal guidelines on the foot divide the body horizontally and are used by reflexologists to locate the reflex points accurately, whatever the shape and size of a person's feet. The first one follows the gentle arch running immediately below the ball of the foot and represents the diaphragm separating the abdominal and thoracic cavities. The second one runs roughly halfway down the foot, from the bottom of the upper bulge on the outside of the foot, extending directly across to the other side; this denotes the waist line.

Reflexologists use maps of the feet (see p.204) that show how different zones of the feet are thought to mirror various parts of the body. It is thought that illnesses reveal themselves as tender spots on the reflex areas of the affected organs. By massaging the correct points on the feet, the reflexologist can treat virtually any organ in the body.

THE BENEFITS

A reflexologist is not trained to diagnose or treat any specific medical conditions. In fact, qualified reflexologists do not claim to cure medical problems. Instead, they treat the person holistically so that, through improving the general

By applying pressure to one of the reflex points on the feet, a reflexologist aims to stimulate 1 of the 10 zones, which are said to flow through the body.

health of the body, it is then in a better condition to heal itself.

Among the many benefits claimed by reflexologists, perhaps the most obvious one is that it relieves stress by making you feel more relaxed. Relieving tension in the body helps improve circulation, aids the elimination of wastes, and generally rebalances and re-energizes the body.

Because of the effect of gravity, the flow of blood around the feet and back toward the heart tends to be sluggish. Perhaps this is why inorganic waste products that cannot be broken down, such as uric acid and calcium crystals, can accumulate in the feet. An experienced reflexologist will aim to locate and break up these crystals, aiding their elimination from the body.

Reflexologists claim to help hormonal problems, such as those related to the menstrual cycle, as well as allergies, hypertension, arthritis, back and neck problems, digestive problems, ear, nose and throat disorders, headaches and skin conditions. However, there is not yet scientific evidence to back this up.

THE FIRST SESSION

At an initial meeting, the reflexologist will ask you a series of questions. She will want to know about your lifestyle and health history and about any medication you are on so that she can build up a complete picture of you as an individual. You will be lying down or seated with your feet raised, with the reflexologist sitting facing the soles of your feet.

The feet, not the hands, are usually worked on: the hands are considered to be less sensitive because the reflexes are located at a deeper level. However, working on the hands can be valuable when a particular health problem makes working on the feet too painful for the patient to reap any benefits.

THE FOOT MASSAGE

Before the reflexologist begins treatment, she will dust your feet with talcum powder or cornflour, which makes the skin of your feet softer and easier to massage. The reflexologist will then do some form of massage routine on your

Reflexology offers the patient the opportunity to talk about herself with the therapist, which, in turn, allows the therapist a deeper knowledge and understanding of the patient and her needs.

feet to make them more supple and relaxed, which makes them easier to treat. This will also introduce you to the feel of the reflexologist's hands and allow her to adjust the pressure of touch to suit you.

The degree of pressure required varies from person to person. For example, some people have ticklish feet and require a firmer touch, while others find that a firm touch is uncomfortable or even painful. Once the reflexologist has established the degree of pressure suitable for you, she will massage all the reflex areas of both feet, feeling for areas of tenderness. The forefinger and thumb of both hands will be used to treat each foot in turn. A particularly tender area will indicate a part of the body that is tense and congested. Such an area will receive special attention in order to break up any crystals. Apart from the odd tenderness, the treatment should feel pleasurable and relaxing. There are no side effects, but some people report feeling physically drained, tired or emotionally stirred after treatment.

The first reflexology session will last about an hour, and subsequent ones should last between 30 and 45 minutes. The length of a course of treatment will depend on the patient, although an average is typically about six to eight weekly treatments. ∎

REFLEXOLOGY FOOT MAP

The location of the reflexes for every organ in the body can be seen on the reflexology foot map. Some reflexes, such as the heart on the left foot and the liver on the right, appear on only one foot. This is because there is only one of each organ and they lie on that side of the body. In many instances, there are matching points on both feet. The points on your right foot identify those parts on the right side of your body, while the ones on your left foot correspond to those on the left side of the body.

RIGHT FOOT

LEFT FOOT

1 Brain/top of head
2 Sinuses/brain/top of head
3 Side of brain and
   head/neck
4 Pituitary gland
5 Spine
6 Neck/throat/thyroid gland
7 Parathyroid gland
8 Thyroid gland
9 Trachea
10 Eyes
11 Eustachian tube
12 Ear
13 Shoulder
14 Lung
15 Heart
16 Solar plexus
17 Stomach
18 Pancreas
19 Kidney
20 Liver
21 Gall bladder
22 Spleen
23 Ascending colon
24 Descending colon
25 Small intestine
26 Bladder
27 Sciatic nerve

RELAXING THE FEET

This sequence – and variations of it – is recommended for relaxing the feet before beginning a treatment. Your therapist will start by doing a step on one foot, then move to the other foot, before proceeding to the next step. The last two steps are used to relax the feet after a massage. You can follow these steps if treating a friend.

BEFORE A MASSAGE

1 To loosen up your feet, the therapist will begin by applying firm pressure with her thumbs down the complete length of your foot.

2 After placing the palms of her hands on either side of your foot, she will gently but rapidly rock the foot by pushing it back and forth, maintaining contact between her hands and your foot.

3 While holding your toes with her supporting hand, the therapist will use her right thumb on your right foot (or left thumb on your left foot) and firmly press into the diaphragm and solar plexus reflex, located at the arch just below the ball of your foot.

4 To apply additional pressure on the diaphragm and solar plexus reflex, the therapist will gently bend your toes toward her, which pulls your foot against her thumb.

5 She will then support the heel of your foot in her hand, with her thumb between your ankle and heel. Using her other hand, she will grasp the top of your foot and gently rotate the whole foot a few times in one direction, then the other.

AFTER A MASSAGE

1 While holding your foot in one hand, the therapist will grasp your big toe with the other hand. She will rotate it for 5 seconds, then gently pull it; then she will proceed to the next toe until they have all been manipulated.

2 While supporting the top of your foot with one hand, the therapist will gently rotate the back of the fingers of her other hand against the ball of your foot six times.

Massage

The oldest of the "hands on" therapies, from which every other branch of physical therapy has evolved, massage probably first developed out of our instinctive response to soothe aches and pains by rubbing the affected area. It is a highly enjoyable therapy, is suitable for all ages and can be tailored to suit individual needs.

Massage has been in use for many centuries. For the Chinese, Greeks and ancient Romans, it was part of everyday life. Devotees included Hippocrates, who wrote in the 5th century BC that "the way to health is… an oiled massage every day", and the emperor Julius Caesar, who had therapeutic massage to treat his neuralgia.

Until the 19th century medical text books frequently referred to massage, but it lost its appeal with the development of drug therapy. It is only recently that it has regained popularity and is increasingly seen as a valuable form of therapy by the medical and nursing professions.

Cultures around the world have developed their own distinct forms of massage. They can be divided into two main categories. The first is the holistic or "intuitive" form of massage, which aims to treat the whole person. It tends to be slower, more rhythmical and relaxing, with a greater emphasis on the tactile communication between the therapist and the person who is being massaged. One example of the holistic approach can be found in traditional Indonesian massage with aromatic oils.

The second type of massage is more Western in character and concentrates on treating specific conditions or parts of the body. The Swedish massage system, which was first developed in the early 19th century by the Scandinavian practitioner Professor Peter Henrik Ling, is one example. Another example is Hellerwork, which is an intense form of massage that is designed to improve posture; this technique also has a strong psychological dimension.

THE BENEFITS

A well-executed massage of any kind has many benefits, both physical and mental. On a physical level, it relaxes and tones the muscles, stretches the tendons to

---

TRY IT YOURSELF

A relaxing head and face massage can ease a headache. How long you spend is up to you, but 15 minutes is usually enough time.

- Wash your hands, dry them, then rub your hands together to warm them if they are cold.

- Lie down and shut your eyes.

- Using the flats of your fingers and your palm, massage your face from the centre of the forehead outward with long stroking movements. Use the left hand to work on the left side of your face, the right hand for the right side. Using the same strokes, move to the cheeks, working from the top to the jaw.

- Using both hands in a small circular motion, massage the temples, jawbone and ear lobes. Move to the scalp, working from the crown, in increasingly larger circles, to the hairline.

- Rest for a couple of minutes before slowly getting up.

make them more supple, improves the flow of blood throughout the body – especially in the muscles and skin – and encourages the drainage of lymphatic fluid, which aids the removal of waste products and toxins.

On a mental level, massage reduces stress and increases your body awareness so that you begin to notice those areas of your body where you store tension. For example, if you have a sedentary job, you may find that you store tension in your neck, back and shoulders – tension headaches can be the result. Massage can be invigorating if the energy wasted as muscle tension is released by relaxation.

THE HANDS – THE TOOLS OF THERAPY

Fingers The "flat" of the fingers and the fingertips are used in light, sensuous strokes such as feathering and can work at a deeper level too, as in petrissage.

Thumbs The strength and size of the thumbs make them ideal for working on small areas of tense tissue. The thumbs are also involved in grasping strokes, such as kneading.

Palms The palms are used in gentle stroking and gliding movements, such as effleurage, and to grasp and hold various areas of the body.

Heel of the hand This part of the hand helps in stretching and manipulating tissue. The heel can also be useful for working on deeper tissue levels.

At the other extreme, you may have a job in which you spend a great deal of time on your feet, or you may even have to perform strenuous physical tasks. In this case, you may be prone to aching legs, exhaustion and muscle strain and may be at risk of injury. Whatever your particular occupation or lifestyle, massage can be a great preventive help in dealing with the physical and mental stresses that it imposes on you.

IN SPECIAL CIRCUMSTANCES

Massage can be valuable during pregnancy to relieve backache and other physical discomforts associated with changing posture and weight. It can also help with pain relief during labour and even reduce the amount of pain-killing drugs needed.

Touch is the very first sense that a baby possesses, and it is largely through touch that it arrives at its perception of the world. In India and the Far East, baby massage is part of everyday childcare and mothers find that it helps soothe fractious infants. Baby massage is now gaining in popularity in the West, and there is strong scientific evidence that touch is vital to a baby's healthy development.

In later life, when the human body loses its strength and vigour and functions less efficiently, massage can help relieve the effects of rheumatic and arthritic aches and pains. It can be a comforting form of therapy, too, for those who feel depressed or lonely, as well as for the seriously or terminally ill. Many hospices for the dying and some intensive care units now use massage.

THE BEST TECHNIQUE FOR YOU

The type of massage therapy that is best for you depends, to a great extent, on what you want from it. If you are looking for relaxation and a release from stress, the more gentle, holistic forms of massage are likely to be appropriate. If you have a musculoskeletal injury or postural problem, the Swedish approach or a sports massage would probably be of greater benefit. However, many massage practitioners can offer either approach.

It is important that you feel a rapport with your massage therapist. If not, it is unlikely that you will relax enough to enjoy the experience.

WHEN TO AVOID MASSAGE

If you have any doubts about the state of your health and whether you will benefit from massage, you should, of course, consult your doctor. Massage for people with cancer or serious psychiatric illness requires particular expertise and, in many cases, could be inadvisable. Professional advice is important if you are pregnant or if you have any of the conditions listed below:

- cancer
- psychiatric illness
- epilepsy
- HIV or AIDS
- severe back pain or injury
- skin infections, inflammations, bruising or recent scar tissue
- fever
- varicose veins, phlebitis or thrombosis
- undiagnosed lumps or bumps.

THE DIFFERENT STROKES

Massage uses a variety of strokes, some of which are shown on the facing page. Some therapists like to start with the back and work from head to toe before doing the same on your front. Others work from the extremities toward the heart. The massage therapist may use a pure vegetable oil or baby oil to help his hands slide over your skin, enabling the strokes to be performed more smoothly. ∎

THE DIFFERENT TECHNIQUES

Effleurage This technique uses the flat of the hand in long, slow, flowing strokes. It is a relaxing stroke, which can be used at any time in the massage and after all deeper strokes.

Knuckling A type of friction stroke, knuckling is performed with the hand curled into a loose fist, moving in small circling strokes. It is often used on the shoulders and chest.

Kneading A stimulating and invigorating action in which both hands alternately grasp and release the flesh, kneading aids the elimination of wastes, improves the elasticity of connective tissues and helps break down fatty tissue. It is used on soft, well-padded areas such as at the waist, the thighs and the bottom.

Skin rolling This technique involves kneading the flesh to stimulate the circulation. Using the thumbs and index fingers, the skin is picked up, rolled and released.

Hacking This percussion technique involves rapidly and vigorously striking a part of the body with the sides of the hands to increase circulation and tone up muscles. The fingers should be relaxed. These strokes are energizing instead of relaxing. Hacking should not be used on bony areas or on broken veins or bruises.

Cupping A type of percussion stroke, cupping is performed with the hands – as the name suggests – in a cup shape. The hands are alternately moved up and down rapidly, with the fingertips and the heel of the hand contacting the skin. The stroke is suitable for a fleshy area without broken veins or bruises.

SEE ALSO

Massage	206–209
Acupuncture	212–213
Acupressure	214–215

Shiatsu

A unique form of pressure massage, shiatsu hails from Japan and has much in common with the Chinese therapies of acupuncture and acupressure. Shiatsu means, literally, finger pressure, but this is not accurate – as well as fingers, therapists use the palms and heels of their hands and their elbows and knees to apply pressure.

The key to understanding shiatsu is the concept of *ki,* or *chi* in Chinese. This is the vital life force within the body on which health and wellbeing are said to depend. According to traditional Chinese and Japanese medicine, *ki* runs throughout the body along invisible energy channels, or meridians, each linked with certain organs of the body and aspects of health. When these pathways become obstructed or overstimulated, which can be caused by factors such as stress, injury or an unhealthy diet, the flow of *ki* is disrupted and illness results.

The aim of the shiatsu therapist is to rebalance the flow of *ki* by using special techniques to work the *tsubos* – hundreds of surface points scattered all over the body on the meridians, where it is possible to contact *ki.*

Shiatsu is a safe and effective technique. Similar massage techniques have been practised in Japan for centuries, passed down from one generation to another, and they are still used in the home where family members practise on each other. However, shiatsu itself was not formulated as a therapy until the 20th century.

WHAT CAN IT HELP?

Although shiatsu cannot cure diseases, the symptoms of stress-related conditions seem to respond particularly well to the therapy, as they do to most manipulative therapies. For example, people with asthma, muscular aches and pains, tension headaches, migraines, toothache, depression, insomnia, digestive problems and stomach ulcers can all benefit.

Shiatsu is also claimed to be especially good for restoring individuals to their best possible state of health. Many people, while not actually ill, are often run down in some way, which lowers the immune system's ability to defend the body (see pp.26–27). They may suffer from repeated colds, mood problems such as irritability, feeling low or depressed, stomach upsets, and so on. Shiatsu is helpful in fine-tuning a person's general health, which helps keep the immune system at its best – therefore, shiatsu is largely a preventive therapy.

THE FIRST SESSION

When you go to the therapist for a first session, he will start by questioning you about your medical history. He will also take notes on certain relevant observations about your physical appearance, including your facial colour, your body structure, your posture and sometimes your tongue, which practitioners believe can indicate to them valuable information about your state of health.

The therapist will then perform a *hara,* or abdominal, diagnosis. To do this he will kneel down beside you as you lie on

SHIATSU SELF HELP
Using your thumb, press the *tsubo* on the back of your hand between the thumb and index finger for five seconds. An indentation along the bone of your index finger will indicate the spot; it may feel slightly tender. Stimulating it in this way, on both hands, can help relieve headaches, toothaches and the stuffiness of a head cold.

a futon (a type of Japanese mattress) or mat on the floor. He will place the palm of one of his hands on your lower abdomen. Using the other hand, he will then use his fingertips to palpate the abdomen, which is where the body's principal energies are thought to reside. The therapist's goal is to locate any areas of overactivity or weakness in the flow of *ki*. The *hara* diagnosis should take only a couple of minutes.

THE MASSAGE

The shiatsu therapist does not require special equipment or oils to give a massage, just a warm but airy room and a hard surface on which to work. To have a shiatsu massage, you should wear loose, comfortable clothing so that your body movement is not restricted. You will be asked to lie down on the floor, with your arms resting by your sides.

The therapist often begins the massage by gently stretching parts of the body. This is meant to stimulate the flow of energy and to bring meridians to the body surface so that they are easier to reach and less pressure is required to work on them. Generally, two meridians are selected for treatment. Which areas are worked on will depend on where the *tsubos* that need stimulation are located. The massage could involve treating the head, trunk, legs, arms and the hands and feet.

After the stretching procedure, the therapist will apply pressure to the *tsubos*. It should be deep but pleasant and not painful. Therapists will adjust the level of pressure, which they apply mostly with the ball of the thumbs, to the individual.

The therapist's goal is to free blockages or relieve areas of overactivity, thus rebalancing *ki* so that the body is able to heal itself. A blockage along a meridian can result in either deficient *ki*, which is known as *kyo*, or excessive *ki*, which is known as *jitsu*. *Tsubos* that feel soft and yielding are called *kyo* – they will usually feel pleasant when pressed because of the energy the therapist supplies to rectify the deficiency. *Tsubos* that feel resistant, tense and stiff are called *jitsu*. Don't be surprised if they produce a twinge of discomfort when pressed. By working on the energy-deficient *kyo* areas, the therapist also encourages the *jitsu* meridians to relax.

A complete session will take between an hour and an hour and a half. You should feel relaxed after the session is over. A course of shiatsu usually lasts between 6 and 10 sessions. ∎

CAUTION

Shiatsu should not be performed on anyone who has just drunk alcohol or eaten or on anyone with a high fever, an infectious disease, heart disease or cancer. Avoid areas of inflammation, wounds or scar tissue.

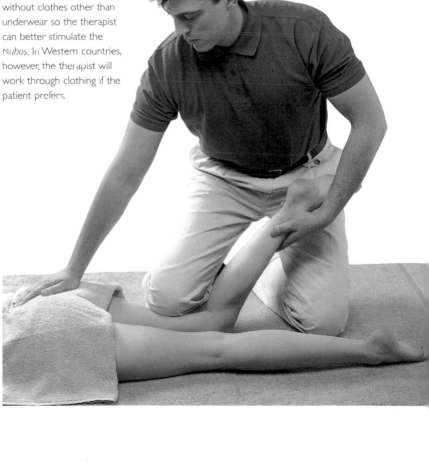

Both patient and therapist should be as comfortable as possible. Shiatsu is traditionally performed without clothes other than underwear so the therapist can better stimulate the *tsubos*. In Western countries, however, the therapist will work through clothing if the patient prefers.

Acupuncture

The practice of acupuncture, which has a 3,500 year history in China, is part of Traditional Chinese Medicine (TCM). Acupuncture heals and revitalizes by rebalancing the flow of energy, known as "chi", within us.

In Traditional Chinese Medicine, it is thought that *chi* flows in the body by using 14 invisible channels, known as meridians (see p.214). If *chi* becomes blocked, unbalanced or too active or weak at a point on a meridian, the person can become ill. Factors that can disturb the flow of *chi* include poor diet, hereditary factors, infections, injuries, illness, stress, emotional upset, seasonal changes, the weather and even the time of day.

An acupuncturist tries to influence the flow of *chi* by making contact with it via acupoints – these points are located where the *chi* travels closer to the surface. He can stimulate the acupoints with a variety of methods: by inserting fine needles into them, applying warmth in the form of smouldering dried herbs, tapping them with a rounded probe, treating them with laser techniques or applying thumb and finger pressure. The number of treatments needed varies. Sometimes the results are achieved in one session, but more often a course of treatments is necessary, once or twice a week or less frequently.

WHAT CAN IT HELP?

Health problems that can respond well to acupuncture include painful arthritis, headaches, migraines, trigeminal neuralgia and neuralgia following shingles.

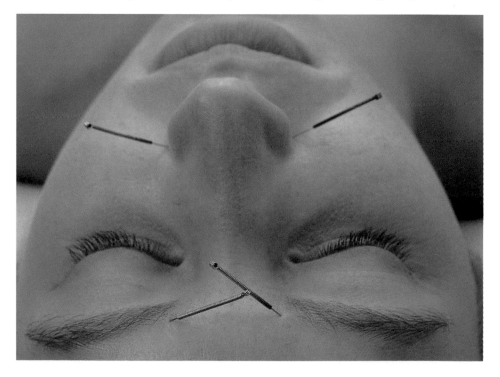

To treat a patient for hayfever, the acupuncturist inserts needles into the skin of the face at points on the bladder and large intestine meridians. He rotates the free ends to stimulate the energy flow.

Acupuncture can help disorders as diverse as sprains and fractures after the bones have been set, sports injuries, depression and anxiety, physical drug addiction, allergies, sinusitis and conditions aggravated by stress. It can also prove effective preventive medicine when people are feeling run down but do not have a physical disease. However, treatment by acupuncture is less likely to be successful where disease has produced long-term damage to tissues and organs, which may impede the flow of *chi*.

YOUR FIRST CONSULTATION

Expect your first consultation with a traditional Chinese acupuncturist to last an hour or longer. He will take a detailed medical history and evaluate all aspects of your lifestyle. During the consultation he will take note of your nails, skin colour, voice, tongue, eyes, breathing, posture, emotional state and body odour. Taking the pulses – six in each wrist, which correspond to the 12 paired meridians and their related organs – is an important part of the diagnosis. Pulses can reveal where the flow of *chi* is compromised.

This whole body approach provides a detailed picture. The acupuncturist can establish the exact nature of the imbalance you are suffering from and how best to restore harmony and encourage healing. However, acupuncture can also be used locally for symptom relief, for example, to alleviate acute pain. In this case, a full diagnosis is unnecessary, as only the acupoints localized to the painful area need stimulating.

INSERTING THE NEEDLES

Once the therapist decides which acupoints to work on, he inserts fine, sterile needles into them. They may go just into the surface of the skin or penetrate 7.5–10 cm (3–4 in). Depending on the treatment, the needles will stay in place for a second or two or for 20–30 minutes. The acupuncturist may rotate them or move them up and down to increase stimulation. Or he may leave them alone if the *chi* needs calming and sedating. Sometimes, he will apply gentle electrical stimulation through the needles to make them vibrate slightly.

It is likely that you will notice when the needles are inserted, but it is usually not more than a pinprick. Once in, you may experience a warm, heavy, dull or tingling sensation, but it should not feel painful. While the needles are in place you may sense a heaviness in the limbs and a pleasant feeling of drifting and relaxation.

AURICULAR ACUPUNCTURE

The ear offers a full set of points that correspond to all the areas of the body. Auricular acupuncture, as it is known, is often used to reinforce full body acupuncture. It is also used for patients who want to give up smoking. Studs resembling miniature drawing pins can be left in place in auricular points. The patient can press them to reinforce treatment between sessions. ∎

WHAT IS MOXIBUSTION?

Like all acupuncture practice, moxibustion does not hurt. It is used to introduce heat at an acupoint where there is a deficiency of *chi*, thus enhancing its flow. The acupuncturist inserts a needle, then places a small cone of dried moxa – the Chinese herb mugwort – or a moxa stick on the head of the needle and lights it. The heat travels to the needle and feels pleasantly warm to the patient. The moxa can also be applied directly without needles by placing a slice of ginger or onion skin under the moxa to protect the skin from burning.

SEE ALSO
Acupuncture   212–213

CAUTION

You should not attempt acupressure on any area of broken, inflamed or infected skin, on or near varicose veins or when the patient is pregnant, has a fever, has recently consumed alcohol or is feeling particularly weak or exhausted.

Acupoints (they are the same for both acupuncture and acupressure) are located along 14 meridians. The twelve major meridians are paired: they are the bladder (Bl), gall bladder (Gb), heart (He), kidney (Ki), large intestine (Li), liver (Lv), lung (Lu), pericardium (Pe), small intestine (Si), spleen (Sp), stomach (St) and triple warmer (Tw). The other two – the conception vessel (Cv) and governing vessel (Gv) – are unpaired and run down the midline of the front and back of the body. Some acupoints have a precise effect on an organ or body system; others exert a general influence.

Acupressure

Working on the same principles as acupuncture, acupressure provides an alternative to it for those who fear needles. The other advantage of acupressure is that you can learn to use it on yourself to treat minor ailments. However, as it is less precise and direct than the needles used in acupuncture, the results are usually slower and less dramatic.

Essentially a form of acupuncture, but without the needles, acupressure stimulates *chi* (the flow of energy within your body) at points, or acupoints, on the meridians (invisible energy channels) by using thumbs and fingertips. Practising acupressure properly requires a thorough knowledge of anatomy and the traditional Chinese system of medicine.

The main disadvantage of acupressure is that it is not so easy to stimulate the deeper lying acupoints with pressure alone. Although acupressure is not as effective as acupuncture, for some people it seems to work extremely well.

You can learn to use the technique of acupressure in a limited way to relieve some everyday minor ailments; for

THE MERIDIANS

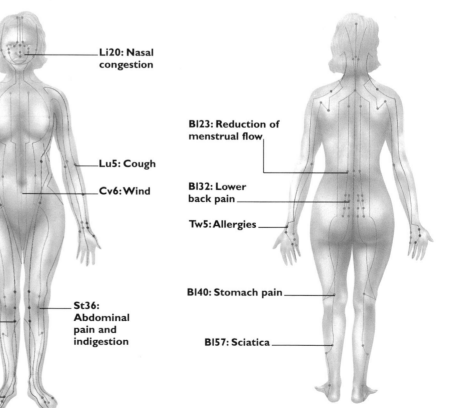

Li20: Nasal congestion

Lu5: Cough

Cv6: Wind

Pe6: Nausea

Lu10: Sore throat

Sp8: Premenstrual syndrome

St36: Abdominal pain and indigestion

Lv3: Menstrual cramps

Bl23: Reduction of menstrual flow

Bl32: Lower back pain

Tw5: Allergies

Bl40: Stomach pain

Bl57: Sciatica

example, it is suitable for self treatment of tiredness, constipation, headaches and colds. More serious and long-standing health problems should be treated by a properly qualified acupressure practitioner and it is best to see your doctor, too.

Acupressure is especially useful for patients who have a phobia of needles and, consequently, do not like the idea of acupuncture. It is also more suitable for babies and small children. Some acupuncturists prefer to use acupressure on pregnant women, the elderly and patients who are at risk of infection when their skin is pierced or broken.

Sessions are normally brief: a few minutes to an hour is all that is required for adults and 30 seconds for a baby is enough. They may be repeated several times a day – little and often is the key.

LOCATING THE ACUPOINTS

Most acupoints lie between bones, muscles or tendons, often in natural indentations. Each acupoint is named and numbered according to which meridian it is on and which organ corresponds to it, for example, Lung 5.

The direction of the flow of *chi* along a meridian can be ascertained by the numbering: it flows from acupoint 1 to the highest number. Pressure is normally applied with the flow, but occasionally it is given in another direction when a sedating and calming effect is desired. It helps to imagine the flow of energy during acupressure.

Deep thumb pressure is often the most effective way of stimulating the acupoints, although some people may respond to a lighter touch. Small rotations of the thumb can help boost the flow of *chi* along the meridian. The practitioner may also press the acupoints by using small wooden sticks, which have either rounded ends or rollers on the ends to cover several points at once.

Most people can tell when an acupoint has been successfully located, because it feels tender or sensitive to pressure. Fingertips – not fingernails – are used to apply gentle pressure, which should be applied gradually until you feel a mild sensation but not necessarily pain. The acupoints should never be jabbed.

Some people feel a tingling, which peaks and then disappears. If this occurs, stop treating the acupoint when the feeling disappears, because it shows that the rebalancing has already taken place. If an acupoint does not feel particularly sensitive, the practitioner will apply more pressure until you start to feel a slight discomfort, which should soon pass. Generally, the more sensitive an acupoint feels, the more indicative it is of an excess of *chi*. A lack of sensation suggests that there is a *chi* deficiency. ∎

RELIEVING COLDS

You can press Lu7 on the lung meridian to relieve cold symptoms. The point is located on the thumb side of the inside of the wrist, two fingers' width from the wrist crease, in the hollow behind the bone. Use the thumb on the opposite hand to press the point, angling it toward the wrist and thumb for 30 seconds. Repeat on the opposite wrist.

THE ENERGIZER

Ki1 on the kidney meridian is called "the bubbling spring" by the Chinese. It is a useful point to press when you are suffering from fatigue and lethargy. Work both feet together, using the left hand to treat the left foot and vice versa. Apply firm pressure with the thumbs to the point located just below the ball of the foot for 30 seconds to a minute. (Do not use this point if you have low blood pressure.)

SEE ALSO

Yoga   218–223

CAUTION

Meditation is not suitable for everyone. Some people find the process disturbing or uncomfortable. People with persistent mental health problems should seek advice before working with a meditation technique.

Meditation

One aim of meditation is to revitalize the mind by providing it with a rest from continuously processing information and responding to the world around us. Meditation can improve your wellbeing, encourage more positive thoughts and feelings, lift self-esteem and help you to develop a more tolerant and stable attitude toward life.

For thousands of years, meditation has been associated with religion – from Christianity in the West to Japanese Zen in the East. Only recently has it been removed from this context and practised by many people as a spiritual means of relieving mental and physical stress. Whether prompted by religion or not, all types share the characteristics of resting, often with the eyes closed, and performing mental exercises to focus the mind and relax the body.

Stress is a key contributing factor to many health problems, from anxiety to irritable bowel syndrome. Research has shown that people with stress-related conditions can derive great benefits from practising meditation. This has led scientists to look more closely at what happens to the body during meditation. Among their findings are that blood pressure falls, the metabolic rate slows and brainwave patterns alter to become more synchronized.

HAVEN OF PEACE

There are many ways to meditate. Most involve sitting comfortably in a peaceful place and breathing rhythmically while you focus your attention on one thing. This could be your breath, a physical object such as a candle or the repetition of a "mantra" – a neutral word or a few lines from a poem, hymn or prayer.

The following visualization technique draws on your imagination to quiet your mind. It will be easier on some days than others, depending on your underlying state of mind.

Sit comfortably with your back erect and eyes closed and concentrate on your breathing for a few moments. Now imagine your haven of peace. It could be a palm-fringed beach in the tropics, an alpine meadow, a boulder by the side of a waterfall or watching rain fall on the

At any level, meditation has a calming effect on your mind and body and provides an antidote to stress. As you continue to practise, you will gradually find it easier to be aware of the flow of your thoughts and feelings and to let your mind settle into deeper levels of consciousness.

garden. Alternatively, hold an apple in your hand, feeling its shape and texture and studying its colour. Smell it, put it down and close your eyes. Capture all you have seen and felt in your mind.

If you want to use a mantra, choose a simple word that contains an "o" sound such as "one". There is no need to move your lips – just silently repeat the word in your mind with each breath. Or you could meditate by using a positive thought. A well-known affirmation is "Every day and in every way, I am getting more and more relaxed."

MAINTAINING FOCUS

It can seem as if there is nothing much to meditation. However, it takes practice and perseverance to achieve the contemplative state where the mind remains alert, yet empty of thought. It is common at first to find unwanted thoughts repeatedly intruding or to become so relaxed that you drift off to sleep.

As you sit, you will notice many things: minor discomforts and tensions, the rhythm of your breath, sounds in the room. You will also find that you lose your focus as thoughts drift in. This is natural. Simply return to your word or thought. There is no need to force your mind to become empty. The secret of simple meditation is to be comfortable, to provide your mind with something to focus on and, in a nonjudgmental way, to let go of thoughts as they drift back in.

Many people find that simple stretching exercises and awareness of breathing will help them to be more aware of their body, making comfortable relaxation easier to achieve. These simple body techniques plus meditating on a word, thought or an image, even on the rhythm of the breath itself, is often all that is needed to achieve useful and healing periods of relaxation.

Continue meditating for five minutes. When you notice your thoughts drifting, simply bring your focus back. This will happen many times, so just accept it. Do not try to block out intrusive thoughts. Acknowledge them briefly, then return to your meditation. Over a period of months, gradually extend your meditation period to 20 minutes.

When you are ready to come out of meditation, place your hands over your eyes and blink a few times, then open them and look around you. Slowly stretch and take a deep breath.

If you want to learn more about meditation, you should find a teacher. There are many groups, some of them associated with a religion, including Christian groups. Other groups are entirely secular, although their meditation techniques will probably have been derived from an Eastern tradition. ■

TIPS ON MEDITATING

■ Choose a quiet place where you will not be distracted. Take the telephone off the hook or put the answering machine on.

■ Make sure your environment is warm. Before beginning, go to the toilet if necessary.

■ Wear loose comfortable clothes.

■ To prevent your body energy being taxed with the processes of digestion, make sure you do not eat for two hours or drink for an hour before beginning.

■ Breathe through the nose all the way down to the abdomen, slowly and regularly without forcing it.

■ Try to release any obvious tension in your body, particularly around the neck, shoulders and upper back.

■ Find a method of meditating that suits you, whether it involves focusing on an object, an imaginary scene, a word or phrase or simply your breath.

■ Practise a minimum of three times a week but, preferably, daily.

SEE ALSO
Meditation   216–217

Yoga

As practised in the West, yoga provides a comprehensive workout for the mind and body. The form most familiar to Westerners is "hatha" yoga, which combines physical postures, breath control and relaxation.

Originally developed as a Hindu religious discipline, yoga is thought to rebalance the mental, physical and spiritual aspects of a person's life. In the East, yoga is practised as a way of working toward the ultimate goal of spiritual realization. However, it is perfectly possible to practise yoga simply as a means for relieving stress or improving overall health, with no special knowledge of the philosophy that lies behind it.

EXERCISE FOR EVERYONE

The enormous advantage of yoga is that it can be safely undertaken by almost anyone, from children to the elderly, and even those who are unfit or overweight. The yoga postures, known as *asanas,*

slowly move all the major joints through their range of motion, reducing stiffness. They stretch and tone almost every muscle and tendon in the body, eventually making them strong and supple.

The *asanas* work on the inner body, too. Certain postures improve the blood circulation to specific organs, replenishing them with fresh oxygen and nutrients. For example, the force of gravity is employed in the shoulder stand to increase blood flow to the thyroid gland in the neck, and the head stand can do the same for the brain. Some *asanas* – for example, the forward bend – gently compress the digestive organs within the torso. This has a massaging effect, promoting a healthy digestive system and encouraging the elimination of wastes. Others, such as the so-called corpse pose, enhance mental and physical relaxation during a yoga session.

BENEFITS OF BREATH CONTROL

Breathing exercises known as *pranayama* are practised at the same time that the *asanas* are performed. Research has shown that *pranayama* leaves people feeling more energized, both physically and mentally, and more positive in outlook than other forms of relaxation.

In the West, we generally take little notice of how we breathe. However, breathing in the way that yoga teaches has been found to reduce the levels of the body's stress hormones – adrenaline, noradrenaline and cortisol. When these hormones are continually raised, as is the

THE COMPLETE BREATH

Sit comfortably, with your back straight but relaxed. Place your hands on your abdomen, just below your ribcage, with the middle fingertips just meeting above your umbilicus (belly button). As you count to five, take in a deep breath through your nose. Fill your lungs from the bottom to the top. You are achieving this correctly if your middle fingers no longer touch as your lower chest expands. Hold the breath briefly, then slowly breathe out to a count of 10. Repeat 10 to 15 times. Remember that your abdomen should expand as you inhale and contract as you exhale.

case in a person who is under stress, they can upset the smooth running of the body. A hormonal imbalance that is linked to stress can interfere with digestion, increase muscle tension and raise blood pressure. This may be why yoga breathing exercises are valuable for treating conditions that can be exacerbated by stress such as anxiety, panic attacks, hyperventilation, asthma, hypertension and digestive upsets.

WHAT TO EXPECT

A typical beginners' class will start with a period of relaxation, followed by a sequence of *asanas* that work on every part of the body. While performing each posture, you will be taught to breathe in a controlled way, as well as how to stretch your body slowly, to the point where you feel the stretch but never any pain or discomfort. Each *asana* is held for a few seconds or more before relaxing and moving into a different pose.

Try not to feel disheartened if your attempts at various postures fall far short of what is demonstrated: yoga is not competitive. You will still reap benefits, whether or not you attain the full posture. You should never force your body into an uncomfortable posture because this could be harmful. As a beginner you will not be expected to attempt advanced postures. In any case, some of the more advanced *asanas,* such as the scorpion, are likely to be impossible to perform until you are experienced at yoga. However, with regular practice, it is often astounding how quickly a stiff and inflexible body becomes more supple.

During the yoga session a variety of different relaxation *asanas* will probably be used to take short breaks. A longer period of deep relaxation, designed to re-energize the body, will finish the session.

HOW TO PRACTISE

A full yoga routine takes 45 minutes to an hour to complete. Ideally, it should be performed every day at least two hours after your last meal and half an hour after your last drink. If you do not have the recommended amount of time available, it is better to do yoga little and often than a full session infrequently.

A good standby, for when you have little time to spare, is the Salute to the Sun (see pp.222–23). It stretches all of the major muscles and flexes the main joints. The Complete Breath (see facing page) is also quick and easy, can relax you if you are upset and can be practised as often as you like throughout the day.

It is much better to go to a yoga class run by a properly qualified teacher than to attempt to learn yoga out of books. The teacher will ensure that you have the correct posture, and that you are breathing appropriately and moving at the right pace and flow.

There is an increasing number of *ashrams* – centres that are devoted to the teaching and practice of yoga – around

---

LIFESTYLE CHANGES

People who regularly practise yoga often discover that they automatically begin to embrace a healthier lifestyle. Because they are generally more relaxed they may not feel the same need to smoke or drink alcohol. Similarly, perhaps because yoga makes people more aware of their bodies, they find they prefer to eat lighter, more energizing foods and fewer heavily spiced or rich meals which are harder to digest.

A lactovegetarian diet is recommended for those practising yoga: it contains plenty of easily digested natural foods, especially fruit, vegetables, grains, nuts, seeds and dairy products such as cheese and yoghurt. These are so-called *sattvic,* or purifying, foods. Foods that should be largely avoided include meat, alcohol and stimulants such as hot spices, coffee and tea.

the world. You can attend short courses at such centres. They are free from the stresses of everyday life, so it is often easier to concentrate on your yoga, combined with periods of meditation.

CLOTHING AND EQUIPMENT

When practising yoga, you should wear comfortable, nonrestricting clothes that give you complete freedom of movement. It is best to have bare feet to prevent your

feet from sliding while practising certain postures. During the longer relaxation periods, when your body should be motionless, you may want to keep a sweater, pair of socks or blanket to hand to prevent you from becoming cold.

Practise yoga in a room that is warm but not stuffy, with plenty of space and a quiet environment. You will need a yoga mat, towel or blanket as cushioning for your body as you perform the postures. ∎

THE CAT POSTURE

This posture, which is known as *chakravakasana*, can increase spinal flexibility. It is one of several *asanas* that can be performed as a warm up before starting a routine.

I Start in a kneeling position, with your back straight, arms at your side and looking in front of you. You should keep your legs and feet together.

2 Bend over, placing your hands on the floor. They should be directly under your shoulders, with the fingers together. Your arms and back should be straight, with your head in line with your back.

3 Keep your elbows in and feet together as you raise and arch your spine as far as is comfortable. You should use your arms to support yourself, not to push up on. Lower your head as you raise your spine. Hold the position for a few seconds.

4 Gently lower your spine and push your buttocks up, raising your head. Repeat steps 3 and 4 up to six times. Once you have mastered the posture, try it inhaling as you raise your spine and exhaling as you lower it.

THE WARRIOR

There are several versions of this easy posture, the *virabhadrasana*, which firms the muscles of the chest and back, as well as strengthens legs and hips.

1 Stand comfortably, with your feet spread apart – initially in line with your shoulders, but as you progress you can move them farther apart. Relax your arms at your sides and look forward. Keep your back straight.

CAUTION

If you have any doubts about your health, consult your doctor before taking up yoga and make sure you find a qualified teacher. If practised incorrectly, yoga can induce back disorders, and hypertension, as well as glaucoma.

2 Raise your arms until they are parallel to the ground, with palms facing down and fingers together. At the same time turn your right foot to the side, at a 45 degree angle. Turn your left foot slightly to the right.

3 Keeping your arms in the same position, twist your torso to the right and look in that direction. Bend your right knee until the lower and upper parts of the leg are at a right angle. Return to the beginning position and repeat on the opposite side.

RESTING POSTURES

These positions can be used to rest between *asanas* and at the end of your yoga session.

Kneel down with your legs and feet together. Slowly bend forward with your chest resting on your knees, your head resting on the floor and your arms stretching in front of you. Rest the palms of your hands on the ground. After several seconds, slowly rise up and return to the kneeling position.

Alternatively, kneel down and slowly bend forward, resting your chest on your knees and your head on the floor, but keeping your arms by your side. Stretch them behind you, palms facing upward. After a rest, slowly return to the kneeling position.

SALUTE TO THE SUN

This exercise is normally performed in a continuous motion 5 to 10 times. It is particularly valuable for stretching the spine and hamstrings. First concentrate on learning the postures. Then incorporate the breathing rhythm. If you have any concerns about your health, do not attempt this exercise without first consulting your doctor.

2 Inhale as you stretch your arms back so that your hips move forward, your back arches and your head is tilted back. Your palms should face upward.

YOGA THERAPY

This therapy is designed to be preventive medicine and to keep you healthy. Yoga therapists have undergone additional training in how to use the discipline to treat and manage specific ailments.

Basic yoga routines have been adapted to emphasize those posture, breathing and relaxation exercises that are particularly beneficial to the ailment in question. At the same time, the routines avoid postures that might not help the specific problem.

1 Stand with your weight evenly distributed and your back straight. Exhale as you place your palms together, aligned below your chin, in the "prayer pose".

10 Exhale and move your left foot next to your right and slowly roll up. Inhale, stretching your arms back as in step 2, and repeat the cycle. End after 5 to 10 complete repetitions by standing straight and relaxed with your hands by your sides.

9 Inhale as you move your left foot forward between your hands, allowing your right knee to bend to the floor, and look up.

3 Exhale as you stretch forward. Slowly stretch your fingertips to your toes as far as you can comfortably go, bending your knees if necessary. If you are flexible, keep your knees straight and rest your palms on the floor.

4 Inhale as you extend your left leg behind you, resting the knee on the ground as you raise your chest and head.

5 Hold your breath as you bring your right foot back. Raise your body in a press-up position, with your head in line with your neck and back.

6 Exhale as you lower your knees, chest and chin to the floor, but keep your buttocks and hips raised off it.

8 Exhale and push yourself up on your feet. Raise your buttocks up so that your body forms a "V", keeping your arms and legs straight.

7 Inhale as you slide your chest forward and up and lower your hips. Keeping your shoulders down, arch your back and look forward. This is the cobra position.

CAUTION

Never strain at yoga postures. Keep your eyes shut if you are tempted to compete with classmates. Breathing correctly helps to avoid strain: inhale on upward movements and exhale as you come down.

Tai chi chu'an

The ancient Chinese exercise system of tai chi chu'an, or simply tai chi as it is usually known in the West, promotes a long healthy life, rejuvenates the body, strengthens the immune system and speeds convalescence.

With its long-established sequences of slowly performed, flowing movements, tai chi chu'an is a particularly graceful and gentle form of exercise that can be performed by young and old alike. Like other traditional Chinese therapies and forms of medicine, such as Chinese herbal medicine and acupuncture, tai chi is founded on the ancient Taoist philosophy, which seeks to find the natural harmony in what is around and within each person.

According to Taoist beliefs, everything, even inanimate objects, can be classified as *yin* or *yang*. *Yin* is the dark, receptive, contracting feminine principle, while *yang* is the light, active, expanding masculine principle. Good health is only achievable when a balance has been maintained between these complementary opposites.

In China, it is common for people to practise as a group outdoors. Ideally, tai chi should be performed in the open air and on grass, either under trees or near water, where there is considered to be more natural energy (*chi*) around.

MOVEMENT WITH MEDITATION

Tai chi chu'an combines movement and meditation to balance *yin* and *yang*, thereby strengthening your inner energy, or *chi*. The aim is to cultivate *chi*, which makes it more potent and focused, and to harness it to stay healthy, for self healing or for self defence.

As well as helping you remain physically strong, fit and supple, tai chi can improve the performance of the whole body. On mental and spiritual levels, it centres the mind, putting it in touch with the body and encouraging a state of inner calm. Yet it is also energizing, aiding concentration and freeing creativity.

Tai chi is an ideal form of exercise for people at any level of fitness and of any age because the movements do not require strength or exertion. They are carried out almost as if you were wading through water, with the body weight frequently shifting from one leg to another. The sequences work on virtually every muscle, joint and tendon, improving body control. Tai chi is not aerobic so it will not increase your heart rate and make you out of breath. However, you may find you sweat, not through physical exertion but because of the heat generated by your circulating *chi*.

CONTINUOUS MOTION

Separate movements involving the whole body are grouped together to make up a "form". Each of these movements has a symbolic meaning and special name such as Repulse the Monkey. When they are performed effortlessly, *chi* is strong and moving freely in the body. There are form variations such as the Eight Pieces of Brocade (see pp.226–27). The popular Yang short form (named after a master teacher) lasts several minutes; the long one takes 20 minutes to complete.

The way you breathe during the form is important. Inhalation occurs during the *yin* aspect of a movement, when the body is "gathered in". Exhalation occurs in the outward and expanding *yang* aspect. You cannot consciously learn the breathing or your mind will be too focused on it and not the movements. Correct breathing will come automatically with practice.

LEARNING TAI CHI CH'UAN

You should learn tai chi from a teacher, who can ensure you carry out the exercises with your body properly aligned. When you attempt, or "test", the movements, your teacher will observe how easily you can perform them. Any difficulties you encounter, such as stiffness or lack of balance, indicate areas of the body where *chi* is not flowing as it should. With practice, you will become aware of these.

It takes six months of regular practice to learn a form; practice then concentrates on improving it. Daily sessions should take 20 minutes, but try to practise a few times a day. The ideal time to practise tai chi is at sunrise or sunset, when *yin* and *yang* are best harmonized, preferably outside. However, it is more important to practise regularly than to restrict sessions to the ideal time and place. According to Chinese tradition, "perseverance furthers".

CHI KUNG

Closely related to tai chi is chi kung, which translates as "cultivation of *chi*". Even older than tai chi, chi kung was once a secret practice reserved for the elite in Chinese society. Compared with tai chi, the accent is on the meditative aspects more than the physical ones.

There are numerous chi kung exercises, and many of these have been brought together and given poetic names such as Soaring Crane chi kung. All forms of chi hung involve meditation, controlled breathing techniques and specific movements, with visualization of where *chi* is focused or moving in the body.

Chi kung can be performed sitting, standing or lying down and in a moving form. It helps maintain health and relieve many disorders, particularly those which are aggravated or triggered by stress. ■

TIPS FOR TAI CHI PRACTICE

- ■ Remember to relax and switch off from preoccupations and worries. This state of mind is referred to as "cheerful disinterest" in China.

- ■ Keep in the forefront of your mind tai chi's potential for healing. Focus on sensing the flow of *chi* within your body.

- ■ Be aware of your shoulders and neck and try to keep them relaxed at all times.

- ■ In tai chi the centre of gravity, called *tan tien,* is considered to be just beneath the navel and slightly toward the spine. Imagine that your weight is concentrated in this area.

- ■ Try to feel well rooted to the ground, with your elbows and knees soft and flexible and never locked.

- ■ Your spine should always feel relaxed and vertical, as if you were suspended by a cord from the top of your head. Without tension, tuck in your pelvis and gently draw back the chin.

- ■ Use your imagination to work on your mind, as well as your body. The movements have descriptive titles. Use them or other suitable images to mentally visualize what you are doing.

- ■ Do not try to do too much or go too fast or you will lose any benefit from the practice.

EIGHT PIECES OF BROCADE

This set of eight movements (shown in additional steps for clarity) was created during the Sung dynasty (960–1279AD) to improve the health of Chinese soldiers. It is often used today as a warm up before practising a tai chi form, but it can also be performed on its own. Always practise the movements slowly but in a continuous motion, with the body relaxed and the mind focused.

The starting position

This position is often used between movements and is referred to throughout this exercise. With your knees slightly bent – but not protruding beyond the tips of your toes – stand with your feet parallel and spread apart. Your back should be straight and shoulders relaxed. Bring your hands in front of you, with palms facing up and fingertips touching.

1 Start by standing with your feet parallel and spread apart, aligned with your shoulders. Let your arms relax by your sides and look forward; slowly inhale.

2 Slowly exhale as you turn your head as far as you can to the left without straining it. Inhale and return your head to the front. Then exhale and turn your head to the right and, once again, inhale as you bring your head back to the front.

3 Move your hands to the starting position (above). As you exhale, interlock your fingers, raise your arms up and out in front of your chest, then bring them up over your head, with palms facing upward. Inhaling, return to the starting position.

4 Simultaneously, slowly move your left hand upward, with the palm facing up, and your right hand downward, the palm facing down – all the while exhaling.

5 Bring the hands back to the centre position as you inhale, then reverse the sequence, with right hand raised and left hand lowered, as you exhale. Return your hands to the starting position as you inhale.

6 Turn your body slightly to the left as you exhale. At the same time slowly raise your hands until they form a cross in front of your chest, with your palms facing you and fingers relaxed.

7 As you inhale, make a fist with your right hand and pull it back to your shoulder. At the same time, press your left hand forward with the hand flexed back. Return to the starting position and repeat on the right side.

8 From the starting position, bend your knees slightly more. Rest your hands on your thighs, just above the knees, with the fingers inward and without locking your elbows.

9 Without raising your feet, lean as far as you can to your left – keep your hands on your thighs. Then lean back to the centre and repeat on the right side. Return to the centre, then to the starting position.

10 Keeping your knees straight (without locking them), as you exhale bend over and, if you can, touch the floor with the palms of your hands. Do not strain – reaching for the floor with your fingertips is just as good.

11 Raise yourself up and return to the starting position as you exhale, but make fists of your hands and draw them in to your sides. If you have a bad back, rest your hands on your knees as you rise for extra support.

12 Slowly strike to the left and upward with your left fist as you exhale. Follow the movement of the fist with your eyes, moving your head to the left. Return to the final position in step 11 and repeat on the right side. Finally, return to the starting position and let your arms rest by your sides. Move your feet together, and stretch your legs by raising your heels as high as possible as you exhale; inhale as you lower them.

Ayurveda

This all-embracing mind, body and spirit approach to medicine from the Indian subcontinent predates the ideas of the Greeks and Chinese. As with many ancient systems of medicine that are holistic and treat the whole person, the aim of ayurveda is to enhance wellbeing and mental and physical harmony by balancing the flow of the inner energies.

The sanskrit word for "life knowledge" is ayurveda, which has its roots in Indian spiritual philosophy and religion. It is more than a system of medicine: it is a way of life designed to enhance the state of mind and promote a long life through existing in harmony with the environment. Ultimately, those who practise it hope to attain harmony with the consciousness of the universe.

Ayurveda is as much about preventing disease as treating ill health. The state of your body, mind and spirit is perceived to be governed by one of three *doshas* – basic forces which must be in equilibrium for you to be healthy. They each have their own characteristics and are known as *vata*, *pitta* and *kapha*.

DOSHAS AND THE ELEMENTS

Every living organism, including the *doshas,* is made up of five elements – space, air, fire, water and earth – in different combinations. The elements are also manifested in the five senses of taste, touch, sight, smell and hearing, through which we interact with our environment. According to ayurveda, we are each born

CONSTITUTIONAL TYPES

According to ayurvedic medicine, every individual is governed by one dominant *dosha* – *vata, pitta* or *kapha* – although we nearly all contain elements from another *dosha* and some people may be governed by two *doshas*. Certain characteristics, such as physical build, general health, intellectual abilities and personality, are determined by the dominant *dosha*.

Vata	Pitta	Kapha
■ thin and slight in build	■ medium height and build	■ solid, heavy build
■ tendency to have dry skin all over	■ normal skin	■ tendency to have smooth, oily skin
■ food and meals are usually taken irregularly	■ often has moles, freckles and birth marks	■ thick, strong hair
■ tendency to experience constipation and flatulence	■ tendency to overeat and needs regular meals	■ small appetite
■ light sleeper	■ good digestion but usually experiences diarrhoea	■ regular bowel habits
■ a worrier	■ prefers cold or chilled foods	■ dislikes damp and foggy weather
■ enthusiastic outlook	■ dislikes the heat	■ reasoned and methodical
■ restless	■ tendency to sweat	■ calm and stable
■ finds it hard to concentrate	■ quick tempered	■ deep sleeper
	■ logical and intelligent	■ slow learner

with an individual balance of *doshas,* which determines our constitution, temperament and body type. If these *doshas* become imbalanced – for example, because of an unhealthy or inappropriate diet, lifestyle, behaviour, stress or negative thoughts – our health suffers.

REACHING A DIAGNOSIS

An ayurvedic practitioner will question you to establish your constitution and lifestyle. She will note the condition and colour of your skin, hair, nails, tongue and facial lines and take pulse readings.

Ayurvedic practitioners use three main forms of treatment: natural medicines, special diets and advice on behaviour

modifications. All types of treatment are classified by their effect on the *doshas.*

Initially, treatment involves helping your mind, body and spirit rid themselves of impurities in the form of "toxins" and "wastes", inappropriate thought patterns and emotions. This stage may involve fasts, restricted diets, massages, enemas and even therapeutic vomiting.

Regeneration begins once your body is purified. Medicines are based largely on plants, although honey, dairy foods and some small quantities of minerals, such as salt, may be used. Breathing exercises and yoga, chanting and meditation, burning incense and steam baths may all be used in the healing process. ∎

A healthy balanced diet is seen as medicine because it has a profound effect on the *doshas.* It is not just what you eat: how you prepare the food, how you feel when you eat it and how long you spend over meals are also important. Certain foods are recommended for each *dosha* type.

VATA

PITTA

KAPHA

Vegetables: Asparagus, beetroot, carrots, cucumber, green beans, sweet potatoes
Fruit: Ripe bananas, apricots, mangoes, papaya
Protein: Chicken, white fish, milk, yoghurt, cheese, almonds
Carbohydrates: Rice, wheat
Herbs and spices: Basil, cardamom, cinnamon, cloves, ginger, juniper berries
Sugar: Honey

Vegetables: Broccoli, white and red cabbages, Brussels sprouts, chicory, courgettes, mushrooms, potatoes, sweet peppers, peas
Fruit: Apples, sweet cherries, grapes, figs, pineapples, coconut
Protein: Poultry, pheasant, game, cottage cheese, sunflower and pumpkin seeds, chickpeas, mung beans
Carbohydrates: Oats, white basmati rice, wheat
Herbs and spices: Green coriander, dill, fennel, ginger, mint, turmeric
Sugar: Brown or white

Vegetables: Aubergines, broccoli, cauliflower, Brussels sprouts, carrots, celery, okra, potatoes, all salad leaves
Fruit: Apples, pears, guavas, cranberries, pomegranates, fresh dates, dried fruit such as raisins and prunes
Protein: Poultry, prawns, game, skimmed milk, most pulses except soya and white and black beans, sunflower and pumpkin seeds
Carbohydrates: Buckwheat, maize, rye
Herbs and spices: Cardamom, cinnamon, cloves, ginger, black pepper and turmeric
Sugar: Honey

Osteopathy

Using techniques of manipulation and massage, osteopaths work on the bones, joints, muscles and connective tissues of the musculoskeletal system to improve the function and health of the whole body.

In the late 19th century, the American army surgeon Dr Andrew Taylor Still found that he could cure disorders with manual techniques alone, and he put his ideas together to launch a new therapy – "osteopathy". Dr Still believed that good health depends on the proper functioning of the body's framework. The musculoskeletal system supports and protects all the organs of the body, so it must work well for the body tissues to be healthy, the brain and nervous system to be responsive and for the circulatory, lymphatic and digestive systems to operate efficiently.

Dr Still thought that poor functioning of the musculoskeletal system, caused by injury, mental stress, bad diet, lack of or inappropriate exercise and poor posture,

is the root cause of many health problems. Standing upright places continual strain on the system, with gravity pressing on the vertebrae and the cushioning discs in between them. By using manipulation to balance the tensions in the body structure and improve the functioning of the framework, he considered he could boost the health of the whole body. Osteopathy is now recognized by most conventional doctors and is one of the most accepted complementary therapies.

Back disorders that can benefit from osteopathy include prolapsed discs, neck pain, whiplash injuries, misaligned joints between vertebrae and ribs, sciatica, chronic muscular tension and scoliosis, the condition in which the spine bends to one side – providing there is no vertebral deformity. However, some conditions affecting the back are not suitable for osteopathy. These include inflammatory conditions such as ankylosing spondylitis, where the ligaments harden and lock the vertebrae together, and cancer.

NOT JUST FOR BACKS

Most people think of osteopathy as a therapy in connection with bad backs, but it has much wider applications. In cases of osteoarthritis, for example, osteopathy can relieve the pain and stiffness associated with the disorder and improve mobility, although it cannot reverse any joint deformities resulting from the condition. (Osteopathy is not suitable for treating rheumatoid arthritis.)

Although some practitioners favour a particular method of treatment, the osteopath will adjust the technique and amount of pressure he applies to suit your needs.

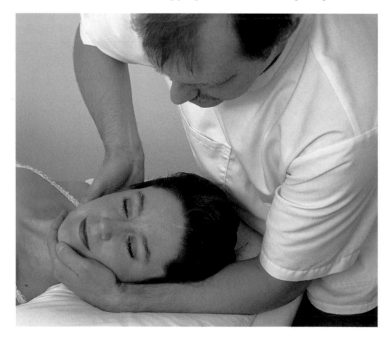

Osteopathy can also help conditions that are aggravated and, in some cases, caused by problems of the musculo-skeletal framework. Examples include premenstrual syndrome, recurrent sinusitis, asthma, migraines and tension headaches. It can aid the recovery from sports injuries and from occupational problems caused by spending long periods at a computer screen, on the telephone or driving, or simply from poor posture.

In pregnancy osteopathy provides a drug-free way to relieve backache, which often occurs because of the change in posture and weight gain, as well as heartburn and constipation. Later on, osteopathy can help relieve musculo-skeletal problems triggered by the birth such as stress incontinence.

WHAT TO EXPECT

During your first visit to an osteopath, he will take a detailed medical history. You should explain in depth your health problems and how they affect you. The osteopath will check your posture and the way you move when sitting, standing and walking, and he will take into account your lifestyle, what physical activity you do and what your work involves.

An examination will follow, in which the osteopath will use his hands to assess tension and stiffness in the muscles, joints and connective tissues and identify the source of your problem. The osteopath may then ask you to perform a series of movements, bends and stretches to see how mobile and supple you are and to reveal any weakness, tension or injury.

Osteopaths are qualified to carry out orthopaedic, neurological and circulatory system examinations, so your practitioner may perform tests on parts of your body other than the bones and muscles. He may take your blood pressure and test

your reflexes. In addition, he may request X-rays, magnetic resonance imaging (MRI scans), blood or urine tests.

There is no standard therapeutic procedure for a particular health problem; osteopathic treatment is geared to the

THE MUSCULOSKELETAL SYSTEM

Collar bone

Spine

Vertebra

Gluteus maximus: one of over 600 muscles

Although osteopathy looks at the body as a whole, treatment focuses on the musculoskeletal system, particularly the spine. The upper back, shoulders and neck are common problem areas. The lower back and hips are frequently affected by stiffness and pain.

individual. Your osteopath has a wide range of techniques to draw on that are generally aimed at loosening and freeing elements, rather than repositioning them. These include different methods that gently stretch the muscles and ligaments and osteopathic soft tissue massage. Other methods are rhythmical movements of joints or high velocity thrust techniques, which can cause joints to click and are designed to improve the range of motion. Gentle release techniques are also widely used, especially on children and the elderly. At times, osteopathy may feel uncomfortable, but it should not be painful. You may feel slightly stiff for a day or two after a treatment. Heat and a mild painkiller will help. Avoid strenuous activity until the stiffness disappears.

The initial consultation and treatment may take up to an hour. Each subsequent treatment lasts for about half an hour, but this varies among practitioners. You can expect to undergo treatments three or more times before you begin to notice any improvement in your condition. You may need six sessions or more if you have long-term problems. Some patients continue to have regular, more infrequent sessions, as a preventive measure.

You will probably be given advice on how to help your problem in other ways. The osteopath may suggest dietary alterations, relaxation techniques or exercises to practise at home to improve suppleness and relieve muscle tension.

CRANIAL OSTEOPATHY

A special branch of osteopathy, cranial osteopathy was developed in the 1940s. Cranial osteopaths claim that compression and moulding of the cranium, or skull, can occur during childbirth or as the result of trauma or long-term tension. This can lead to health problems because they can affect the rhythm of the cerebrospinal fluid in the cranium and spine. These osteopaths believe they can sense pulsations of the cerebrospinal fluid, which are known as the cranial rhythmic impulse. By manipulating the bones of the cranium, they can restore the fluid to a balanced rhythm.

This gentle therapy is suitable even for newborn babies, as well as for children and adults. Problems are diagnosed and treated with a range of manipulative techniques. Difficulty feeding, colic, wind, disturbed sleep, headaches, ear, nose and throat problems, asthma and behavioural disorders can all respond to treatment. It is usually imperceptible, so you may be unaware that anything is happening, apart from feeling the osteopath's hands. Sometimes you may experience a warm sensation as tension is released from the body. It is a therapy that leaves people feeling deeply relaxed. ▪

THE ALEXANDER TECHNIQUE

Developed in the late 19th century by the Australian actor Frederick Matthias Alexander, the Alexander technique is based on the premise that if you are relaxed in everyday life, natural postural reflexes will allow you to move without great effort. Young children have this ability, but as you go through life, physical, emotional and mental stresses result in a build up of tension. This dulls the reflexes and leads to bad postural habits.

Teachers of the Alexander technique help you learn how to move once again with natural reflexes. During the first lesson, the teacher will observe you, noting how you move, sit and stand. By making adjustments to your body at rest and while going about everyday activities, such as standing up from a chair, the teacher increases your awareness of how you move and puts you in closer touch with your body. The aim is to replace bad postural habits with good ones. By releasing tension and improving breathing, the Alexander technique can help relieve ailments such as back pain, headaches and hyperventilation.

Rolfing

The aim of Rolfing is to restructure the body so your posture and the way you move become balanced and free of unnecessary tension. Though similar in its goals to the Alexander technique, the method is different.

Sometimes called structural integration, Rolfing systematically reorganizes the habitual patterns of tension. It changes body alignment by manipulating muscles and the supporting soft tissues, and teaches you movement so that you work with gravity instead of being dragged down by it. It may be helpful for long-term postural pain or tension.

Rolfing was developed by Ida P. Rolf, an American doctor of biochemistry. She became interested in discovering how the body could function more efficiently as a result of personal and family health problems. Through years of research and painstaking observation of the healthy and sick, she developed and refined her method in the 1960s.

According to Dr Rolf, posture becomes distorted over the years for numerous reasons. Children subconsciously mimic their parents' bad postural habits, and they sit for long periods at uncomfortable school desks. She believed that injuries, and even wearing nappies, affect your body alignment.

The result of a course of Rolfing is a lengthening of the body because of improved vertical alignment and a rebalancing of it horizontally so that you do not feel lopsided. Other benefits are relief from tension-related disorders, such as backache and other chronic musculo-skeletal pain, and improved breathing, circulation, digestion and sleep patterns.

WHAT TO EXPECT

A course of Rolfing usually lasts about 10 sessions. Each time the practitioner works on a different part of the body and builds on the session given beforehand. The first session aims to "free the breath" and realign the ribcage; the final treatment integrates all the structural work of the previous sessions. They take between an hour to an hour and a half and are carried out weekly or biweekly.

During a Rolfing session, sensations you may experience range from a warm feeling to momentary discomfort and even pain, although it is described by Rolfers as "good pain". Afterward, you may have a sensation of lightness and, if there is any residual soreness, it should fade after a day or so. ∎

MANIPULATION

The Rolfer first manipulates the superficial levels of soft tissue and gradually goes in deeper. As she manipulates you, she may ask you to breathe "into" the area being worked or to make movements synchronized with her own.

Chiropractic

Emphasis is placed on the spine and nervous system in chiropractic, a therapy in which the musculoskeletal system is manipulated by a trained practitioner. The name chiropractic comes from the Greek. Cheir *means "hand", while* prakitikos *translates as "done by" – an excellent description of how this therapy is performed.*

When the Canadian healer Daniel David Palmer, a man fascinated by bones and how the body works, cured a janitor who had been deaf for years by manipulating a vertebra in his spine, he stumbled on what was to be a new branch of medicine – chiropractic. It is now one of the complementary therapies that is the most accepted by the conventional medical establishment, although it was initially ill-received at its inception in the late 19th century. Research in both Great Britain and the United States shows that chiropractic is effective in treating lower back pain.

A chiropractor treats the musculoskeletal system – the bones, joints, muscles, ligaments and tendons – by using a series of manipulative techniques. Chiropractic and osteopathy are similar in theory and treatment; however, there are differences between the two therapies. For example, a chiropractor aims to perform a number of individual joint manipulations, while an osteopath prefers to work on the soft tissue of larger areas. The chiropractor also makes greater use of diagnostic procedures such as X-rays.

WHO CAN BENEFIT?

Chiropractic can treat many musculoskeletal disorders, including sciatica, sports injuries, a slipped disc, asthma, constipation and other digestive problems and menstrual disorders. Back and neck pains account for most of the visits to a chiropractor, and headaches are often treated by releasing tension in neck muscles. Strains, sprains and knee problems can also be treated.

The therapy can be practised on anyone, from babies to senior citizens. In fact, chiropractors believe that an accident in early childhood, whether a fall from a cot or taking a tumble while learning how to walk, can jolt the spine and cause musculoskeletal problems later on in life. Chiropractors recommend periodic check ups with a member of the profession (as

THE HUMAN SPINE

The spine is a remarkable mechanical structure. It provides the central support system for the human body and is involved in almost all its movements. Up to 34 bones make up the spine, among them the 24 vertebrae that are cushioned between cartilage discs. In addition, the spine encloses and protects the spinal cord, the tube of nerve tissue that relays information to and from the brain and the rest of the body, including its many internal organs.

The nerves emerge from the spinal cord at various points. If there is inappropriate tension at any one point in the structure, it can, according to chiropractic theory, interfere with the function of the body. By correcting the misalignment through manipulation, a chiropractor aims to restore normal function to the musculoskeletal system and even the internal organs.

well as routine visits to the general practitioner) to correct any problems.

Older people suffering from joint pain or back pain are usually given medication by doctors to treat the symptoms. The cause of the pain may be muscle tension, an imbalance between groups of muscles and stiff joints. Chiropractic can be successful in alleviating pain without using medication. It can also be used to relieve some of the back pain that can occur during pregnancy.

HOW A CHIROPRACTOR WORKS

The initial consultation will begin with the chiropractor taking the details of your medical history. You should let her know of any health problems, previous injuries and past surgery, as well as describe any current symptoms or disorders.

After noting your movements and posture, she will perform an examination in which she will feel for areas of pain, tenderness and muscle spasms. She may ask you to move in certain ways or move parts of your body herself. She will be looking for "subluxations", or misalignments of bones in the joints, as well as "fixations", or abnormal movement. The chiropractor will probably take an X-ray of your spine, in which she may detect any signs of arthritis or bone deformities. She may test your muscle strength, which can detect nerve problems, and order tests on blood or urine samples.

Treatment may not begin until your second visit, after the chiropractor has had time to examine your history and test results and to devise a treatment plan. If your neck is being treated, you may be asked to sit on a stool. Otherwise, you will be asked to remove your outer clothes and to position yourself on a table or couch especially designed for chiropractic use. How you are positioned – for

example, lying on your stomach or side – will depend on the course of treatment.

Chiropractors are trained to use a wide variety of adjustments. Each one typically takes only seconds to perform, and will usually be performed after you complete a deep breath. With each adjustment you may hear a "click", but it should be painless. The chiropractor wants to minimize any discomfort, so she will adjust the amount of pressure used for each person, and she may precede an adjustment with massage.

You may feel slightly sore for a day or two after treatment. How many sessions you need will depend on the problem. An acute condition, such as a sprain, may require only two visits in a week, with a follow-up visit the following week. More serious conditions may call for 12 or more treatments over eight weeks, and chronic disorders can take even longer. Some people return for maintenance or preventive treatments. ■

Direct "thrust" techniques, in which small, rapid, forceful movements are used, are typical of chiropractic treatment. Deep massage may also be used to relax tense muscles.

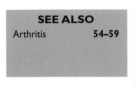

SEE ALSO

Arthritis   54–59

CAUTION:

Avoid wet and dry heat treatments if you have high blood pressure or heart problems. Do not have steam treatments or sitz baths in the first three months of pregnancy.

Hydrotherapy

The Romans appreciated the health and social benefits of bathing and the Greeks believed that water was healing. More recently, interest has resurged in using water to promote health and wellbeing, detoxify the body or stimulate an immune response. If you cannot put your full weight on a limb, hydrotherapy can allow you to exercise without pain.

Many different treatments use water for its health benefits, and these are all encompassed in hydrotherapy. There are saunas, hot tubs, whirlpools, sitz baths, foot baths and thalassotherapy – the therapeutic use of sea water. Depending on the treatment, the water itself may be hot, cold, lukewarm or tepid, and it may be applied to the person as steam or ice.

Germany has a keen tradition of hydrotherapy, and it was the 19th-century monk Father Sebastian Kneipp from Bavaria who pioneered modern methods. He took a less spartan approach than his predecessors, whose harsh treatments included drenching patients in cold water from great heights with such force that they needed to steady themselves by holding on to a bar. Father Kneipp's ideas

were followed wherever natural spring water was available, and spas were opened throughout Europe.

Today's specialized hydrotherapy clinics are found mostly in Germany and Eastern Europe. Modern equipment is computer controlled. Treatments involve directing water at various body parts, with the temperature changing at precise intervals.

AS PHYSIOTHERAPY

For those with a fracture, arthritis, muscle or joint aches and pains, and those who are overweight, bathing in pools and exercising in warm water can help to ease stiffness. The natural buoyancy of the water relieves the stress that body weight puts on the joints, allowing the bather to exercise her muscles. The presence of natural minerals such as sulphur in water can enhance these effects.

PROFESSIONAL TREATMENTS

Health farms and spas usually include whirlpool baths, in which the bather is immersed in water with pressurized bubbles directed at different parts of the body to soothe and massage the muscles. Whirlpool treatment is also a natural balm for circulation disorders. High-powered jets are another option, directed at the back for a few minutes. This treatment is thought to stimulate circulation and internal organs.

TURKISH BATHS

In a traditional Turkish bath, the aim is to flush impurities from the system. Wrapped in a towel, the bather starts off in the cool room (frigidarium), then moves to the warm room (tepidarium), where the heat is 37.4–44°C (100–112°F). The bather stays there until he begins to sweat. At that point, he enters the caldarium, where the heat is intense – up to 65°C (150°F). After sweating for about half an hour, he is thoroughly massaged to remove dirt and impurities from the pores dilated by the heat. The bather finishes off with a plunge in cold water to close the pores.

HYDROTHERAPY AT HOME

Instead of going to a health farm or spa, you can have hydrotherapy treatments in your own bathroom. However, if you have a health problem or are concerned about your health, you should not undertake any of these treatments without first consulting your doctor. You should always test the water temperature in hot treatments before fully immersing your body to avoid burning yourself.

SHOWERS

Hot showers are relaxing and are better at cleansing than cold. They are excellent for relieving muscle tension and can make you feel tired and lethargic, so they are best taken before going to bed. You can direct a hot jet of water at aching or stiff areas of the body. It provides relief because it locally stimulates the circulation and relaxes the soft tissues.

Preceding the shower by rubbing your body with moistened sea salt helps to improve the texture of the skin and draw out impurities. Concentrate on the limbs and, if you have some assistance, on the back. Avoid the face and tender areas of skin such as the breasts.

Cold showers are stimulating and energizing. They can help to constrict overdilated blood vessels such as varicose veins, and there is evidence that over six months or more, they can reduce the frequency and severity of colds.

Try alternating hot and cold showers. Start by standing under a hot shower for two minutes, followed by brief bursts of cold water lasting for 15 seconds. Repeat the sequence twice more, finishing with a cold shower. It combines the beneficial effects of both hot and cold water, relaxing the muscles and soft tissues and toning the circulation, and leaves you with a wonderful glowing sensation.

BATHS

An Epsom salt bath will help to relieve rheumatic aches and pains. Climb into a half-full warm bath to which you have added two handfuls of Epsom salts (magnesium sulphate). Lie in the water for between 10 and 20 minutes, topping up from the hot tap as necessary. Towel dry yourself without rinsing off the salts. Alternatively, you can add a fine blend of oatmeal or bran to the water to soothe the skin or mineral extracts to nourish it.

A hot sitz or hip bath is particularly beneficial for painful periods and inflammation in the pelvic area, as well as haemorrhoids, cystitis and incontinence. Ideally, you should take it in a purpose-built tub, but you can have one in your own bathtub. Fill the bath with hot water, but make sure that the level reaches no higher than where your navel would be. Sit in the water with your knees bent out of the water for up to 10 minutes. From time to time you should let a little water out and refill the bath with hot water to maintain the temperature. ∎

Exercising in a pool of water is used to treat patients suffering from a lack of mobility. It may include the use of water jets to massage the body.

Chapter 3
HEALTHY EATING

MOST PEOPLE HAVE SOME IDEA OF WHAT constitutes a good diet but are confused by the claims some food manufacturers make about their products. Understanding the food groups and the nutrients found in them will set you on the right road to a healthy diet. Eating a properly balanced diet has its advantages: you will feel better, it can help prevent certain disorders or control their symptoms and, along with exercise, it is the best way to maintain your correct weight.

How you eat can be as important as what you eat, and regular satisfying meals can do much to cure psychological bad habits connected with food. Using the wrong cooking techniques can turn healthy food into an unwholesome meal, but there are simple ways to create tasty, appetizing meals without destroying nutrients or adding unnecessary fats, sugar and salt. Wisely chosen, convenience foods can help a busy cook.∎

You are what you eat

Proper eating is fundamental to health. The typical Western diet, with its emphasis on meat, dairy produce, refined carbohydrates and processed food, contributes to many of today's ills, from cancer, heart disease, diabetes and arthritis to bowel disorders, premenstrual syndrome, hyperactivity and frequent colds.

Foods can be separated into groups. Half of your food intake should be complex carbohydrates such as pasta and wholemeal bread. Eat five portions of vegetables and fruit a day: choose a multicoloured range for a variety of nutrients. Meat, eggs, dairy products and nuts should be eaten in moderation; sugar, butter and oils should be limited.

Nutrition is playing an increasing role in medicine, as food contains many different substances vital to your health. Most people know about vitamins and minerals, but what about essential fatty acids and bioflavonoids? Understanding the variety of benefits in food and relating these to the food groups is the first step in creating a healthy diet for yourself.

Many people think that vitamin and mineral supplements can compensate for an inadequate diet. They do have a role to play at times of stress or when taking certain medicines, which can interact with foods (see p.244), as well as when treating a few rare disorders. In the long term, however, a wholesome diet gives you the complete range and balance of nutrients that you need. Specialists believe that there are many as yet unknown nutrients essential to health, and these are not provided in supplements.

The key to a diet that makes you feel healthy is not just to vary what you eat, but also to increase the proportion of plant foods you eat while you decrease your intake of meat products. Grains and pasta are loaded with complex carbohydrates, and whenever you eat a mixture of fresh fruit and vegetables, you treat yourself to a cocktail of nutrients.

HOW YOU EAT

It is better to eat several light meals a day, rather than a large lunch and dinner, which are hard to digest and can make you sleepy. Little digestion occurs during sleep, so try to eat your evening meal at least two hours before going to bed and give your metabolism time to wake up in the morning before having breakfast. Carbohydrates from fruit, toast or cereals are much easier to digest than a high-protein, cooked breakfast.

Grazing is more natural than gorging. Stave off hunger pangs with fruit or nuts in the mid-morning and afternoon. Eating little and often keeps your blood sugar levels even and stops you having mood swings and peaks and troughs in energy and concentration. Exercise helps to stabilize your appetite, too. Combined with suitable eating habits, it is the best way to maintain your correct weight.

Follow these dietary guidelines:
■ Eat three or more pieces of fresh fruit and a salad each day, varying their colour.
■ Choose whole, organic items rather than refined, processed foods that are full of additives. However, it is better to eat inorganic fruit and vegetables than none at all; peel or remove outer leaves, then wash the items to reduce chemical residues.

NUTRITION FOR CHILDREN

The basics of nutrition apply whatever your age or sex, but children and teenagers usually need more nutrients than adults do to help them grow. Boys and girls need more zinc, calcium, magnesium, biotin, essential fatty acids and vitamins A, D and B_6. Adding a tablespoon of ground seeds to cereal provides zinc, magnesium and the essential fatty acids; eating five portions of fresh fruit and vegetables daily in place of sugary, fatty, salty foods should supply the other nutrients. Your doctor can advise you on giving children supplements.

The best way to instil good eating habits in children is to set an example yourself; the visible results of a healthy diet – vitality and healthy hair, skin and nails – can help prove your point. Home-cooked meals eaten together promote enjoyment of food and are much less expensive than take-aways. Follow these suggestions for children:

■ Put a jug of water on the table so that children drink that, or diluted fruit juice, rather than sugary fizzy drinks.

■ Food manufacturers overload breakfast cereals with sugar. Prevent your children from developing a sweet tooth at an early age by giving them oats or sugar-free cornflakes or muesli; most health-food shops sell organic versions.

■ Bananas, dates and dried apricots are nutritious snacks that satisfy children's desire for sweetness. Unsalted nuts are also healthy – and popular.

■ Provide appetizing vegetables with each meal such as strips of red, yellow and green peppers, cucumber chunks, baked potatoes, roast parsnips or grated red cabbage or carrots.

■ To preserve nutrients, buy small amounts of fresh food often.
■ What matters is what you do most of the time – there is no need to worry about the occasional lapse. Aim to enjoy your food without becoming obsessive.

TYPES OF DIET

In the face of epidemic proportions of "diseases of affluence" in the West, such as strokes, asthma and various cancers, there is a greater interest in foods that nourish

Japanese cookery – like that of Indian, Thai and Korean cultures – follows the tradition of eating family meals based on carbohydrates and vegetables, with meat as a flavouring rather than a staple ingredient. Diet is thought to be a factor in the low rate of heart attack among the Japanese; however, with Western influences, it is catching up on those living in Great Britain and the United States.

the body and mind. The growing number of ethnic restaurants and shops and international ingredients in supermarkets mean that everyone can benefit from cuisines from other countries.

Mediterranean eating habits result in populations with a lower incidence of heart disease and cancers, and much research has been done on the diet. People in the Mediterranean region eat large quantities of fruit, vegetables and salads – their climate allows them to grow, for example, aubergines, tomatoes, figs and peaches. They also eat more fish and seafood and less red meat than their northern counterparts; and olive oil is used for cooking instead of butter or hydrogenated fats. The population eats fewer processed and refined foods. Dishes are flavoured with lashings of garlic, which protects the heart and helps ward off cancer, and garnished with leafy basil.

By the time pasta and rice dishes are adapted in northern Europe and the United States, the proportion of sauce, often meaty, to carbohydrate increases. Take a leaf out of the Mediterranean cookbooks and be generous with the pasta and sparing with the sauce, basing the latter on olive oil, vegetables, herbs and garlic rather than animal protein.

Equally nutritious dishes come from the other side of the Mediterranean, for example, Turkish hummus and stuffed vine leaves and Moroccan couscous. All the ingredients are in supermarkets to make at home or buy ready prepared.

FREE RADICALS

One consequence of an unhealthy diet that includes fried or burnt foods, is the production of free radicals – unstable molecules that are responsible for causing cancer, artery damage, aging and inflammation. Free radicals are by-products of normal metabolism and are part of the body's natural defence against disease. However, they are dangerous when the body makes too many of them as a result of oxygen oxidizing molecules. It is not just poor nutrition that oxidizes free radicals. Pollution, such as exhaust fumes from petrol, radiation, sunlight, cigarette smoke, illness or excessive exercise can also take their toll.

ANTIOXIDANTS

The body protects itself from free radicals by producing chemicals known as anti-oxidants to mop them up and make them harmless. Balancing the two can protect your health. Improving your diet can tip the balance in your favour.

Some antioxidants are known essential nutrients. These include vitamin A, betacarotene and other carotenoids, which protect the body against digestive and lung cancers, and vitamin C, which defends against cancers of the mouth, throat, cervix and breast; hence, the advice to eat so much fresh fruit and vegetables, which are loaded with this vitamin. Vitamin E seems to stave off heart disease, so eat more "seed foods" such as sunflower oil, nuts and broad beans. Low levels of vitamins A and E are associated with Alzheimer's disease; a lack of vitamins C and E, with cataracts.

Minerals such as selenium, copper and zinc (all three are in shellfish and can be found in avocados, nuts and seeds) also neutralize free radicals. Watermelon contains zinc, selenium, betacarotene and vitamins C and E, so it is an excellent choice when available. Alternatively, take a supplement, especially if you are middle aged or older, live in a city or polluted area, you smoke or have sunbathed.

Antioxidants also boost your immune system and, therefore, your resistance to disease. They have been shown to reduce the symptoms of AIDS (see pp.150–51). Antioxidants increase fertility, reduce colds and respiratory infections and play a part in myalgic encephalomyelitis (ME).

BIOFLAVONOIDS

Some antioxidants belong to the group known as bioflavonoids. Apart from citrus fruit, good sources of bioflavonoids include rosehips, berries, cherries, grapes, papaya, melon, plums, tomatoes, broccoli, tea and red wine. They have many roles in maintaining good health:

■ Bioflavonoids boost the activity of vitamin C and strengthen the walls of the tiny blood capillaries. They can help rectify bleeding gums, varicose veins, haemorrhoids, bruises, strain injuries and thrombosis.

■ They bind to toxic metals and escort them from the body.

■ They have anti-infection and anti-carcinogenic properties. Bioflavonoids in cucumbers stop cancer-causing hormones binding to cells.

Bioflavonoids and other antioxidants – over 100 have been discovered and there are bound to be more – are called phyto-chemicals. Although our lives may not depend on them, they affect the body's biochemistry and, like vitamins, are not stored. The best way to benefit from these semi-essential nutrients is to enjoy a wide variety of fresh, raw or lightly cooked plant foods. ■

VEGETARIAN PROS AND CONS

Vegetarians avoid meat products for humanitarian or health reasons. Some do not eat meat or fish but do include eggs and dairy products in their diet; vegans eat only foods of plant origin. These people are about 40 percent less likely to develop cancer at an early age than meat eaters. Vegetarians generally eat more fibre and complex carbohydrates and less saturated fat, so they tend to be slimmer than meat eaters, with lower levels of blood cholesterol and heart disease. The exception, for reasons that are not clear, is the vegetarian Asian population in Great Britain, which has a high rate of heart disease.

Vegetarians following a properly balanced diet do not usually lack nutrients. Mixing cereals and pulses (in a dish such as curried lentils with brown rice) provides as much protein as meat, and iron, calcium and folic acid are available in dark green leafy vegetables, nuts and seeds. Vegans may lack vitamin B_{12} and should eat foods fortified with it, such as soya milk and yeast extract, or take a supplement. So long as they are exposed to sunshine they should get enough vitamin D.

Macrobiotic diets are based on the Japanese Zen philosophy and aim to balance the yin (feminine) and yang (masculine) properties of food. In its purest form, the diet consists solely of brown rice, which can result in malnutrition. Less extreme versions do reduce the risks of obesity, raised blood pressure and cholesterol, constipation and cancer, but these benefits can be obtained, without loss of vital nutrients, from vegan or vegetarian diets that are not so restrictive.

HOW MEDICATION INTERACTS WITH DIET

Some medicines can deplete certain nutrients. Conversely, certain foods in your diet can have a negative effect on some medicines. Always consult your practitioner or chemist about any possible dietary concerns.

Type of drug and its use	Potential deficiency	Foods to eat or avoid
Antacids Indigestion, heartburn and stomach ulcers	Can interfere with the absorption of phosphate and other minerals.	Eat meat, fish and eggs. Take medicine an hour after eating.
Laxatives Constipation	May cause dehydration and deplete potassium; reduce absorption of almost every nutrient.	Instead of medicine, eat a fibre-rich diet that includes prunes and figs or use a bulk laxative such as bran, psyllium seeds or ispaghula.
Anticoagulants Stroke, thrombosis and blood-clotting disorders	Reduce levels of vitamin K.	Do not take vitamin A or C supplements, which can reduce effectiveness, or vitamin E, which can cause bleeding problems.
Lipid-lowerers Reduce cholesterol levels	Can lower levels of iron and folate.	Take iron and folate supplements; reduce saturated fats and cholesterol.
Antibacterials and antibiotics Bacterial infections	Destroy beneficial bacteria found in your digestive system.	Eat yoghurt containing live cultures (but first check with your doctor).
Antifungals Candidiasis (thrush)	Reduce amount of vitamins B_2 and B_6.	Eat wholegrains, meat, eggs and dairy produce.
Antimalarials Malaria	Reduce folate; do not take if pregnant or elderly.	Take folic acid supplement; eat green leafy vegetables and pulses.
Diuretics Fluid retention – increase output of urine	Reduce levels of minerals such as potassium and calcium.	Take mineral supplements (but first check with your doctor).
The oral contraceptive pill Contraception and endometriosis	Reduces the absorption of folate, vitamin B_6 and other nutrients.	See "Antimalarials" above for folate; eat eggs and dairy products.
Nonsteroidal anti-inflammatory drugs Rheumatoid arthritis	Lower amount of folate.	See "Antimalarials" above for folate; do not take iron, calcium or vitamin C supplements.
Steroids Long-term anti-inflammatories	Can cause deficiency of calcium, vitamin K, potassium and protein.	Eat dairy products and meats, green vegetables, beans, potatoes, nuts, pulses and seeds.
Anticonvulsants Epilepsy and psychiatric disorders	Lower amount of folate and other B vitamins.	Take supplements or eat oily fish, eggs, dairy produce and leafy vegetables.
Drugs for Parkinson's disease such as L-dopa (levodopa)		Avoid supplements of vitamin B_6 or phenylalanine (an amino acid).
Cytoxics Cancer – chemotherapy		Eat a nourishing well-balanced diet; avoid folic acid supplements.

CAUTION

If you are ill or recovering from an injury such as a broken leg, you need extra protein to repair the damage. Breast-feeding women also need extra protein. Ask your doctor for specific advice.

Protein

One of the necessary components of your diet is protein, and experts recommend that it should make up 10–15 percent of your daily food intake – whether from meat or by combining vegetarian products.

Every cell of the body relies on protein for growth, maintenance and repair. Enzymes, an important group of proteins, also play a role in triggering energy release, in helping the digestion of food, in producing hormones and antibodies and in the excretion of waste.

Protein is composed of amino acids, themselves made up of carbon, hydrogen, oxygen and nitrogen, the four elements vital for life. Protein molecules consist of various arrangements of amino acid units, each with a specific function. For example, collagen makes hair and skin strong and elastic, and haemoglobin is an oxygen-binding protein in the blood.

PROTEIN IN THE DIET

Although the human body can make many of the amino acids itself, eight of them can be obtained only from food. The food sources are divided into two categories: high-quality sources provide complete protein; low-quality sources have only some of the amino acids. However, combining low-quality sources can supply complete protein.

Meat, poultry, fish, eggs and soya beans are classed as high-quality sources. Nuts, pulses, bread, rice, pasta and potatoes are considered low-quality sources. There are many traditional dishes that successfully combine vegetable proteins such as the Indian dahl and rice, the Asian dishes combining tofu, rice and vegetables and the Mexican refried beans and corn tortillas. These all have as high a quality of protein as meat, but without the undesirable saturated fat.

Males require 55 g (2 ounces) of protein a day, while females need about 45 g (1½ ounces). Two servings of a plant-based protein, or one portion of animal protein provides these needs.

In the West, consuming too much protein is more of a concern than eating too little. The body cannot store it, so the liver converts the excess into glucose. The process can strain the liver and kidneys and lead to acidic urine. The loss of calcium involved may increase the risk of osteoporosis. High-protein foods are rich in calories and fats, so too much leads to unwanted weight gain. ∎

FOOD COMBINING – THE HAY DIET

Food combining, developed by the American Dr Hay in the 1930s, works on the premise that you should eat proteins and carbohydrates separately because they have different digestive requirements. You could eat a baked potato with butter, for example, but not with cheese; chicken with broccoli, but not rice.

Dr Hay also divided foods into alkaline – vegetables and salad, most fruit and milk – and acidic types: animal protein, nuts and citrus fruit. He recommended including four times as many alkaline foods as acidic, which has the benefit of reducing the amount of refined and processed products and saturated fats in the diet. The basic rules are:

■ Eat carbohydrates separately from protein and acidic fruit.

■ Form the bulk of your diet from vegetables, salad and fruit.

■ Eat small amounts of protein, carbohydrate and fat.

■ Leave four or more hours between meals.

SEE ALSO
You are what you eat
240–244

CAUTION

Liver is a rich source of retinol (vitamin A). However, pregnant women should avoid eating liver because excessive amounts of retinol are associated with damage to the foetus. Pregnant and would-be pregnant women should not take doses of vitamin A in excess of 3000 mcg.

Vitamins and minerals

You need some of at least 30 identified vitamins and minerals to stay mentally and physically healthy. Most people absorb enough vitamins and minerals through a varied diet – deficiencies are usually rare.

The World Health Organization and other agencies have come up with a list of recommended daily allowances (RDAs), also called reference nutrient intakes (RNIs), but nutritionists advise that these levels are only the minimum necessary for most people. To be truly healthy you may need selected nutrients in greater quantities – but just how much is open to vigorous debate. The ideal amount of a particular vitamin or mineral for you will depend on your physical and mental state, age and sex.

Your body cannot function without vitamins. Although they are needed in only small amounts, they are vital to trigger enzyme functions, which prompt other activities in the body.

The B complex vitamins (a group of vitamins) and vitamin C are water soluble (they dissolve in water). Apart from B_{12}, they cannot be stored by your body. Antibiotics, alcohol and stress inhibit absorption of these vitamins.

Vitamins A, D, E and K are fat soluble and can be stored by your body. They are

VITAMIN SOURCES AND FUNCTIONS

Vitamin	Role	Found in	Signs of deficiency	RDA
Vitamin A	Vital to growth and night vision; protects the lining of the digestive, urinary and respiratory tracts from infection.	Retinol in liver, egg yolks, dairy products and oily fish. Betacarotene in plant foods, especially green and yellow vegetables, particularly carrots.	Eye disorders, including night blindness, greater risk of infection and skin that is dry and rough.	Women 600 mcg; breast-feeding women 950 mcg; men 700 mcg
Vitamin B₁ (Thiamine)	Helps trigger enzyme function; vital for muscles, nervous system and heart function.	Wholewheat, enriched cereals, brown rice, pasta, beans, pork, eggs and some nuts.	Irritability, tiredness, loss of appetite and sleep problems; high sugar diets and an overactive thyroid can lead to deficiency.	Women 0.8 mg; men 1 mg
Vitamin B₂ (Riboflavin, also called vitamin G)	Helps the production of hormones; triggers various enzyme functions.	Liver, poultry, milk, eggs and wholegrains.	Skin problems; people taking contraceptive pills and antidepressants may be more susceptible.	Women 1.1 mg; men 1.3 mg
Niacin (Nicotinic acid, a B complex vitamin)	Metabolizes carbohydrates and fats; helps nervous and digestive systems; maintains skin.	Oily fish, white meat of poultry, liver, dried beans and nuts.	Skin problems, such as cracking of the skin, tiredness and depression.	Women 13 mg; men 17 mg

VITAMIN SOURCES AND FUNCTIONS continued

Vitamin	Role	Found in	Signs of deficiency	RDA
Pantothenic acid (One of the B complex vitamins)	Helps metabolize energy and triggers enzyme functions; assists nervous system functions; helps produce sex hormones.	Most vegetables, animal products and cereals; especially offal, fish, egg yolks, wholegrains and green vegetables.	Muscle spasms, exhaustion, nausea, abdominal pain, headaches, numbness and tingling.	3–7 mg
Vitamin B$_6$ (Pyridoxine)	Helps enzyme functions; makes red blood cells and antibodies; assists the nervous and digestive systems; maintains skin.	Soya and other dried beans, chicken, pork, fish, wholegrains, bananas and potatoes.	Irritability and depression, weakness, anaemia and skin problems, including cracked lips, and inflamed mouth and tongue.	Women 1.2 mg; men 1.4 mg
Vitamin B$_{12}$ (Cyanocobalamin)	Vital for growth; forms red blood cells; stimulates the nervous system; helps enzyme functions.	Animal foods, including poultry, beef, pork, eggs, fish and milk, and fortified breakfast cereals.	Anaemia, sore mouth and tongue, depression, numbness and tingling, nervous system damage.	1.5 mcg
Vitamin C (Ascorbic acid)	Antioxidant; prevents infection; heals wounds; helps form collagen (for healthy bones, nails, teeth and gums); and assists absorption of iron.	Citrus fruit, potatoes, green peppers, green leafy vegetables, tomatoes and some berries (cooking or processing foods depletes vitamin).	Weakness, swollen gums, aches and pains; if severe, scurvy (symptoms are spongy gums and loose teeth and bleeding into the skin).	40 mg; smokers at least 80 mg
Vitamin D (Calciferols)	Absorbs calcium and phosphorus (for healthy bones and teeth).	Sunlight on exposed skin, oily fish, egg yolks and fortified dairy products, breakfast cereals and margarine.	Rickets (soft, deformed bones in children), weakened bones in the elderly.	Enough made from exposure to sunlight; if confined indoors, 10 mcg.
Vitamin E (Tocopherol)	Protects lungs and other tissues from pollutants; maintains red blood cells and enzyme functions.	Margarines, vegetable oils, oily fish, egg yolks, green leafy vegetables and nuts.	Anaemia; irritability and fluid accumulation in infants.	Women at least 3 mg; men at least 4 mg
Vitamin K (Phylloquinone)	Promotes blood clotting by helping liver produce certain substances.	Green leafy vegetables, egg yolks, cheese, pork and liver.	Nose bleeds, bleeding gums and excessive bleeding from wounds.	1 mcg for each kg (2.2 lb) of body weight.
Folic acid (Folate)	Crucial before and during pregnancy for nerve and brain development; forms red blood cells and helps the functioning of the nervous system.	Green leafy vegetables, dried beans and peas, egg yolks, avocados, mushrooms, liver and wholemeal bread.	Anaemia, exhaustion, depression and skin problems such as sores near the mouth; poor growth in children.	200 mcg; pregnant women 300 mcg (plus 400 mcg supplement in first 12 weeks).
Biotin	Essential for digestion and in triggering various enzyme functions.	Dried beans, grapefruit, bananas, mushrooms, egg yolks and peanuts.	Hair loss, poor appetite, exhaustion, eczema and inflamed tongue.	10–200 mcg

best taken with foods containing oils and fats. They need efficient bile function for good absorption.

Your body will not work without minerals, although they represent only 3–4 percent of your body weight. Many people are often short of vital minerals, especially zinc, iron and calcium. These minerals are plentiful in a diet that con-tains good quantities of dairy products, vegetables and seeds. However, since minerals come from the ground via plants in the first place, it follows that degraded soils (especially when poorly farmed) will be mineral-deficient. Processed foods may have minerals extracted; conversely, they may have them added (sometimes by law, as in the case of breakfast cereals). ▪

MINERAL SOURCES AND FUNCTIONS

Mineral	Role	Found in	Deficiency symptoms	RDA
Calcium	Promotes strong bones; vital for cell, muscle and nervous system functions and for blood clotting.	Dairy foods, green leafy vegetables, sesame seeds and fish eaten with bones such as sardines.	Bone fractures, rickets (soft, deformed bones in children) and osteo-porosis in adults.	700 mg; breast-feeding women 1250 mg
Magnesium	Good for healthy bones, teeth, muscles and nervous system.	Fish, wholegrain cereals, nuts, milk, soya beans and green leafy vegetables.	Muscle twitches, heart palpitations, restlessness and anxiety.	Women 270 mg; men 300 mg
Phosphorus	Vital for healthy bones and teeth and helps maintain body fluids.	Most foods, especially meat, poultry, fish and dairy products.	Bone pain and weakness.	550 mg
Potassium	Maintains water balance and helps heart rhythm, muscle contractions and nervous system.	Avocado, citrus fruit, bananas, wholegrains, green leafy vegetables and pulses.	Fatigue, confusion, muscle weakness and irregular heartbeat.	3500 mg
Sodium	Regulates water balance and heart rhythm; helps muscles and nerves.	Table salt (found in many processed foods).	Muscle cramps, weakness and dizziness.	1600 mg
Selenium	Antioxidant, protects cells from free radical damage.	Dairy products, meat, fish, and wholegrains.	No known adverse effects on health.	Women 60 mcg; men 75 mcg
Zinc	Vital for growth, healing and hormones; promotes many enzyme functions.	Oysters, red meat, whole-grain cereals, wholemeal bread and dried beans.	Appetite loss; if severe, hair loss, inflamed skin, mouth and eyelids.	Women 7 mg; men 9.5 mg
Iron	Helps form haemoglobin, which carries oxygen, and certain enzymes.	Lean meats, green leafy vegetables, nuts, beans and fortified cereals.	Anaemia and fatigue.	Women 14.8 mg; men 8.7 mg
Manganese	Triggers enzymes that produce energy; helps make bones and tendons.	Pulses, nuts and fortified cereals.	No known adverse effects on health.	1.4 mg

SEE ALSO
Vitamins and minerals
246–248

Supplements

Food supplements are vitamins and minerals sold as tablets, liquids, powders or capsules. Sometimes the term is used more widely to include products containing vegetable extracts, herbs, amino acids and fish oils.

If you were born healthy and eat a balanced diet rich in nutrients, drink plenty of water and take regular exercise, you should be able to manage perfectly well without taking supplements. However, all too often the diet and lifestyle of many people living in industrialized countries are less than perfect, especially because a large part of their food is processed, which depletes it of essential nutrients and adds fats and sugars. Wheat is a prime example: 25 nutrients are taken out during refining to make white flour,

but just four – iron, vitamins B_1 and B_2 and niacin – go back in.

Government recommended daily allowances (RDAs) tend to be based on the minimum amounts necessary for survival, with an added margin for safety. The ones given on food labels do not take into account personal circumstances that affect nutritional needs such as age, body size, sex, health, income and stress.

Nevertheless, the claims for the benefits of supplements are increasingly exaggerated. Vitamin and mineral deficiencies are rare, and too much of some vitamins, such as A and D, can be harmful. People on very poor diets or with certain health problems, such as malabsorption, are the ones more likely to need supplements.

Many supplements provide the RDAs of vitamins and minerals or a higher dose. Others include substances known to be important to health, which do not yet have an RDA. In Great Britain look for products that carry the Health Food Manufacturers' Association (HFMA) sign.

Supplements are packaged – coating materials keep out moisture and make them easy to swallow. Colours, sweeteners and flavours make them palatable.

TIPS FOR TAKING SUPPLEMENTS

- Your skin will turn yellow with excess betacarotene. To regain your normal colour, reduce your intake.

- Vitamin C in quantity is a laxative: build up levels gradually. If you have stomach acidity problems, take the alkaline-forming "ascorbate" vitamin C between meals.

- Niacin can make you flushed and itchy at the start; vitamin B_2 (riboflavin) makes your urine bright yellow – this is normal.

- When on antibiotics, increase doses of the B complex vitamins. You should also eat live yoghurt (especially if you have previously experienced thrush problems, pp.142–43) or take "probiotic" supplements.

- If you are on the contraceptive pill or hormone replacement therapy, take B_6, B_{12}, folic acid and zinc supplements.

- If you are on antidepressants, anticonvulsants or drugs to thin your blood, seek medical advice before taking supplements.

- Beware of excessive doses if you are combining multivitamin preparations. Add up your total daily intake in each case.

WHEN AND HOW TO TAKE THEM
Take supplements at regular intervals during the day, with or after meals, so they are absorbed with food and liquids. If you must take them all together, do so after your biggest meal of the day.

If one form of a supplement does not agree with you, try another. Tablets have the longest shelf life, but powders are usually the purest form and most suitable for people with allergies. ∎

Understanding fats

There are good and bad fats. Most people who follow the standard Western diet consume excessive quantities of bad fats, which are saturated, and take in too few unsaturated fats – the good fats.

Fats, which are made of fatty acids, have many functions: among these, they absorb the fat-soluble vitamins (see pp.246–48) and betacarotene (the body converts this into vitamin A), promote childhood development and help to produce sex hormones and regulate the body's metabolism. Although saturated fats (which are solid at room temperature, with the exception of palm and coconut oils) and transfatty acids can raise your blood cholesterol levels, unsaturated fats lower blood cholesterol levels or have no effect on them.

Because fat, at 9 calories per gram, has twice the amount of calories as protein and carbohydrates, a diet high in fat can lead to a weight problem. In Great Britain people consume almost half their calories as fat – and mostly the wrong type. Experts agree that 35 percent of our calorie intake should be from total fats, with most of these from unsaturated fats. Unsaturated fats are broken down into monounsaturates and polyunsaturates.

MONOUNSATURATES

Also known as Omega-9 fatty acids, monounsaturates are considered "good" because they have no negative effect on health and can be used to replace "bad" saturated fats. Olive oil, which is 80 percent linoleic acid (see below), is at the top of the list of monounsaturated fats.

Mediterranean diets use olive oil rather than processed fats, and people from those countries have notably lower rates of cardiovascular disease. Claims for olive oil include reducing gastric acidity, preventing constipation, stimulating bile secretions and promoting bone growth. The best olive oil, in regard to both taste and nutrition, is cold pressed, unrefined oil from a single source.

POLYUNSATURATES

Two families of essential fatty acids make up the polyunsaturates: Omega-6, or linoleic acid, and Omega-3, or linolenic acid. These must be supplied by your diet because they are not made by the body.

Gamma-linolenic acid (GLA) is a substance the body produces naturally by

---

WHAT IS CHOLESTEROL?

There are two types of cholesterol: dietary and blood. Every day the liver makes about 1 g of blood cholesterol, a waxy material that is found in all body cells. This amount is essential, but more can be harmful. Eating large amounts of dietary cholesterol does not necessarily lead to high levels of blood cholesterol, a major cause of heart disease. In fact, heredity plays a far greater part in determining cholesterol levels.

However, if you suffer from heart disease, you should cut back on saturated fats, such as bacon, meat pies, butter and cakes, to lower your blood cholesterol. Instead, eat more foods that contain soluble fibre, such as oats and dried and citrus fruits. Garlic can help, either in cooking or taken as a supplement, because it seems to slow down the liver's production of cholesterol.

Although egg yolks, offal and prawns are high in dietary cholesterol, recent studies suggest that eating them does not raise blood cholesterol levels.

converting linoleic acid. GLA, in turn, is
eventually converted into series 1 prostaglandins, which are vital for health. They
do not survive long, so you need to maintain your levels daily. Benefits include
fewer circulatory disorders, reduced
inflammation and improved sugar and
water balance in the digestive system.

The body makes series 3 prostaglandins
from converted linolenic acid. They are
vital in brain function as well as circulatory problems, vision, water balance, a
sound immune system and many other
aspects of a healthy body. Eating oily fish
rich in associated acids maintains the
levels and helps the body bypass some
of the conversion processes.

BUYING THE RIGHT FATS

Watch out for manufacturers' claims
about the levels of fats in their products,
as they can be misleading. Reduced fat is
not the same as low fat. For the levels of
fat to be reduced, the rules say that there
should be at least 25 percent less fat than
in a normal serving of the food. However,
there can still be a great deal of fat in a
single serving. Bear in mind, too, that less
fat may mean more sugar to add flavour.
Foods can have reduced fat but still have
a high calorie count.

Treat terms such as light (or "lite"),
economy and low fat with caution. Per
100 g (3½ oz), 20 g (¾ oz) is a large
amount of fat; 3 g (⅛ oz) is a little. ∎

A GUIDE TO GOOD FATS AND BAD FATS

Type of fatty acid	Food source	Role
Saturated (Bad)	Butter, hard cheese, cream, palm and coconut oils, hard margarine and solid cooking fats, fatty meat products, such as hamburgers, bacon, sausages, frankfurters, salami and meat pâté, biscuits, cakes, chocolates and pastries.	Not required in the diet because the body can make its own, but it adds flavour to food. Too much saturated fat can lead to obesity, athero-sclerosis, heart disease and cancer of the breast, bowel and pancreas.
Monounsaturated Omega-9 (Good)	Olive oil, rapeseed oil, avocados, nuts and seeds.	Not necessary nutritionally, but many foods that contain monounsaturated fatty acids also have essential polyunsaturated ones; rapeseed oil is one example.
Polyunsaturated Omega-6 (Derived from linoleic acid; **essential**)	Vegetable oils, particularly corn, safflower and soya oils.	Necessary for healthy growth and develop-ment; deficiency can inhibit growth and the functioning of the immune system and lead to skin disorders and blood clots.
Omega-3 (Derived from linolenic acid; **essential**)	Oily fish, such as sardines, mackerel and herrings, walnuts and rapeseed oil.	Needed for early development of the brain and retina of the eye; reduces inflammation and tendency of the blood to clot; can be helpful for treating heart disease, psoriasis and arthritis.
Trans (Bad)	Meat and meat products; dairy products; processed foods such as crisps, biscuits, cakes and sweet and savoury pies; margarines and fats commercially hardened to prevent them from turning rancid.	Not essential to the diet; transfatty acids in processed food have been linked to heart disease. Frying food in transfatty acids, such as margarine, can turn good fats into bad, so use olive or other vegetable oils.

CAUTION

Excessive sucrose contributes to health problems, including obesity, tooth decay, kidney problems, gastrointestinal and cardiovascular diseases, depression or hyperactivity in children, allergy and even some types of criminal behaviour. The only people who benefit from sucrose are those with a low blood sugar condition, which requires medical advice.

Carbohydrates

In all but the most specialist diets, carbohydrates provide the greatest number of calories. They range from "simple" sugars to more "complex" starch and provide energy and bulk.

In the average diet, starch accounts for 50 percent of carbohydrate intake, sucrose (table sugar) 30 percent, lactose (milk sugar) 10 percent and the remaining 10 percent a mixture of other sugars.

Carbohydrates burn at different rates in the body. You gain a quick response from simple carbohydrates, such as brown and white sugar, honey, refined products and sweets, and a slow release from complex carbohydrates, which are found in foods such as vegetables, pasta, rice and grains.

Ideally, complex carbohydrates should provide two-thirds of your calories. They release their sugar content gradually, providing energy over a longer period. They also help keep your blood sugar levels, weight and energy constant. You can receive good quantities of complex carbohydrates from potatoes, parsnips and beans of most sorts (but not baked beans).

Simple carbohydrates have become part of many diets only in the last 150 years, bringing with them new diseases. They are damaging to teeth, and they may take the place of healthier foods loaded with nutrients. If you want a quick boost from healthy simple carbohydrates, try cooked root vegetables or some fruit.

REFINED SUGAR

Table sugar (sucrose) is a refined carbohydrate that consists of two simple sugars: glucose and fructose (sugar from fruit), which are naturally joined. Most sugar in Western diets comes from cane sugar, but high quantities are also present in syrups and fruits such as figs and dates.

An intake of sugary foods gives you calories in abundance. Despite the instant energy boost, you receive no essential nutrients, hence the term "empty calories". White sugar, for instance, has had all but 10 percent of its vitamins and minerals removed. These calories are usually processed by the body into fat for long-term energy supplies, unless you take a great deal of exercise to burn them up.

Sucrose is a major part of many processed foods. It is a preservative, binds foods together and disguises many unpalatable aspects, especially of refined foods. By reducing your sucrose intake you can benefit your health and well-being. These will be further enhanced if you increase your fibre intake instead. ■

THE SUGAR FAMILY

Simple sugars are quickly digested. These simple carbohydrates include glucose and fructose, which can be found in certain foods such as fruit, honey and corn products. They also encompass lactose, uniquely found in milk and derivative products; maltose, which is contained in malt extract and malted wheat and barley; sucrose and dextrose, found in white and brown sugar, many soft drinks, sweets, chocolate and other processed foods (read the ingredients on the label for hidden sugars); and overcooked grains. They have little nutritional value.

Starches and fibre are sugars found in complex carbohydrates, which are slowly digested and have high nutritional value. Grains, potatoes and other vegetables, beans and pulses such as lentils are all examples of complex carbohydrates.

Fibre

A healthy diet will include fibre, a natural part of plant foods. It comes from the cell walls of the plants — the older the plant, the tougher the fibre. The more you cook food, the more you reduce the fibre content.

SEE ALSO

Constipation   88
Irritable bowel syndrome
    98–99

CAUTION

A number of people cannot tolerate high-fibre diets. These include those with diverticular disease, inflammatory bowel disease and certain kinds of irritable bowel syndrome.

There are two types of fibre: soluble and insoluble. Many foods, particularly wholegrains, contain both. Soluble fibre includes most fruits and vegetables, pulses and oats. These foods slow the absorption of carbohydrates and slowly release sugars into the bloodstream. Insoluble fibre includes nuts, bran, rice and fruit peel. It passes through the intestine unchanged, but is a vital link in the digestive process.

Although fibre has almost no nutritional value in itself, it is vital for digestion. The more fibre you eat, the more water your digestive tract is able to absorb. This increases the bulk of the faeces, which can then pass through the body more easily and comfortably. High fibre intake also aids blood sugar control and lowers the cholesterol count by helping the body excrete the substance. As a bonus, fibre is filling, which encourages the health-conscious to resist sugary and fatty refined foods.

Eating plenty of fibre and drinking at least a litre (about two pints) of water a day, combined with a little exercise, can boost a sluggish digestive system. Although the Department of Health suggests we need at least 18 g (⅝ oz) of fibre a day, some nutritionists urge that we eat up to 35 g (1¼ oz) a day from a variety of sources.

Whatever levels you aim for, most healthy digestive systems would benefit from more fibre than they receive in the average Western diet. Diets deficient in fibre can leave you susceptible to diabetes, heart disease and intestinal disorders such as bowel cancer, diverticular disease, gallstones and constipation.

CHANGING YOUR DIET

If you suddenly switch to a high-fibre diet, having habitually eaten little, your body can take time to adapt to its new fuel. You may experience flatulence and digestive discomfort. Increase your fibre intake gradually, beginning with soluble fibre, and drink more water than you think you need, preferably between meals. If you have problems with one type of fibrous food, try another, and keep your diet as varied as possible.

The most common cause of fibre discomfort is wheat bran (which can also reduce the absorption of essential minerals, especially zinc). Children on a high-fibre diet are sometimes found to be deficient in calcium, particularly if they are not regular milk drinkers.

Many people who have problems when they suddenly change to a high-fibre diet are more likely to be dealing with conditions associated with their previous high-sugar, high-fat diet. It can take the body time to adapt, but it is worth persevering for long-term health benefits. ∎

INSOLUBLE FIBRE

SOLUBLE FIBRE

Water

Our most important nutrient, water makes up nearly two-thirds of our bodies. Without sufficient quantities of water, all essential bodily functions quickly come to a halt, followed by death within days.

While the body can survive for long periods without food, the same does not go for liquids. A healthy person on a normal diet might expect to process about 3 litres (5¼ pt) of fluid a day. Up to two-thirds of this may be taken directly, as water, tea or coffee, soft drinks, juices or alcohol. The remaining one-third is contributed to by vegetables and fruits, as well as less obvious sources such as dairy products, bread and cereals and, in small quantities, pulses, poultry, meat and fish. The body also makes its own water as it burns glucose to produce energy.

Climate and activity can affect fluid requirements. Normally the body loses 1.5 litres (2¾ pt) from breathing, sweating, processing food and excreting waste and toxic substances through the kidneys. People sweat more in heat and when they take exercise. But it is also easy to become dehydrated without realizing it when running a fever or in extreme cold.

British water is considered perfectly drinkable. However, anxieties about quality are reflected in the amount of bottled water sold, still and carbonated.

British minimum standards for drinking water are set by the Water Quality Regulations. These establish legal levels of micro-organisms, chemical residues, pesticides and fertilizers. The Regulations also stipulate what the authorities may add legally, such as chlorine for cleanliness, fluoride to harden tooth enamel and prevent decay and aluminium sulphate to remove suspended waste.

Water quality varies according to the area and over a period of time. Hard water seems to be healthier: it contains less salt than soft water and higher levels of calcium and magnesium. If you are worried about water taste or suspected pollutants, contact the Environmental Health Officer or local water supplier.

BUYING OR FILTERING WATER

Bought "mineral" water must by law be taken from "a naturally protected source of constant composition and free from all traces of pollution", so that it needs no further processing before drinking. Even so, the quality is variable. People on low-salt diets should check the label to see if the water contains 20mg sodium per litre or less. Over 200mg is high for anyone.

You can filter water, although many natural beneficial minerals disappear along with the impurities. The simplest carbon filter removes chlorine and any solids, while the most sophisticated deal with almost all bacteria, as well as chemicals and minerals. Use filtered water at once and change the filter regularly. ∎

If you do not wish to drink water from the tap, you can buy it from a shop. Bottled water may not be healthier than water from the mains, but you may prefer the flavour. It may contain higher levels of bacteria than tap water, as well as nitrates and other chemicals in varying degrees.

DEHYDRATION ALERT

Signs of dehydration include very dark urine, nausea, dizziness, headache, poor concentration, exhaustion and disorientation. For those susceptible to a build up of calcium and other chemicals, a shortage of fluids can lead to kidney stones – insoluble crystals that form in the kidney and cause acute pain.

CAUTION

To avoid becoming drunk:
- *Never drink without a food or snack.*
- *Avoid alcohol on an empty stomach.*
- *Dilute strong drinks.*
- *Keep track of what you are drinking.*
- *Finish one glass before you ask for more.*
- *Go for quality rather than quantity.*
- *Avoid binging.*

Knowing the size of one unit can help you determine how much you can drink. One unit of beer or cider equals 300 ml (½ pt); one unit of spirits is a standard measure of 25 ml (¾ fl oz). A standard glass of wine (125 ml/4¼ fl oz) is one and a half units, and a 50 ml (1½ fl oz) glass of sherry is one unit.

Alcohol

If you are a fit adult, alcohol in moderation can benefit your health and encourage relaxation. However, it is packed with "empty" calories and, in excess, gives rise to well-known health and behaviour problems.

The benefits of having a few alcoholic drinks go further than oiling the wheels of social life. Alcohol can encourage relaxation after a hard day, thereby reducing stress. It helps stimulate conversation, which is beneficial over meals because it slows down consumption, which, in turn, helps the digestive system.

Alcohol has been shown to limit the danger of disease-promoting free radicals. The active ingredients in alcohol, found particularly in dark beers and red wine, are antioxidants known as flavonoids. Their properties vary according to grape, soil, area and wine production methods. Some flavonoids attack furred up arteries; others have anticancer properties. Yet others help reduce the incidence of coronary thrombosis. Doctors now advocate alcohol in moderation to those with heart conditions, including angina.

THE PROBLEMS WITH ALCOHOL

After drinking too much alcohol, a drunk is a social nuisance, even a danger to himself and others (see pp.20–21). More immediately, there is the pain of hangover. In the long term a problem drinker may lose his job, friends and family.

Long-term excessive alcohol consumption can cause health problems: it leads to liver damage, as well as to diseased heart muscles and certain cancers. In men it can lead to impotence (reduced testosterone levels); in women there is evidence of more rapidly aging skin and foetal abnormality, as well as miscarriage.

WHAT IS A UNIT?

The Department of Health has recommended a limit of 28 units for men and 21 units for women per week. The recommendations also warn men not to take more than four units in a day and women no more than three. Saving all the units for a weekend of binge drinking is not considered helpful to the body or recognized as responsible socializing.

A unit of alcohol, as measured by the authorities, is the equivalent of 10 ml (8 g) ethyl alcohol by volume. The size of the unit depends on the type of alcohol (see left). A bottle of wine might contain 9 units, one of sherry 13.5 units and one of gin 28 units.

One problem is that the strength of the alcohol is not consistent. For example, wine strength can vary from 9 to 13 percent, beer and lagers from 3.5 (sometimes even less) to as much as 8 percent. Fortified wines such as sherry and port are 20 percent, while gin, brandy and whisky are as much as 40 percent.

So while thinking in units helps you keep abreast of how much you are drinking, bear in mind that measures and strengths can vary widely. The most responsible way to approach alcohol intake is to find what suits your body, weight and other circumstances. Age and gender make a difference, as does the efficiency of your enzyme system, which helps metabolize alcohol. Regular drinkers generally deal with alcohol more efficiently than occasional bingers. ∎

Eating for high energy

The more you exercise, the more you need to eat a balanced diet. The nutritional rules still apply, but with an added carbohydrate intake. The combination of healthy food and physical exertion combats stress, encourages tissue repair, rebalances hormones and releases endorphins and enkephalins. Mood and outlook should improve markedly.

To boost your sporting performance, you need glucose. The body makes glucose from starches and sugars in carbohydrates, including bread, potatoes and rice and stores it in the muscles and liver as glycogen. Like everyone else, sportspeople need protein, obtained mostly from pulses, poultry, red meat, fish, cheese, eggs and seeds, and vitamins, minerals and essential fatty acids (see pp.250–51). Sufficient fluids, particularly in advance of sport, are vital. You should also drink water during (if possible) and after exercise to replenish fluids.

If strenuous exercise and physical fitness are an integral part of your life, you need to think long term and consistently stick to a well-balanced but varied intake of food. Most athletes have a large and nutritious breakfast, especially on the day of an event, and eat a diet permanently rich in complex carbohydrates.

SPORTS DRINKS – GOOD OR BAD?

Many "isotonic" sports drinks claim to rehydrate and boost energy, but any product containing calories will increase your energy levels. The best way to obtain calories is from the complex carbohydrates found in bread, potatoes, rice, pasta and cereals. In fact, the least nutritionally satisfactory way is by eating simple carbohydrates – that is, sugar. However, many sports drinks contain large quantities of sugar – in some cases, as much as 18 percent. Furthermore, such sweet drinks are bad for the teeth and potentially dangerous for diabetics.

Sports drinks also contain caffeine, as well as additives to enhance colour, flavour, sweetness and stability. Although it may give a sense of instant energy, caffeine can act as a diuretic and is more likely to dehydrate than replenish fluids. The additives contribute nothing to performance, although they may make the product more appealing.

The most efficient rehydration drink is a combination of fruit juice and water with a pinch of salt. For a quick surge of energy, snack on fruit such as a banana or dried apricots.

SCALING UP CARBOHYDRATES

Current advice for sportspeople is to obtain a maximum of two-thirds, or 67 percent, of their energy requirements from complex carbohydrates. The more glycogen the body can store, the more long-term energy it has available to put into sustained exercise. Glycogen is the main fuel that muscles use to move. Rice, pasta, potatoes, pulses and seeds are all high in complex carbohydrates, which are converted into glycogen.

Aim to obtain 10–15 percent of your calories from protein, 20–30 percent from fats and the rest from complex carbohydrates. Remember that low fat does not mean no fat – you need essential fatty acids. Your fat intake is best gleaned mainly from vegetable oils, oily fish and nuts and partly from dairy products, with a limited intake of red meat to keep your consumption of saturated fats down.

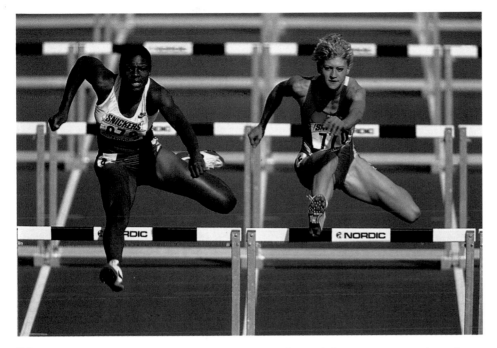

The demands of competing in an active sport require gradual training and a diet that produces enough glycogen, or muscle fuel, to allow the athlete to perform sudden bursts of aerobic activity at her peak.

NORMAL PROTEIN INTAKE

In the past, nutritionists recommended extra protein to boost energy during sports training. But 1 g of carbohydrate and 1 g of protein generate the same number of calories – four – and a high-protein diet can make the body produce too much acid. To counteract the effects of this acidity, the body uses up its supplies of sodium and calcium (which is alkaline), so high intakes of protein can have a serious effect on calcium levels. In turn, this can lead to osteoporosis, a condition that weakens bones (see p.179).

VITAMINS AND MINERALS

If you participate in sports that burn high levels of energy, make sure that you obtain the vital nutrients from your diet.
- Choose foods containing vitamin B_1 (or thiamine), such as fortified breakfast cereals, porridge, muesli, potatoes, nuts and pulses, to help digestion and for good muscle condition.
- Vitamin B_6 (or pyridoxine), found in lean meat, fish, eggs, yeast extract and soya beans, helps prevent anaemia and muscle spasms or cramps.
- Potassium in avocados, fresh and dried fruit – especially bananas – mushrooms and potatoes regulates muscle function and body fluid levels.
- Magnesium contributes to nerve and muscle function, so choose green vegetables, sesame seeds, wheat germ, pulses and nuts.
- Zinc is lost continually through sweat and blood. To counteract this, you can consume shellfish, red meat, peanuts and sunflower seeds.
- Foods rich in vitamins A, C and E, such as oily fish (herrings and sardines), vegetable oils, dairy products, citrus fruit, potatoes and red and green vegetables help your body use oxygen efficiently.

Some athletes regularly take vitamin and mineral supplements to boost their performance. There is no need to exceed the recommended daily requirements – it is much better to gain the necessary nutrients for strength, stamina and suppleness from a healthy diet. ■

Your best weight

There is no such thing as an ideal weight, even for people of the same height. It is best to regard your "optimum weight" as falling within a band rather than being a specific measurement.

Your weight is influenced by a range of factors, such as age, sex and body frame. The easiest way of calculating your ideal weight range is with the body mass index, or BMI (see box, below). However, this measures only total mass. If you exercise and put on muscle – which is desirable – you will appear to be heavier because muscle weighs more than fat. Experts use other methods, such as calipers to measure skin-fold thickness, but these cannot be used at home, so the BMI remains the best alternative.

Most people are concerned about their weight, and with good reason. The incidence of obesity in the industrialized world has increased sharply in recent years. In some countries, it has doubled between 1980 and 1990, and more people are now overweight than of normal weight. This is far from being a merely cosmetic problem, as most people think

BODY MASS INDEX

The body mass index (or BMI) is the measurement used by doctors to assess weight and health risks. It is calculated by dividing your weight in kilogrammes by your height in metres squared (round off the numbers to a decimal point). For example, if you weigh 60 kg and are 1.6 m tall, follow this equation: 1.6 x 1.6 = 2.6; then 60 ÷ 2.6 = 23.1. To convert from imperial measurements, multiply your weight in pounds by 0.45 to get kilogrammes and your height in feet by 0.3 to get metres.

BMI
Under 20   Underweight
20 to 25   Desirable healthy weight
25 to 30   Overweight
Over 30   Obese

Doctors may also take into account your "waist to hip ratio", because carrying weight centrally around the stomach and abdomen is associated with an increased risk of heart disease, high blood pressure and diabetes.

Research shows that a person with a BMI of 27 has twice the risk of developing heart disease, hypertension and gallstones and 14 times the chance of becoming diabetic. The risks increase dramatically if you have a BMI over 30.

Obesity is an adverse condition in anyone, but it is particularly undesirable in children. Apart from the health risks and pattern of poor eating, their self-esteem is easily damaged by being overweight.

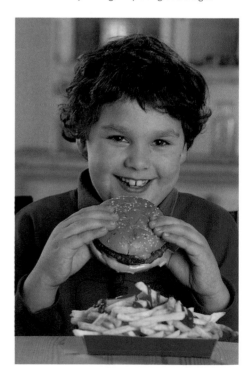

of it. Obesity increases the risk of a range of diseases. The most widespread and serious are heart disease, hypertension (high blood pressure) and diabetes. Obese people also have more joint problems, gall bladder disorders, hernias, cancer and fertility problems.

People with a family history of any of these conditions are advised to maintain their weight at a healthy level and to reduce it if it rises too far above the desired level. Decreasing your weight by just 5–10 percent can substantially reduce all these risks.

OBESITY IN YOUNG AND OLD

Fat children are much more likely to become fat adults, and the risks of related diseases multiply with the duration of obesity. Some studies have shown that if children grow into fat teenagers – even if they subsequently lose weight – they retain a higher than average risk of these diseases in adulthood.

Reducing children's food consumption is complicated because they have a greater need for nutrients than adults. Because treating overweight children is only about 50 percent successful, prevention by establishing good eating habits in toddlers is the key to making sure children reach adulthood at a desirable weight.

Obesity can cause special problems in the elderly. They run a greater risk of joint injury because the additional weight puts increased pressure on their joints, which are weaker than those of younger people. They have a greater risk of heart disease, which also increases with age.

BEING UNDERWEIGHT

Underweight people run far fewer dietary-related risks and have a greater life expectancy than their fat peers, but being underweight can still carry some risks. It reduces fertility in women of child-bearing age and increases the likelihood of developing osteoporosis in later years. However, only if it is severe or you have an eating disorder, will you need to consult your doctor. Most people can put on weight by making minor changes to their diet and lifestyle (see box, below). ▪

GAINING WEIGHT DELIBERATELY

Because obesity is so much more widespread, there is little information available for those people who need to put on weight. It is not as easy as the overweight may think – simply reversing the slimming rules typically results in an unhealthy high-fat diet and inactive lifestyle. Before addressing your diet, you should visit your doctor to rule out any medical causes of your low weight such as a thyroid problem.

Take a look at how much you eat. Researchers have found that, just as overweight people underestimate the amount of food they eat, underweight people often overestimate it. Many people who are underweight eat "on the run" and are unaware of what they do – or don't – eat. The only way to be sure of your consumption is to keep a food diary for a week or two. A normal adult requires 1800–2200 calories a day, depending on frame size and gender. If you are consuming less than this, you need to eat more.

Eating complex carbohydrates is the healthiest way to gain weight. You should increase both muscle and fat mass as you put on weight, so it is important to also eat foods high in protein (p.245 and pp.284–91), which is necessary for muscle growth. Increasing fat consumption raises calorie intake more quickly, but men over 40 years of age and post-menopausal women must be careful not to eat more foods containing saturated fat than normal, because they increase the risk of heart disease. Mono-unsaturated fats, which can be found in olive oil, are healthier.

It helps to set aside enough time to eat so that you can properly chew and digest the food. Instead of eating a lot at each meal, increase the frequency of meals. Snacks should be made up of nutritious food – for example, a sardine or cheese sandwich – to ensure that you are receiving the nutrients you need to metabolize food and turn it into body fat. If you do not put on weight within a month, you should see your doctor.

CAUTION

Although extremely low-calorie diets can produce rapid and significant weight loss, they encourage the body to consume its own muscle tissue, which reduces metabolism and strength for exercise. They can also cause extreme hunger, which encourages people to binge on high-fat foods if their resolve weakens.

Losing weight

More than half the population of many Western countries have tried to lose weight before reaching 50 years of age. But only a minority manage to achieve their target weight and keep it off in the long term.

The theory behind losing weight is simple: you need to expend more energy than you consume – but this is more difficult to do than it sounds. In addition, the conflicting messages from food manufacturers and self-styled slimming experts have confused many people. However, there are only two golden rules for losing weight effectively: eat less fat and exercise regularly.

The number of overweight people has increased so fast in recent decades that experts refer to it as an obesity epidemic.

For long-lasting weight loss, develop an exercise routine that you enjoy. Jogging is one form of aerobic exercise that speeds up the metabolism. Combined with less fat in your diet, this dual attack will slim and tone your figure – and help you keep it that way.

Yet they have calculated that we are eating about 20 percent less than people did in the 1960s. The only conclusion is that we are expending a lot less energy. This is supported by the observations that people spend more than twice as much time watching television and that car ownership has more than doubled.

MORE EXERCISE

The only real answer is to place greater physical demands on your body by exercising regularly (see box, facing page). Do this not only with a view to losing weight, but also with the aim of continuing throughout life. You will both sustain a healthy weight and reduce the risk of heart disease, diabetes and high blood pressure. Ideally, exercise should be encouraged in childhood because there is evidence to show that active children become energetic adults.

CARBOHYDRATES – NOT FAT

The second rule of weight loss is to eat less fat. Dietary fat is responsible for a whole range of biological responses that encourage the body to store fat.

Fat, in whatever form, is rich in calories. It contains twice as many calories as carbohydrates of the same weight. What is more, the body expends little energy converting dietary fat into body fat, but turning carbohydrate into fat tissue uses almost twice as many calories.

Nature has designed humans to store fat efficiently as a survival mechanism. Our ancestors needed fat stores to use during times of famine. Although we no longer need this biological security system, we are still programmed to desire fat.

We can easily eat a lot of it, too. When you have eaten enough carbohydrates, a message is efficiently sent to the brain to tell you to stop. However, this satiation signal is delayed when responding to fat, so the brain does not tell you to stop eating until you have consumed more than your body needs. Furthermore, studies have shown that the more fatty foods people eat, the more they want.

The average diet in the West contains 30–40 percent fat. To lose weight, reduce your fat intake to less than 30 percent. Choose foods that are naturally low in fat, select low-fat processed foods that are not high in sugar and eat plenty of complex carbohydrates – this is easier than it may sound. It is certainly much simpler, and more effective, than calorie-counting.

An extra incentive for minimizing your intake of fat is that this also reduces your risk of developing high blood pressure and heart disease. Increasing your intake of complex carbohydrates may have another benefit. They are thought to affect a hormone in the thyroid gland that both raises the metabolism and tells the body to consume its fat stores for energy.

Although losing weight following this two-pronged approach will take time – you should not lose more than ½–1 kg (1–2 lb) a week – it will put you in control of your body and offer lasting health benefits.

WEIGHT LOSS GIMMICKS

If exercising and reducing fat is effective, why are so many other systems devised and publicized? One obvious reason is that they make money for the manufacturers. The other is that they promise instant or effortless results. Crash diets may work for a few days, but they do nothing to help you to change bad eating habits in the long term. Once you return to your normal habits, the weight will return quickly and you may end up fatter than when you started.

Various pills, supplements and mechanical devices are sold as weight-loss products. The best you can do is ignore them. Even if some have a marginal effect, exercising and reducing fat is a more sustainable way of losing weight. ∎

TAKING MORE EXERCISE

There are two kinds of exercise – aerobic and anaerobic. Both accelerate the metabolism (the rate at which the body burns up energy), which helps to use up fat stores. Otherwise, they benefit the dieter in different ways.

Aerobic exercise increases the heartbeat and raises the amount of oxygen in the blood, leading to increased energy and stamina. It also raises the metabolism quickly. Swimming, running, cycling and dancing are all aerobic forms of exercise. Half an hour's swimming burns up about 300 calories and, if you practise such sports regularly, your metabolism will remain higher even when you are not exercising.

Anaerobic exercise, such as weight-lifting, builds muscle. The more muscle you have relative to fat, the faster your body burns energy. Anaerobic exercise also strengthens bones, which helps prevent osteoporosis; this is important for women, especially ones on a low-fat diet and cutting down on dairy products.

For the body to reap these benefits, you need to do a half hour of aerobic exercise three times a week and two short sessions of anaerobic exercise. It need not be vigorous. It is better to do a longer session of moderate exercise in which you can talk than a short, strenuous one that leaves you breathless.

As you develop a routine of exercise, you should find that your appetite becomes better regulated. When starting any new programme, proceed gradually and build up your strength and stamina over time to reduce the risk of injury. If you have been inactive or have a family history of heart problems, consult your doctor before beginning to exercise.

Good eating habits

Many people today have poor eating habits. This is mainly because changes in our lifestyles mean we have less time to prepare food when we need it and are faced with an increasing supply of unhealthy processed foods. We also tend to eat in a sporadic way, alternately ignoring conventional mealtimes and gorging on high-fat snacks.

Surveys have shown that many people now skip breakfast. Yet breakfast is an important meal. It enables the body to replenish its energy after a long break without food and raises the metabolism, which drops during sleep, and the blood sugar level, which increases alertness. Studies have shown that people who eat a good breakfast have better short-term memory and higher spirits in the morning than those who go without.

People often skip breakfast because they have consumed a large, heavy meal the night before, yet this habit can lead to excess weight. Some dieticians believe that food eaten late in the evening may be laid down as fat during the night. In some people, a habit of large, late suppers can also increase the risk of heart attack. Harmful fats circulating in the blood may encourage clots to form in the arteries after hours of immobility. Perhaps this is why heart attacks are most common in the early hours of the morning.

LITTLE AND OFTEN

It is much better to spread your calorie intake evenly throughout the day, with a good breakfast, a moderate lunch, a light supper and snacks mid-morning and mid-afternoon. Preferably, supper should be eaten at least two hours before going to bed to allow time for digestion.

Researchers have shown that people who divide their food intake into five to seven "episodes" a day take in a greater variety of essential nutrients and tend to eat less fatty food. Such an eating pattern can help prevent many of the common diet-related diseases – so long as you are discriminating about what these snacks contain. Sweet biscuits, for example, can raise your fat and sugar intake above the desirable level. The sugar, in particular, can curb your appetite so that you do not eat well at mealtimes. But with the right choice of foods (see box, left), snacking is a healthy option.

It is a good idea to plan meals in advance and to have a ready range of

HEALTHY SNACKS

There is a huge range of snack foods available in shops and cafés but many are unhealthy, especially if eaten often. Try to select snacks based on natural, healthy foods such as the ones below:

- fresh fruit (bananas, apples and pears)
- crispbreads, breadsticks, rice cakes, crackers
- popcorn (unsweetened, unsalted and unbuttered)
- plain yoghurt (low fat for adults)
- raw vegetable sticks (carrot, celery, cucumber, baby sweetcorn)
- nuts
- dried fruit (but clean your teeth afterward to remove sugar)
- breakfast cereal (with reduced-fat milk for adults).

Sitting down to a family meal of nutritious dishes instils good eating habits in your children, and it combats the unhealthy trend of grabbing whatever is available "on the run" or eating excessively large meals at inappropriate times of the day. It also allows your family to spend more time together.

healthy snack foods available wherever you are, whether at home or work. This prevents you from relying on convenience foods, which are not always nutritionally balanced, or grabbing a quick but unhealthy snack. It may also give you more time to eat and relish your meal.

ENJOYING YOUR FOOD

Taking pleasure in eating is important and, as long as you choose healthy foods, it reinforces good habits. Equally, it helps to put aside time to eat. This not only lets you enjoy the experience more, but also gives you the opportunity to chew and swallow your food properly, preventing digestive problems. Eating slowly is also good for appetite regulation. If you bolt down your food, there is not enough time for the satiation signals to reach the brain and tell you when to stop (see p.261).

Give yourself the opportunity to listen to your body before a meal and while you are eating. Studies have shown that obese people and those with eating disorders such as anorexia and bulimia nervosa override their body's appetite control mechanisms. Try not to turn eating into a distraction or a reward. Eat only when you need food, and concentrate on what you are doing as you eat. This will help keep the mechanism finely tuned.

THE RIGHT DRINKS

As well as eating, you should drink fluids regularly. Water is needed for all bodily functions and most people do not drink nearly enough. Try to drink about 2 litres (3½ pints) a day. It is easy to become dehydrated without being aware of it. Symptoms of dehydration include lack of concentration, tiredness and lethargy. Many people's reaction to these feelings is to eat, when in fact what their body needs is water to unlock energy in cells.

Drink water or diluted juices and not alcoholic or strongly caffeinated drinks: these are diuretics and cause more water to be lost from the body (as urine) than normal. Many people use caffeinated drinks as a "pick-me-up" when they are short of energy. The effect is temporary and such drinks provide no nutrition. It is much better to snack on starchy, unsweetened foods such as bread or bananas for sustained energy release. ∎

SEE ALSO
Convenience foods
270–271
You are what you eat
240–244

Adjusting your diet

To maintain good health and to prevent future diseases, everyone needs a variety of nutrients. These come from a range of foodstuffs, which are required in different proportions.

The diet of our ancestors (and of those who still live off the land) contained much more starch and plant foods and far less fat and animal protein than our own. Although it may not have been perfect nutrition, it probably prevented the premature deaths related to dietary diseases that have become so prevalent today in the industrialized world.

Experts are now advising us to return to a more basic diet that is rich in plant produce and grains and low in fats and sugars. They recommend that starchy foods, such as potatoes, bread, rice and pasta, together with fruit and vegetables, should constitute about 70 percent of our daily calorie intake. We need a smaller volume of meat, fish and other proteins, such as soya, and slightly less of dairy products such as milk, cheese and yoghurt. Last of all are foods based on fat and sugar, of which we need little.

SHOPPING TIPS

It is worth thinking about the food you typically eat to see if it fits into this pattern. You will find it easier to decide on any necessary alterations to your diet if you make a list of what you need before you go shopping. Once in the store, don't be tempted by the huge increase in processed food products. There is plenty in the majority of supermarkets to distract even the most focused shopper.

Concentrate on buying the types of food that are the cornerstone of a healthy diet: starchy foods, fresh fruit and vegetables, fish, lean meat, nuts and dairy products. Milk should be reduced fat for adults. However, children under three years old should not be given reduced-fat foods at all: they need the energy for growth and require more of certain fats than adults for brain development.

Try to buy local fruit and vegetables that are in season. They will be cheaper, as well as richer in vitamins and better tasting because they will not have spent time in storage or travelling across the world. Organic fruit and vegetables are preferable, although more expensive (see box, facing page). If you cannot buy truly fresh plant foods, choose frozen vegetables instead. Because they are

Stir-frying is a healthy method of cooking food quickly. As in steaming, stir-frying retains the shape, colour and nutrients in food, especially vitamins that are destroyed by heat. As well as vegetables, try stir-frying meat, fish and shellfish.

frozen right after being picked, which preserves the vitamins, they will be more nutritious than so-called "fresh" ones that are losing vitamins as they wilt.

The style of supermarket shopping encourages us to buy infrequently and in bulk, but it is much better to buy your fruit and vegetables every few days to ensure you gain maximum nutrition from them. At home, always store vegetables in a cool, dark place to retain the vitamins.

Wholegrain foods are preferable to those containing refined grains. They not only increase the amount of fibre in our diet, helping to prevent constipation and cancers of the digestive tract, but also contain more nutrients. Items to look for include wholemeal bread, brown rice and pasta. Young children, however, should not have too much fibre in their diet, so give them the white equivalents.

HEALTHY COOKING METHODS

It is possible to buy healthy produce but to convert it into unhealthy food by your method of cooking. Some of the least healthy cooking methods are the most appealing because they are quick and convenient. For example, potatoes are an excellent source of dietary fibre and vitamin C. But if you make them into chips by frying them in oil, you increase the amount of fat more than 150 times, making them an unhealthy option. Cooking foods, particularly vegetables, for too long can destroy some of the water-soluble vitamins. Even simpler and healthier is not to cook vegetables at all.

There are other techniques that do not rely on fat and so do not contribute to obesity and circulatory diseases. Most vegetables can be steamed, which does not add calories and retains the nutritional quality and attractive colour of the vegetables. Using vegetables in stock-

---

ORGANIC PRODUCE – A SAFER OPTION

Foods grown or reared without the aid of artificial chemicals such as pesticides, fertilizers and growth hormones are described as being organic. Fruit, vegetables, cereals, eggs, dairy products and meat can all be produced organically.

The full impact that powerful agricultural chemicals may have on our health is not yet known, but they are suspected of causing cancers among other diseases. Research is expected to reveal further damage caused by the "cocktail effect" of these chemicals, when they react together in the body. There is also concern about the use of antibiotics on livestock. There is some evidence that they can contribute to antibiotic resistance in humans so that common antibacterial medicines may not work.

Although the government sets limits on the permissible amounts of such chemicals, some critics claim that these are too high and that many farmers exceed the established limits. Pesticides and fertilizers do ensure that fruit and vegetables are produced to a uniform size and shape and with fewer blemishes, which consumers are thought to want. However, the lack of uniform appearance in organic alternatives is compensated for by improved taste and better health.

---

based soups is another healthy, low-fat option. Try grilling or casseroling meat or fish rather than frying it. Many fish can also be poached or stir-fried.

Salads are a reliable source of vitamins and fibre: try to eat them at least three times a week, either as an accompaniment to a main dish or in sandwiches. Make up a low-fat dressing with lemon or tomato juice, a little oil and seasoning. Herbs are a healthy way to season food and can be used in main dishes as a substitute for some of the salt or to replace it entirely.

KITCHEN EQUIPMENT

Investing in a few new kitchen appliances can make cooking easier and healthier.
- Buy stainless steel or glass cookware.
- For steaming, buy an expandable metal steamer that fits into any size of saucepan.

A main course of poached salmon, new potatoes steamed in their skins and a fresh salad with a citrus dressing combines healthy ingredients with preparation methods that maximize their nutrients – and gives the dish an appetizing appearance. Follow with a piece of fresh fruit.

■ A food processor is ideal for quickly chopping vegetables for stir-fries, soups and salads.

■ Microwave ovens are good for cooking fish succulently without using fat. They are useful, too, for cooking some vegetable dishes such as baked potatoes more quickly than in a conventional oven.

■ Pressure cookers are useful for rapid pulse dishes and soups, and slow cookers are excellent for soups and stews, which can be made with little fat and nutritious stocks. With either of these methods, take care not to overcook the food.

HEALTHY SUBSTITUTES

There are several foods that are common in a Western diet that experts now advise us to cut down on. Most, like salt, are easy to replace. Instead of red meat, try substituting poultry, game or fish, which are equally high in protein but lower in fat. You can also use pulses and nuts instead of animal protein.

For some, if not all of the time, you should replace full-fat cheese, cream and yoghurt with their reduced-fat equivalents. However, it is best not to rely on processed convenience or snack foods that have had the fat removed from them, but to get used to eating foods that are naturally low in fat and sugar (both of which have little or no nutritional value).

MEDICINAL DIETS

Certain substances found in everyday foods can help protect us from disease (see chart, below). Incorporate them into your diet if you have a family history of a particular disease or disorder. However, they should be regarded as an insurance policy and not a substitute for medical treatment. The efficacy of some is still debated, but you can do yourself no harm by increasing the proportion of nutritious foods in your diet. ■

FOOD AS MEDICINE

Disease	Good nutrients	Food sources	Foods to avoid
Cancer	Vitamin A	Offal, oily fish, egg yolk, cheese, carrots	Fatty foods
	Betacarotene	Brightly coloured fruit and vegetables	
	Vitamin C	Blackberries, broccoli, oranges, peppers, watercress	
	Vitamin E	Seeds, nuts, sweet potatoes, wheat germ, oily fish	
	Fibre	Wholegrains, fruit and vegetables	
	Glucosinolates	Members of the cabbage family (p.277)	
	Selenium	Meat, fish, brazil nuts, avocados, lentils	
Osteoporosis	Calcium	Dairy products, tinned fish with bones (such as sardines), sesame seeds, leafy green vegetables	Excessive protein Alcohol
	Vitamin D	Dairy products, oily fish, fortified cereals	

FOOD AS MEDICINE continued			
Disease	**Good nutrients**	**Food sources**	**Foods to avoid**
Heart disease and stroke	Vitamins A, C and E	See Cancer, facing page	Fatty foods
	Selenium	Meat, fish, brazil nuts, avocados, lentils	
	Omega-3 fatty acids	Oily fish, tofu, soya beans, rapeseed oil	
	Allium compounds	Garlic, onions, leeks, chives	
Rheumatoid arthritis	Vitamin E	Seeds, nuts, sweet potatoes, wheat germ, oily fish	Refined foods Saturated fats Sugar and salt
	Potassium	Bananas, celery	
	Omega 3 fatty acids	See Heart disease and stroke, above	
	Bromelain enzymes	Pineapple	
High blood pressure	Vitamins A, C and E	See Cancer, facing page	Saturated fats
	Magnesium	Brazil nuts, almonds, soya beans, peanuts	
	Calcium	See Osteoporosis, facing page	
	Potassium	Bananas, celery	
	Dietary fibre	Wholegrains, fresh fruit and vegetables	
Infertility	Vitamin C (men)	See Cancer, facing page	Tea and coffee Alcohol
	Selenium (men)	See Heart disease and stroke, above	
	Manganese (women)	Oats, wheat germ, rye bread	
	Vitamin B_6 (women)	Wholegrains, leafy green vegetables	
	Zinc	Seafood, red meat, nuts, sunflower seeds	
	Essential fatty acids	Oily fish, polyunsaturated oils	
Alzheimer's disease	Vitamins A and E	See Cancer, facing page	Alcohol Food cooked in aluminium pans
	Betacarotene	See Cancer, facing page	
	Co-enzyme Q10	Soya beans, potatoes, offal, spinach	
	Silicic acid	Kelp, alfalfa, cabbage, lettuce	
Urinary infections	Anthocyanins	Cranberries, blackcurrants, bilberries	None known
Menopausal hot flushes	Phyto-oestrogens	Soya beans, rhubarb, fennel, cabbage	None known

An immune-boosting diet

The health of the immune system is influenced by many factors. One of the most critical, and easiest to influence, is your diet. Vitamins and minerals are the key ingredients.

It is preferable to obtain immune-boosting nutrients from your diet – not from food supplements. You can overdose on some antioxidants in supplement form, but this is unlikely from food sources in a balanced and varied diet.

L ike any other type of major biological system, your immune system can work efficiently only if it is supplied with the right nutrients. The nutritional needs of the immune system appear to increase under certain conditions that are common today. For example, stress, excessive alcohol and caffeine consumption, air pollution, smoking and heavy metals in the air and water are all thought to exert extra demands on it.

The best way to keep your immune system working well is to eat a wide variety of foods in as natural a state as possible. Not only will this provide the nutrients that are known to be necessary, but it will also supply other less known nutrients that may be beneficial.

ANTIOXIDANTS

The main nutrients that help the immune system fight off bacteria and viruses are the antioxidants, including betacarotene (the plant form of vitamin A), vitamins C and E, selenium and zinc. Antioxidants can neutralize free radicals – chemicals generated by the white blood cells to fight infection. When free radicals are produced in excess, they cause harmful cellular changes that can lead to disorders such as cancer and heart disease. Smoking, illness and excessive exposure to environmental pollution or sunlight can all stimulate free radical production.

Vitamin C is the best known antioxidant and performs many immune functions. It destroys bacteria and viruses

Carrots for betacarotene

Salmon for essential fatty acids

Shellfish for selenium

Kidney beans and other pulses for calcium

Citrus fruit, strawberries and broccoli for vitamin C

Brown bread and wholegrains for minerals and the B vitamins

Lentils for iron

and boosts the level of immunoglobulins (blood proteins that act like antibodies). It increases prostaglandin E production (which boosts beneficial T-lymphocytes) and interferon, a naturally occurring antiviral agent. It also aids phagocytosis, the process in which cells in the blood or lymph system destroy foreign invaders.

Vitamin E is a fat-soluble vitamin stored in fatty tissue. It is released to kill free radicals and is thought to protect our bodies from air pollution. It slows down the process of atherosclerosis, too. Betacarotene is another fat-soluble vitamin and strengthens the cell membranes to keep out infection. It also keeps the thymus gland active.

Selenium helps the white blood cells to recognize and destroy invaders and aids antibody production. Good sources are nuts, seeds, seafood and wholegrains. Zinc is essential to the thymus and enables new immune cells to be produced quickly in the presence of a new invader. It is found in offal, shellfish, eggs and seeds.

STRIKING A BALANCE

Health-food producers have capitalized on the qualities of antioxidants and claim that antioxidant supplements increase overall protection from infection and heart disease. But too much can be counterproductive. Excessive vitamin C, for example, may encourage the cells to produce more free radicals. Conversely, if taken during an infection, it can neutralize the free radicals produced to kill the bacteria. It also acidifies the urine, which can lead to renal stones. High doses of vitamin E increase the risk of a brain haemorrhage and excessive vitamin A can accelerate the development of lung cancer in those with cancerous cells.

Eating plenty of fruit and vegetables increases your antioxidant intake to a safe level and also ensures you have plenty of bioflavonoids. These are substances in plant foods that act like antioxidants in stimulating the body's defences.

OTHER IMMUNE BOOSTERS

Lesser known nutrients also boost immunity. Calcium is necessary for phagocytosis and enables white cells to manufacture enzymes. (Overconsumption of coffee, chocolate, fatty foods and bran interferes with calcium absorption.)

Vitamins B_5 and B_6 are essential for phagocytosis and antibody production. Folic acid, another type of B vitamin, is essential during pregnancy for the proper development of the foetus.

Essential fatty acids also regulate immune reactions. Magnesium helps maintain the thymus and supports antibody production. Iron is necessary to produce antibodies and enable the white cells to work; however, avoid iron-rich food during bacterial infections, as it helps the bacteria to reproduce. ∎

HERBS TO BOOST IMMUNITY

Many herbs are reputed to strengthen the body's resistance to disease. Listed here are just a few:

- Aloe vera applied externally is an antiviral and antiseptic.

- St John's wort has long been used as a general immune system tonic and is taken for its antibacterial properties.

- Cat's claw (*Uncaria tomentosa*) is an antiviral containing certain alkaloids that are thought to boost immunity.

- Echinacea is traditionally used in many countries as a general antiviral and antibiotic. It is thought to increase white blood cell count and is usually taken in the form of a tincture.

- Garlic contains allicin, which has antiviral, antibacterial, antifungal and antioxidant properties.

- Ginger is thought to boost resistance to infection.

SEE ALSO
You are what you eat
240–244
Good eating habits
262–263

CAUTION

■ *Additives can be harmful to babies and children and have been linked with "attention deficit disorder" or "hyperactivity".*
■ *Asthmatics and people with allergies may have a bad reaction to certain additives.*
■ *Nitrates and nitrites are carcinogenic.*

Convenience foods

Food is more nutritious the fresher it is and the less that is done to it before it reaches our plates. Convenience food is prepared to save you time and processed so that you can store it, but it may not be as healthy.

Whether convenience foods are partially or completely prepared, many nutrients may be lost from them as they are processed, as well as flavour and texture. Colour additives, sugar, salt, fat, water and chemicals are added to the food to compensate and to preserve it further.

The key to using these foods is to read the label. Ingredient information can help you choose the best out of the vast range of convenience foods now available in supermarkets, as well as in health-food shops – where more nutritious alternatives can be found.

ADDITIVES TO BEWARE OF

Type	Use	Ingredient on label
Artificial colours	Drinks, cakes, biscuits, jams, puddings, sauces, soups, tinned vegetables, smoked fish, cooked meat products (such as Scotch eggs, burgers, pies), cheese, ready-crumbed food	Tartrazine (E102), quinoline yellow (E104)*, sunset yellow (E110), cochineal (E120), carmoisine (E122), amaranth (E123)*, ponceau (E124)*, erythrosine (E127)*, red (E128, 2G)*, indigo (E132), carmine, brilliant blue (E133), caramel (E150), black (E151, PN)*, brown (E154, FK)*, brown (E155, HT)*
Preservatives	Soft drinks, sweets, bottled sauces, pickles, beer, prepared fruit products (such as desserts and jam), cooked meat and some cheeses	Benzoic acid and its derivatives (E210-219), nitrates and nitrites (E249-252)
Antioxidants	Oils and fats, prepared fried foods and snacks, raisins, bottled sauces (such as mayonnaise), ice cream, margarine, cakes, biscuits, breakfast cereals	Butylated hydroxyanisole (E320, BHA), butylated hydroxytoluene (E321, BHT)
Flavour enhancers	Savoury snacks, soups and meat products	Monosodium glutamate (E621, MSG), monopotassium glutamate (E622), calcium glutamate (E623)

* Banned in the United States.
The "E" numbers relate to the European approval system.

ADDED INGREDIENTS

Sugar and added salt (also called sodium) are unnecessary in the diet and harmful in quantity. Both may be added in large amounts to processed foods, and often where you least expect them – sugar in savoury products such as crisps, soup and baked beans, salt in cakes and biscuits and both sugar and salt in ready-made salads.

Ingredients are listed in quantity order, so avoid any product which lists sugar near the beginning. Beware of sugar in supposedly healthy foods such as breakfast cereals, fruit yoghurts and fruit juices. Sugar may be listed as glucose, fructose, dextrose, lactose, maltose, sorbitol and invert syrup. Malt extract is another form of sugar, but slightly more wholesome as it is less refined (and, therefore, takes longer to digest) and contains small amounts of vitamins and minerals.

Bear in mind that tinned soups and meat products often have a high amount of salt added. Foods advertised as "low-salt" may contain monosodium glutamate (MSG), another form of sodium, and "low-sugar" products may contain artificial sweeteners such as saccharine or aspartame. Try to avoid foods containing artificial flavourings or sweeteners.

FAT CONTENT

Pastry, biscuits, cakes and meat products contain large amounts of fat, particularly saturated (animal) fat. Vegetarian sausages and burgers may also be fatty. Vegetable fat is nearly always subjected to a process called "hydrogenation", which destroys the essential fatty acids and may impair your ability to absorb them from other foods. All margarine, unless labelled "nonhydrogenated", is made from hydrogenated fat.

Avoid ready-fried products because oils produce toxins if overheated. When frying at home do not let the oil become so hot that it smokes. Use it only once; olive, sunflower, peanut (groundnut) and rapeseed oil withstand heat best.

CHOOSING AND COOKING

Where possible, choose frozen, dried or bottled products: tins, certain plastics and foil can leach harmful chemicals into food. Refrigerated ready-meals that come in plastic or foil containers and fresh soup in cartons are expensive, but they are healthier than their tinned equivalents.

Frozen vegetables are more nutritious than fresh ones that are more than a few days old. They are already partially cooked, so simply add them to boiling water and bring the water back to a simmer. ∎

HEALTHY CONVENIENCE FOODS

Instead of...	...Substitute
Meat pies, pasties, sausages, burgers	Vegetarian sausages and burgers and ready-made meals (check labels)
Meat stock cubes	Herbs, spices and low-salt vegetable stock cubes
Meat pâté	Vegetable and fish pâtés and dips; hummus (chickpea pâté)
White pasta	Wholewheat pasta
Custard, sweetened fruit yoghurt	Plain "live" yoghurt (add your own honey or fruit)
Crisps	Unroasted nuts, pumpkin and sunflower seeds
Biscuits, cake, desserts, sweets, chocolate	Fruit, fresh or dried
Fruit squashes, fizzy drinks, sweetened fruit juices	Unsweetened fruit juices diluted with still or carbonated water; fruit or herb teas (made from real fruit or herbs, not flavourings)

Food allergies

When a food activates the body's immune system, the response is known as an allergy. Symptoms can be immediate and serious – even life threatening. It is nearly always possible to detect the offending food, but avoiding it is not always easy. Food allergies should not be confused with food intolerances: different mechanisms cause the symptoms.

CAUTION

Anaphylactic shock – a severe life-threatening reaction in which the respiratory and circulatory systems collapse – can occur within minutes or a few hours after eating the offending food. Symptoms include swelling of the tongue and mouth, an itchy rash covering the body, abdominal pain and diarrhoea. This condition requires an immediate injection of adrenaline – call an ambulance right away.

For unknown reasons, a food allergy occurs when the body's immune system treats a particular food as a foreign invader and attacks it. Heredity may play a role. If both parents have allergies, their children will, too; however, the symptoms and the food that they are allergic to may be different. Symptoms may not develop until after the person eats the offending food, or allergen, a number of times.

THE SYMPTOMS
In some cases the symptoms are mild; for example, a tingling of the lips and tongue after eating an apple or tomato. Yet, they can be severe in other cases, causing swelling in the mouth or throat that can block the airways. If the symptoms are acute, there will be a reaction within a few minutes to a few hours after eating the food, although in rare cases it can take up to two days for them to appear. Chronic symptoms such as asthma and chronic rhinitis can occur when the unsuspected allergen is consumed daily.

Common acute symptoms include a skin rash, swelling in the mouth or throat, red itchy eyes, sneezing and a runny nose, abdominal pains, vomiting, diarrhoea, swelling of the joints, confusion, breathing difficulties and anaphylactic shock. Chronic symptoms include eczema and urticaria (rash), asthma, a runny nose, catarrh, excess fluid in the middle ear and, in babies, diarrhoea and vomiting.

The allergen usually triggers the same symptoms each time it is eaten, but other factors will affect their intensity, including stress, how the food was prepared, whether the food was combined with other foods and the amount of the food. Small amounts may cause no reaction. Conversely, even a minute trace of the allergen can cause a severe reaction; this can occur in people allergic to peanuts.

The food does not necessarily have to be ingested; for example, touching the skin of an orange, which contains an oil, can trigger a reaction in some people. Having someone else peel the orange allows susceptible people to eat them.

LIVING WITH ALLERGIES

- If you have a food allergy, also investigate if you have an environmental allergy such as one to pets or dust mites.

- Avoid introducing the most common offending foods (see facing page) into a child's diet until she is at least 12 months old. If you or your spouse's family has a strong history of allergies, avoid any offending food when pregnant and breast-feeding, and avoid any food causing an allergic reaction in a previous child.

- Increase your intake of betacarotene, vitamins A, C and E, zinc, selenium and essential fatty acids to help your immune system.

- Try homeopathy and herbal medicine, to see if they help.

DETECTING THE ALLERGEN

A food allergy can be obvious if the symptoms occur immediately after the food has been eaten. Otherwise, a food diary, listing foods and the symptoms, may help reveal a pattern. In difficult cases, a blood test can detect the problem if it is a true allergy (not an intolerance); it has the advantage of the person not coming into contact with the allergen. Sometimes, skin-prick tests are used but they are less reliable: food extracts are placed on the skin, which is then pricked so that a small amount penetrates it. However, a hypersensitive person can react severely. If these tests fail to find the allergen, an elimination diet (see pp.274–75) may be the only answer.

Once you determine the allergen, the only option is to avoid eating it. When shopping for food, always check the ingredients on food labels, and don't be afraid to ask about the ingredients in the dishes when eating at a restaurant.

MEDICATION

Drugs do not cure allergy. The symptoms will return once treatment is stopped and the medicines themselves may cause unpleasant symptoms. However, they can give temporary relief. The main types are:
■ antihistamines in pill form: these must be stopped several days before taking any skin tests because they mask the results
■ steroids as inhalers, pills and creams
■ bronchodilators in the form of inhalers and pills: they help ease breathing difficulties, which can be triggered by a food allergy in people who have asthma
■ adrenaline injection, which is necessary for anaphylactic shock (see facing page). A severely allergic person should carry adrenaline with her at all times in case she accidentally eats her trigger food. It is wise to wear a medical alert tag, too. ■

PROBLEM FOODS

Although they are not the only ones, the following foods are the most common triggers of allergies and often cause the symptoms listed:

■ Milk and other dairy products (including cheese, yoghurt, cream and ice cream): constipation, diarrhoea and vomiting; less often rashes and breathing problems.

■ Eggs (especially egg whites): rashes, swelling and intestinal problems. They can trigger eczema and asthma attacks.

■ Fish (fresh, tinned, smoked or pickled, as well as fish-liver oils and caviar): rashes, itchy eyes and a runny nose. Fish can also trigger an asthma attack, diarrhoea and anaphylactic shock.

■ Shellfish (including prawns and shrimps, crab, lobster, clams, oysters and scallops): vomiting, intestinal problems, rashes, migraines and anaphylactic shock.

■ Wheat and wheat products: diarrhoea and other intestinal problems, migraine and eczema.

■ Corn: rashes, diarrhoea and other intestinal problems and breathing difficulties.

■ Peanuts and other nuts: intestinal and breathing problems and anaphylactic shock.

■ Citrus fruit, melons and fruit with seeds (especially strawberries): rash on the face and tingling sensation in the mouth.

■ Chocolate: rashes.

Food intolerances

The typical IgE antibodies produced by true food allergies cannot be found in cases of food intolerance, although the symptoms may be similar. The intolerance may be caused by a metabolic problem, such as the inability to digest wheat or dairy products, but in many cases the causes are unknown.

There is much controversy about food intolerances. While several of them, such as a reaction to wheat or dairy products, are accepted by doctors as recognizable intolerances, others have less established causes and may be looked upon with scepticism. One school of thought is that environmental pollution and the increased use of processed and mass-produced fresh food may be linked to some types of food intolerances.

Some practitioners blame the oral contraceptive pill, antibiotics, viral illness, giardia infection, candidiasis (thrush), a poor diet and stress. They claim a vast range of symptoms, including craving certain foods, an inability to maintain your correct weight, diarrhoea, irritable bowel syndrome, constipation, cystitis, wind and bloating, rheumatoid arthritis, aching muscles or joints, psoriasis, water retention, nausea, stomach and duodenal ulcers, headaches and migraines, mouth ulcers, hyperactivity in children, fatigue, depression and premenstrual syndrome.

GLUTEN INTOLERANCE

One recognized type of food intolerance is gluten intolerance, which is also known as coeliac disease, or coeliac sprue, and it tends to run in families. It occurs when a person cannot absorb gluten, which is the protein found in wheat, rye and barley – an ingredient of some common foods such as bread and pasta. The protein damages the lining of the small intestine, making it difficult to absorb nutrients, which can lead to malnutrition.

The symptoms usually appear in babies within six months of giving them foods containing gluten. They include bulky, greasy, pale and foul-smelling stools, weight loss, listlessness, irritability, a swollen abdomen and wind. In adults, the symptoms are diarrhoea, abdominal

COMMON TRIGGERS

With the exception of gluten and lactose intolerances, the most common causes of food intolerances are given below. However, there are many other triggers suspected of causing intolerance.

- Histamine: found in fish, including tuna and mackerel, it can cause chest and abdominal pain, diarrhoea, nausea and vomiting, a rash and swelling and a drop in blood pressure.

- Sulphite: a food additive in prawns, dried fruit, processed potatoes, wines, beer and some restaurant foods, sulphite can cause severe, allergylike reactions. Always check food labels, especially if you have asthma.

- Methylxantine: this compound, which causes headaches, palpitations, vomiting and anxiety attacks, occurs naturally in coffee, tea, colas, chocolate and cocoa.

- Migraines: these can be triggered by alcohol, strong or aged cheeses such as Cheddar, cured meats such as ham and bacon, chicken livers and pickled herring and mackerel.

pain, vomiting, fatigue, breathlessness, weight loss and swollen legs. They occur more gradually, over months or years.

A jejunal biopsy, in which a sample of tissue is taken from the lining of the small intestine, can confirm a diagnosis. The only treatment is a gluten-free diet. Health-food shops sell substitute foods such as gluten-free bread.

LACTOSE INTOLERANCE

The enzyme lactase, which is produced in the small intestine, breaks down milk sugar, or lactose. Sometimes the enzyme is deficient, causing lactose intolerance. The deficiency may be present at birth, or it may not occur until adulthood. It develops in 80–90 percent of blacks and Orientals and 5–15 percent of whites. It sometimes occurs after a bout of gastroenteritis, but it often disappears after recovery from the disease.

Symptoms include wind and bloating, stomach cramps and diarrhoea. Mild sufferers can drink up to half a litre (a pint) of milk without symptoms, but this can cause severe symptoms in others. Enzyme drops or tablets are available to help you digest dairy products.

THE ELIMINATION DIET

Other food intolerances can be traced by following an "elimination" diet. This takes commitment and requires guidance from a practitioner or nutritionist. Restricting foods in the wrong way can lead to a deficiency of nutrients and many of the symptoms can have other causes.

Before embarking on the diet, you will be asked to eat healthily for three to four weeks, cutting out tea, coffee, chocolate, food with additives, smoking and drugs. This prepares you for the restricted diet to come and shows whether stimulants or poor diet are the cause of your ill health.

If you feel better after this preliminary diet you do not have to go any further.

The next phase is exclusion. During this period you should only eat foods that rarely cause problems, such as lamb, rice, cabbage and pears, and drink mineral water for from four days to two weeks.

During either of these phases, you may suffer unpleasant "withdrawal" symptoms, such as headaches, nausea, an infection or depression, or an increase in the symptoms you are trying to reduce. These are a sign that your body is detoxifying and should last three to four days.

The next phase is to reintroduce food groups, one at a time, at intervals of a few days and note your reactions. Once the offending foods have been discovered measures are necessary to stop symptoms returning. If the symptoms are mild, a "rotation" diet can be followed. In some cases, however, severe symptoms may mean completely eliminating the offending food from your diet. ∎

THE ROTATION DIET

A food intolerance may be avoided if you don't consume the same food too often and, therefore, do not strain the particular digestive and detoxifying processes that the food demands of the body. One way to avoid this problem is to follow a rotation diet. Eat a wide variety of foods, and eat each type of food or food group at intervals of four or more days. This interval gives the body time to recover.

Some people can follow a rotation diet without having pinned down their food intolerances and find that their health improves. People who have been through an elimination diet are usually advised to stop eating their offending foods for several months but then to reintroduce them gradually and in rotation. The rotation diet then becomes a part of their life for good. Some people, however, once their health is restored, can be more relaxed about what they eat and when.

Vegetables

According to the World Health Organization (WHO), we should eat five portions of vegetables and fruit a day. Vegetables provide us with fibre, minerals, vitamins, especially A, B, C, E and K, and some protein. They also provide other substances such as bioflavonoids and enzymes, which contribute to the healthy functioning of the body.

Because vegetables have different nutrients, eating a wide variety of vegetables is the best way to ensure a healthy intake of all the nutrients. Most vitamins are destroyed or depleted by the cooking process and nutrients can leach into cooking water, so vegetables are best eaten raw, lightly steamed, roasted, baked or casseroled – not boiled.

FROM LOCAL TO EXOTIC

It is best to eat vegetables in season and locally grown. Eating vegetables in season ensures that they are fresh. Some nutrients begin to dissipate as soon as the vegetable is picked. This is why frozen vegetables can be more nutritious than fresh ones. The farther vegetables are transported, the more time they take to reach your table – and the more time nutrients have to be depleted. To keep vegetables as fresh as possible, store ones from a warm climate, such as aubergines, beans, peppers, marrows, courgettes and tomatoes, at 10°C (50°F). Other vegetables are best stored at 0°C (32°F), but avoid storing potatoes below 4°C (40°F).

At the same time, take advantage of the fact that formerly luxury items such as avocado pears are now readily available in supermarkets. Avocados are rich in nutrients and convenient to store and eat. Another exotic option is sea vegetables. They are exceptionally rich in minerals and a rare vegetable source of vitamin B_{12}. If you live near the sea you can gather your own – wash them well and eat raw, stir-fried and in soups or stews. Otherwise, Japanese varieties such as nori, arame, kombu and wakame are available dried from specialist shops.

USING HERBS

Like vegetables, herbs come from the leaves or roots of plants. Herbs and spices add flavour, reducing the need for salt, sugar or artificial additives. Many have medicinal value as well. Plenty of types are on sale but they are also easy to grow outdoors or in pots on the windowsill. ▪

VEGETABLES AND THE SEASONS	
Season	**Vegetables available**
Spring	Broad beans • sprouting broccoli • green cabbage • new carrots • cauliflower • spring onions • peas • radishes spinach • watercress
Summer	Beetroot • broad beans • carrots • French beans runner beans • courgettes • cucumber • lettuce mangetouts • peas • new potatoes • radishes spinach • tomatoes
Autumn	Sprouting broccoli • green, red and white cabbage carrots • cauliflower • celery • corn on the cob leeks • marrows • spinach • tomatoes • watercress
Winter	Broccoli • Brussels sprouts • green, red and white cabbage • celery • leeks • parsnips • swedes

A GUIDE TO THE VEGETABLE FAMILIES

Vegetable	Nutritional value	Other benefits	Hints on using
Onion family Onion Garlic Leek Spring onion (scallion) Chives Asparagus	Provide minerals such as potassium, selenium, manganese and iodine; increase assimilation of the B vitamins. Spring onions, leeks and asparagus contain vitamin C. Leeks supply calcium; spring onions are more nutritious than ordinary onions.	All members, especially garlic, destroy harmful bacteria, fungi and parasites in the body, enhance your ability to withstand colds and flu, reduce blood pressure, lower blood cholesterol and inhibit tumours. Asparagus benefits the liver and kidneys and is recommended for people with arthritis (but not gout). Leeks are cleansing, diuretic and good for gout.	Garlic is most nutritious eaten raw; eating raw parsley at the same time can help stop breath smelling. Nutrients in onions are enhanced by frying. Some people develop an intolerance to this family.
Cabbage family Cabbage Cauliflower Broccoli Kale Chinese leaf Watercress Mustard and cress Brussels sprout Kohlrabi Turnip Radish	These green leafy vegetables are rich in vitamins A, C, E and K, the B vitamins, folic acid and betacarotene. Cabbage is rich in iron. Broccoli has almost as much calcium as whole milk, twice as much vitamin C as oranges and more vitamin B_2 than any other vegetable. Watercress has iodine, calcium, iron and phosphorus.	Cabbages and turnips contain sulphur compounds, which combat respiratory infections. Radishes are valuable for the liver and gall bladder. Turnips are bactericidal and recommended for gout. Watercress is a powerful antibiotic.	Eat radish tops if they are fresh, as well as the roots. Chinese leaf is a useful alternative to lettuce. Eat the bulb (swollen stem) and tops of kohlrabi; young bulbs can be grated and eaten raw.
Potato family Potato Tomato Aubergine Bell pepper Chilli pepper	Potatoes are a good source of vitamins C and B_6, potassium and other minerals. The other members of this family, except aubergine, are high in vitamins A and C and betacarotene.	Potatoes provide complex carbohydrates (which are good for long-lasting energy) and fibre. The skin contains much of the nutrition so leave it on. Chillies (in moderation) benefit the heart and circulatory system and boost digestion. They also thin mucus, making them good for coughs and colds.	To preserve vitamin C, eat raw, except potatoes, which are more nutritious baked. Potatoes are treated with chemicals, so try to buy organic ones; green patches are poisonous. This plant family is not recommended for people with joint problems. Some people develop an intolerance to these vegetables.
Pea and bean family Pea, mangetout and sugarsnap Bean, runner, French and broad	High in protein, calcium, iron and manganese, and a good source of vitamins A, C, E and K and the B vitamins.	Provide complex carbohydrates (like pulses, which belong to same family). Peas contain as much protein as meat and provide nicotinic acid, which is believed to reduce blood cholesterol.	Eat raw or cooked, with the exception of broad beans, which should be cooked.

A GUIDE TO THE VEGETABLE FAMILIES continued

Vegetable	Nutritional value	Other benefits	Hints on using
Pumpkin family Pumpkin Squash Courgette Marrow Cucumber	Pumpkin and squash are exceptionally high in betacarotene. The family is a good source of vitamin C.	Cucumbers are good for the digestion and for gout and contain silicon (which is good for nails and hair). Courgettes, marrows and cucumbers are low in calories.	Cucumbers lose vitamin A content if peeled but are sprayed with pesticides and may be waxed, so try to buy organic ones. There is no need to peel courgettes.
Parsley family Parsley Carrot Parsnip Celery Celeriac Fennel Coriander Dill	Parsley is high in vitamins and minerals. and is a good source of iron and vitamin C, as well as other vitamins and minerals. Carrots are high in betacarotene. Celeriac contains iron; fennel, vitamin A and calcium. Celery contains calcium.	Parsley and coriander enhance digestion. One carrot supplies a day's intake of vitamin A. Fennel has antibacterial agents and is high in protein.	The vitamin A content of carrots is easier to digest if they are cooked. Peel carrots if nonorganic – they retain high pesticide levels. Eat parsley in moderation in pregnancy. Eat celeriac raw or cooked. Both the fennel bulb and tops can be eaten; the aniseed taste is reduced when cooked.
Lettuce family Lettuce Artichoke, globe Artichoke, Jerusalem Chicory Endive Salsify Dandelion Tarragon	Globe artichoke, dandelion leaves, tarragon and some varieties of lettuce contain vitamins A, C and E and minerals, especially calcium and iron. Chicory and endive are high in vitamins C and K, the B vitamins and minerals.	Lettuce in large quantities helps cure insomnia. Globe artichokes act as a tonic for the liver and are recommended for arthritis and gout. Chicory, endives and dandelions benefit the liver and kidneys. Dandelions, particularly the roots, detoxify the body and have antibiotic, antitumour and anti-inflammatory agents. Tarragon stimulates the heart, liver, appetite and digestion.	Jerusalem artichoke can be eaten raw or cooked, but it causes severe flatulence in some people. Cultivated dandelion leaves are less bitter than wild ones. The root is usually made into a coffee substitute. Salsify is a little-known, underrated root vegetable that should be eaten cooked.
Beet family Beetroot Swiss chard (sea-kale beet) Spinach	A good source of vitamins A, C and K, minerals, especially iron and calcium, and protein; the leaves contain folic acid.	Beetroot enhances digestion, the liver and the immune system, and it has anticarcinogenic agents. Oxalic acid in the leaves of this plant family prevents much of their mineral content being absorbed by the body.	You can eat beetroot leaves (cooked like spinach), as well as the root. Beetroot's nutritional qualities are enhanced when eaten raw; grate it into salads. Cook stems and leaves of Swiss chard separately. Young spinach can be eaten raw.
Avocado	Rich in essential fatty acids, protein and potassium. Also supplies vitamin A, C and E and some of the B vitamins, especially folic acid.	It has antibacterial and antifungal agents and contains substances that counteract skin aging. The fats are easily digestible.	They are ripe when they yield slightly to pressure. Keep unripe avocados at room temperature to ripen; store cut ones with the stone in the refrigerator.

A GUIDE TO THE VEGETABLE FAMILIES continued

Vegetable	Nutritional value	Other benefits	Hints on using
Sprouted beans, seeds and grains Alfalfa Mung beans Buckwheat (unroasted) Adzuki beans Chickpeas Brown lentils Corn (maize) Sunflower seeds (hulled)	Most vitamins and minerals, in large quantities.	These are, gram for gram, the most nutritious food available, full of protein, vitamins (including B_{12}), minerals and enzymes that boost the body's metabolism.	Eat raw to gain maximum benefit. Some varieties are available in supermarkets, others in health-food shops, or you can grow and prepare your own – the varieties listed are the easiest to grow. (For more information on sprouting, see pp.284–86.)
Mushrooms Field (button, cup or flat) Chanterelle Truffle Oyster Shitake Cep Dried Chinese	Some protein and moderate source of minerals.	Organic and wild varieties are most likely to contain minerals.	Eat with grains: mushrooms are rich in an amino acid (a source of protein) that grains do not provide. People on yeast-free diets should avoid them. Edible varieties can be gathered from the wild as long as you can distinguish edible ones from poisonous ones (but do not overpick, jeopardizing future stocks).

HERBS AND SPICES TO COMPLEMENT VEGETABLES

Name	Benefits	Hints on using
Basil	Calming and good for digestive problems, colds and headaches.	Only eat fresh; tear leaves rather than cutting them. Delicious in salads and tomato dishes.
Curry	Helps thin mucus, aids digestion and counteracts flatulence.	Adds interest to vegetable and pulse dishes, especially lentils.
Ginger	Counteracts nausea and colds.	Root delicious grated into stir-fry dishes.
Marjoram/ oregano	Has a sedative quality, fights infection and accelerates healing.	Best used dried in tomato dishes.
Mustard	Used medicinally to treat rheumatism, arthritis and, in China, bronchitis.	Try in salad dressings or, instead of cheese, in sauces.
Pepper	Stimulates appetite and digestion; a source of the mineral chromium.	Best bought as whole corns. Grind into salads, or into cooked dishes at the last minute.

CAUTION

Citrus fruit peel is coated with a fungicide. Use untreated fruit when making candied peel or marmalade. Or scrub the fruit under clear running water before use.

Fruit

An essential part of a healthy diet, fruit provides fibre, vitamins and minerals. In fact, it is our main source of vitamin C. Fruit is also high in potassium, which balances our sodium (salt) intake. Eating several portions of a variety of fruits each day is one of the easiest and most delicious ways to improve your diet.

Each day, we should eat five portions of a combination of fruit and vegetables. A portion of fruit can be a single piece of raw fruit, such as an apple or banana, a saucerful of berries or grapes or a glassful of pure fruit juice. Dried, tinned and frozen fruit count, too, but eating fruit raw preserves the vitamin C.

Citrus fruit, such as oranges and grapefruit, has the highest vitamin C content. Dried fruit, including figs and apricots, and citrus fruit is a good source of both soluble and insoluble fibre, which helps prevent constipation, reduces the risk of colon cancer and keeps blood cholesterol levels in check. Betacarotene in orange-coloured fruit such as apricots may protect against cancer.

The best time to eat fruit is when it is in season and fresh. However, local fruits such as raspberries and pears are available only at specific times during the year, so imported, frozen and dried fruit is useful when local produce is not available. Unless you grow your own, organic fruit is hard to come by, but there are many delicious wild fruits that can be gathered in season such as blackberries in autumn.

If you want to cook fruit, simmering gently (and reserving the juice) or baking destroys the least number of nutrients. You can sweeten a fruit dish with concentrated fruit juice (available from health-food shops) or honey and flavour with spices. If you buy tinned fruit, choose those canned in their own juices or apple juice, without added sugar.

TEAS, JAMS AND JUICES

The benefits of fruit can extend to beverages and jams. Fruit teas are a nutritious alternative to tea and coffee, but buy tea made with real fruit, not fruit flavour. Make or buy jam sweetened with fruit juice or honey rather than sugar.

Fruit juice lacks the fibre of the whole fruit, but if you press your own, you can scrape the pulp back into the drink. If you are buying fruit juice, be sure to choose pure juice without added sugar or artificial additives. Vitamin C (ascorbic acid) is sometimes added as a preservative, which is fine. Try using fruit juice instead of milk in baking. ∎

LOCAL AND IMPORTED SEASONAL FRUIT

Season	Fruit
Spring	Rhubarb
Summer	Peaches • apricots • nectarines • cherries strawberries • raspberries • blackberries blackcurrants • gooseberries • melons
Autumn	Apples• pears • plums • grapes • raspberries blackberries • blackcurrants
Winter	Citrus fruit • cranberries • bilberries

THE NUTRITIONAL ROLE OF FRUIT

Type	Nutritional value	Other benefits	Hints on using
Tree fruits Apple Pear Quince Medlar Loquat	High in minerals such as calcium and magnesium; some vitamins A and C.	Apples lower blood cholesterol markedly, aid digestion and have antiviral properties.	Most of the nutrients are found near the skin, but apples are sprayed with pesticides and may be waxed, so peel if nonorganic. Cook and purée quinces (do not eat raw). Loquats can be eaten raw or cooked, in sweet or savoury dishes. Medlars have to be picked and fermented before they are eatable. Susceptible people may become intolerant of some of these fruits.
Soft fruits Raspberry Strawberry Blackberry Loganberry Tayberry Boysenberry Blueberry Bilberry Huckleberry Blackcurrant Redcurrant Whitecurrant Gooseberry Cranberry Cloudberry	High in vitamin C, especially blackcurrants; good source of vitamin A and calcium. Both raspberries and strawberries are high in iron.	Blackcurrants have more vitamin C than any other fruit. Cranberry juice is good for preventing or treating cystitis (see pp.146–47). Strawberries combat high blood pressure and are good for circulatory problems, and blueberries may help treat diarrhoea.	Strawberries lose their vitamin C quickly so eat as soon as possible after picking them. Blackberries can be picked wild. The vitamin C in blackcurrants and blackcurrant juice is very stable. Cloudberries are usually made into a liqueur but can be treated like blackberries. Soft fruit can cause an intolerance in some people; strawberries can cause an allergy.
Stone fruits Peach Nectarine Apricot Plum Greengage Damson Cherry	High in betacarotene, especially apricots; good source of vitamin C. Plums, greengages and damsons also contain calcium and magnesium.	Good source of fibre.	Some types of plums are dried to make prunes. Damsons are too tart to eat raw. Peaches and apricots keep their betacarotene after being dried – the bright colour is usually retained by treating with sulphur dioxide (see Dried fruit, p.282).
Citrus fruits Orange Grapefruit Lemon Lime Tangerine Mandarin Clementine Satsuma Ugli fruit Pomelo	High in vitamin C and a good source of calcium and betacarotene.	Bioflavonoids, which keep blood vessels healthy, are found in the pith and membranes (so keep pulp when juicing). Lemon juice helps prevent fatty deposits, which is useful if trying to lose weight.	Because vitamin C deteriorates quickly, keep the fruit in the refrigerator and eat it as soon as possible. The peel on citrus fruit is usually waxed to make the fruit look glossy and fresh, even when it is not. Buy fruit marked as unwaxed if you are grating the peel for a dish or using fruit slices to flavour drinks. Lemon and lime juice can be used instead of salt to enhance cooking.

THE NUTRITIONAL ROLE OF FRUIT continued

Type	Nutritional value	Other benefits	Hints on using
Melon Cantaloupe Honeydew Watermelon	A reasonable source of vitamin C, calcium, phosphorus and potassium. Watermelon is high in vitamin A.	Stimulating to the kidneys.	Because it can ferment in the stomach, it is best to eat melon on its own or at the start of a meal. You can test a melon for ripeness by its scent – it should have a deep fragrance.
Tropical fruits Pineapple Banana Date	Pineapples are high in vitamin C and magnesium. Bananas are a good source of the B vitamins and vitamins A and C, as well as potassium, phosphorus, zinc, iron and calcium. Dates are a good source of vitamins A, C and D, the B vitamins, calcium and phosphorus.	Pineapple contains an enzyme called bromelain, which is a powerful protein digestant. Bananas are recommended for constipation and diarrhoea. They reduce allergy symptoms and increase helpful bacteria in the bowel. Dates are a laxative.	Eat fresh pineapple with a heavy or meaty meal (the bromelain will help digestion). Bromelain is not present in pineapple juice or tinned pineapple. Pineapple is ripe when you can easily tug a leaf out of it. Green bananas are indigestible. Ripe bananas are extremely digestible and are good for babies. Dates are usually sold dried.
Mediterranean origin Grape Fig	Grapes are rich in calcium, phosphorus, potassium and some of the B vitamins. Figs are a good source of iron, protein and calcium.	Figs contain an enzyme called ficin, which helps digestion.	Wash grapes well; they are usually sprayed with pesticides. Buy fresh figs when the skin is firm and smooth, not wrinkled, and eat on the same day.
Stems Rhubarb Angelica	Rhubarb is high in calcium and a good source of other minerals; it also has some vitamin C. Angelica contains minerals.	Rhubarb is a purgative. Angelica belongs to the parsley family; it is good for digestion and stimulating the appetite.	In temperate climates, rhubarb is available in early spring. It must be cooked before eating. Throw away all leaves and leaf buds, which are high in oxalic acid. Do not eat the stems in summer; they will also be high in oxalic acid. Use the stem and leaves of angelica to flavour fruit desserts and jams; garnish cakes with candied stem.
Dried fruit Apple Peach Pear Banana Mango Pineapple Prune Date Fig Raisin Sultana Currant	Retain minerals and most of the vitamins of the fresh fruit.	Dried fruit is high in fibre and acts as a laxative, especially dried figs and prunes.	Store well for many months. Eat them raw, use to sweeten desserts and cakes or soak and simmer in water or fruit juice. The sulphur dioxide used to preserve dried fruit may trigger asthma in susceptible people; wash it off in hot water. Mineral glazes stop the fruit sticking together but impede vitamin absorption. "Unsulphured" and organic (unsulphured and unglazed) dried fruit is available. Do not confuse dried fruit with glacé or crystallized fruit preserved in sugar.

UNUSUAL FRUITS

Name		Nutritional value	Hints on using
Kumquat		High in potassium, calcium, phosphorus and vitamins A and C.	Looks like a miniature orange. Eat raw, including rind, in salads.
Mango		Exceptionally rich in betacarotene.	Consume raw, puréed or as juice. Related to cashew and pistachio nuts.
Pawpaw (Papaya)		Full of betacarotene.	Eat as a starter or dessert; underripe fruit can be cooked and eaten as a vegetable.
Lychee		High in vitamin C, potassium and phosphorus.	Available dried or tinned in Chinese food shops, as well as fresh in supermarkets. Eat raw or in sweet and sour dishes.
Physalis (Cape gooseberry)		High in vitamins A and C, phosphorus and calcium.	Remove papery case and use sliced or whole in salads. Can be stored for up to 3 weeks.
Kiwi fruit		Exceptionally rich in vitamins C and E and minerals; contains proleolytic acid, which is said to reduce cholesterol.	If unripe, can be kept in the refrigerator for months. Peel and eat raw or puréed.

SPICES TO COMPLEMENT FRUIT

Name		Nutritional value	Hints on using
Cinnamon		Antiseptic, stimulating and good for the digestion.	Good with apples, oranges, bananas, blackberries and peaches, in hot fruit drinks, in cakes and biscuits made with dried fruit and with stewed dried fruit. Available in stick or powder form.
Nutmeg		Good for wind, nausea and vomiting. More than half a clove can cause rapid heartbeat and hallucination; can be toxic.	Try with lemons, pears and pineapples, with stewed dried fruit and in baking.
Cloves		Antiseptic and good for the digestion.	Go well with apples and bananas and in hot drinks. Available as dried flower heads (use for flavouring only – avoid eating) or powder.
Allspice		Aids digestion.	Use when baking with dried fruit and with lime juice, bananas and other tropical fruit.
Vanilla		Beneficial to the nervous system.	Pods or extract can be used to flavour cooked dishes and in baking.

SEE ALSO
Carbohydrates   252
Good eating habits
                 262–263
Food allergies 272–273
Food intolerances
                 274–275

Pulses, grains and nuts

Many of the wide range of grains and pulses, seeds and nuts provide protein, as well as numerous other nutrients. They are an inexpensive alternative to meat. Most are available organically grown.

Also known as legumes or beans, pulses are high in fibre, complex carbohydrates, minerals such as calcium, protein and the B vitamins and are low in fat. They can cause flatulence if you are unused to eating them, so gradually introduce them into your diet. Pulses are usually sold dried. Larger ones should be soaked for several hours before being cooked. For all pulses, you should destroy a toxin by boiling, uncovered, in fresh water for 10 minutes; then cover and simmer for ½–1½ hours. Alternatively, you can pressure cook them (except for split peas) for 5–20 minutes after boiling.

Grains are a good source of complex carbohydrates. Wholegrains also provide protein, minerals and vitamins.

TYPES OF PULSES

Name		Nutritional value	Additional information
Lentils		High in iron and the B vitamins; moderate source of calcium and vitamin A.	Available in orange, brown, green and blue-grey. Soaking unnecessary; orange types cook most quickly.
Peas, split or whole		Contain vitamin A, and they help reduce blood cholesterol.	They are available in green or yellow. There is no need to soak them before cooking.
Kidney beans		High in calcium and iron; contain some vitamin A.	There are red and black types of this bean.
Chickpeas		Extremely high in calcium; high in iron and protein.	Require a longer cooking time. Cooked chickpeas are used in hummus, a pâté that also includes sesame seeds, garlic, lemon juice and olive oil.
Blackeye beans and peas		A good source of protein and minerals.	These can be cooked without soaking.
Adzuki beans		A good source of minerals.	Small, sweet-flavoured red beans from Japan.
Mung beans		Rich in vitamins A and C and iron.	Used for beansprouts in Chinese cooking. Easy to sprout them yourself.
Haricot beans		A good source of protein and minerals; the usual constituent of baked beans.	Baked beans are high in sugar and salt, but health-food shops sell them sweetened with fruit juice.
Butter beans		Contain protein and minerals.	These are good in soups and salads.
Broad beans		A source of calcium, iron and protein.	Usually available fresh or frozen rather than dried.

Nuts are rich in essential fatty acids, protein, minerals (including calcium), the B vitamins and vitamin E. Eat them raw to preserve nutrients and buy cold-pressed oils. Shelled nuts can go rancid and become toxic, so store them in an airtight container or in the refrigerator. Nut butters are a wholesome spread – health-food shops sell nonhydrogenated unsalted versions sweetened with fruit juice.

Like nuts, seeds are rich in essential fatty acids, protein, minerals and the B vitamins. Although toasting them improves their flavour, it depletes the nutrients. Buy oils that are cold-pressed.

Nearly all the foods in this category, particularly the pulses, can be sprouted – made to grow shoots like beansprouts – which increases nutrients and reduces indigestible ingredients. ∎

CAUTION

When sprouting pulses, do not leave them in extreme temperatures or in direct sunlight. Soak them overnight, drain, rinse and place in jars covered with muslin tops. Leave them in a warm, dark place for a few days, rinsing twice a day.

A GUIDE TO GRAINS

Name		Nutritional value	Additional information
Wheat		High in protein, vitamin E and the B vitamins. Wheat germ and wheat germ oil are particularly good sources of omega-3 essential fatty acids and vitamin E. High in gluten (a protein which people with gluten intolerance cannot digest).	Can cause allergy or intolerance. It may be high in pesticides, so buy organic products. Sprouted, durum or spelt wheat are easiest to tolerate. Bulgar wheat (partially cooked grains) can be used like rice. Additive names are cereal binder, filler, protein, starch and modified starch.
Rice		Rich in B vitamins, calcium and iron.	Choose wholegrain, brown or wild rice. Easily digestible.
Corn/maize		Contains vitamin A, the B vitamins and minerals.	May be genetically modified. See Wheat for additive names. Can cause allergy or intolerance.
Rye		A good source of vitamin E, magnesium, silicone (benefits bones, teeth, nails and hair) and essential fatty acids – and gluten.	Rye biscuits and bread available. Rye groats, or wholegrains, sprout well or can be soaked and cooked like rice. Can cause allergy or intolerance.
Barley		A good source of minerals; lower fat than other grains. High in gluten.	Choose pot type. Roast barley is a coffee substitute. Can cause allergy or intolerance.
Oats		High in protein (including gluten), iron, calcium and the B vitamins. Particularly beneficial for blood cholesterol levels and sugar metabolism.	Types available (from most to least nutritious) are: wholegrain oats (groats), hulled (or gritted) oatmeal, steelcut oats, rolled oats, instant oatmeal. Can cause allergy or intolerance.
Millet		Rich in protein and minerals, especially silicone. Grain highest in iron. Gluten free.	Use like rice. Can be used by those with gluten intolerance.
Buckwheat		High in calcium and contains bioflavonoids, rutin and vitamin C. Gluten free.	Not related to wheat. Can be used by those with gluten intolerance.
Quinoa		A complete protein and rich in calcium and iron.	Use like rice. Can be used by those with gluten intolerance.
Amaranth		A complete protein and the richest vegetable source of iron. Gluten free.	Use like rice. Can be used by those with gluten intolerance.

THE NUTRITIONAL ROLE OF NUTS

Name		Nutritional value	Additional information
Peanut (groundnut)		A good source of iron.	Eat in moderation. They are a common allergen. The oil resists heat well, so it is good for cooking.
Cashew		Contains vitamin C.	Makes an alternative to dairy cream when liquidized. Occasionally triggers allergy.
Walnut		One of the few nonfish sources of omega-3 essential fatty acid.	Can use oil form on salads.
Brazil		Particularly rich in protein.	These can go rancid quickly.
Hazelnut (cobnut, filbert)		Lowest fat content of all nuts; high in calcium.	Also available as an oil.
Pinenut		Richest nut source of protein.	Best lightly cooked to reduce turpentine taste.
Almond		One of the most nutritious nuts; high in calcium and the B vitamins.	Cream can be used instead of dairy cream; available as an oil.
Chestnut		Low in fat and high in carbohydrates.	Best cooked to reduce tannic acid. Can be made into flour.
Coconut		High in saturated fat so use sparingly.	Coconut milk (puréed flesh) can be used in sauces instead of dairy milk.
Pistachio		Contains vitamin A.	The greener the colour the better the quality.

THE VALUE OF SEEDS AND THEIR OILS

Name		Nutritional value	Additional information
Sesame		Particularly high in protein, minerals such as calcium, essential fatty acids and vitamin E.	Seeds are used in tahini and in some breads. Oil keeps well but does not tolerate heat – add as flavouring at end of cooking. May trigger allergy.
Sunflower		High in vitamin E, the B vitamins and minerals.	Seeds are used in some breads. The oil is good for cooking. Some of the ingredients mimic the effect of nicotine – use to help stop smoking.
Safflower		A good source of essential fatty acids.	Use this strong-flavoured oil sparingly in salad dressings or at the end of cooking.
Pumpkin		Source of minerals and B vitamins.	Eat seeds as a snack or with salads. Eaten traditionally as a male hormonal tonic.
Linseed		A source of omega-3 essential fatty acids.	Use food-grade oil in salad dressings or take as a supplement. Oil is not suitable for cooking.

Animal produce

Many people plan meals around fish, poultry and other meat. These foods, as well as dairy products and eggs, provide protein, minerals and some vitamins, but they should be eaten in moderation.

Although an important source of complete protein, meat products also contain saturated fat. Saturated fat and too much animal protein can be unhealthy. In addition, basing too much of your diet around animal produce can stop you from eating an adequate amount of vegetables and fruit, which contain complex carbohydrates and essential nutrients and play an important role in preventing disease. However, some of the disadvantages of animal produce can be mitigated by choosing low-fat varieties and preparing them without adding extra fat during cooking.

Commercially farmed animals may contain residues of the hormones, antibiotics and other drugs used to treat them, as well as pesticides from their feed. You can avoid these by eating fish and organic meat, dairy produce and eggs. Organic options are increasingly available in supermarkets. You can order organic meat from your butcher if he does not stock it. Organic animals arc also raised in far superior conditions – for example, poultry are allowed "free range" and live in as natural a state as possible.

SUBSTITUTE PRODUCTS

Some people avoid meat products for health or humanitarian reasons, and some may avoid dairy products because they are lactose intolerant. As an alternative to these products soya beans are one of the most protein-rich vegetable foods.

Soya beans are not eaten by themselves in their original state because they are difficult to digest; instead, they are made into a variety of products (see box, left), some of which are flavourings. Sixty percent of processed food contains soya in some form. However, soya may be genetically modified, so buy organic products if this worries you. Some people are sensitive to soya products and should avoid them.

SOYA AND ITS PRODUCTS

Soya is available in various forms, some of them as substitutes for dairy products:

- Tofu is soya "curd", a substance with the consistency of soft cheese but little taste; use it in savoury and sweet dishes.

- Soya milk, yoghurt and cheese contain half the fat of dairy products. They may be found in commercial ice cream.

- Tempeh is a cheeselike "cake" made of fermented soya beans. This is a source of vitamin B_{12}.

- Textured vegetable protein (tvp) is used as a vegetarian mince, which is often found in processed foods.

- Soya sauce (shoyu), often used to prepare Oriental meals, has a salty flavour. Buy additive-free and low-sodium versions.

- Miso is a paste similar to soya sauce and is also used in Oriental cooking. It contains vitamin B_{12}, as well as wheat.

- Soya flour is used in numerous processed foods.

- Soya oil is rich in essential fatty acids, including omega-3, but do not use it for cooking at a high heat. It is used in processed foods, but in the nutritionally worthless hydrogenated form.

- Vegetable gum, protein or starch are all names of additives made from either soya or corn (maize).

FISH AND SHELLFISH

As well as providing protein, fish are a good source of minerals, particularly iodine, which may be lacking in other foods. White fish and most shellfish are extremely low in fat and all fish are low in saturated fat – it makes up less than one-quarter of their total fat content. Oily fish are valuable for their essential fatty acids. Fish also contain the B vitamins and oily fish vitamins A and D. Of these, the most important are the B vitamins, which are often lacking in the typical Western diet, especially vitamin B_{12}, which is rare in nonanimal food.

Fresh fish should be firm and pleasant smelling. Aim to eat it on the day you buy it. It is healthiest to grill, steam or poach fish because deep frying adds a lot of fat. However, if you do decide to deep fry, always use fresh oil, and make sure it is hot enough so that it is not absorbed by the batter.

Farmed trout and salmon may contain chemical residues. The purity of other fish depends on the amount of pollution in the sea from which it came.

MEAT

Chicken, beef, pork and lamb are the most common types of meat consumed, but more exotic types, including ostrich and kangeroo steaks, are appearing in the supermarkets. Meat is an excellent source of complete protcin and minerals, such as iron, selenium and zinc, as well as the

THE NUTRITIONAL ROLE OF FISH

Type	Nutritional value	Additional information
Oily fish Mackerel, salmon, trout, tuna, herring, sardine, anchovy, swordfish	Richest food source of essential fatty acids, particularly omega-3. Low in saturated fat and high in protein, iron, some of the B vitamins and vitamin D; contains some calcium and a valuable source of iodine.	Three portions of oily fish a week provide the recommended intake of omega-3 essential fatty acids, but tinned fish contains reduced quantities. Small fish eaten with bones are a good source of calcium. Buckling, bloaters and kippers are smoked herrings; if kippers are red-brown they have been dyed – choose nut-brown or yellow-brown fish.
White fish Bass, cod, coley, haddock, hake, halibut, monkfish, mullet, plaice, skate, sole, turbot, whiting	High in protein and has some calcium and B vitamins. A valuable source of iodine and extremely low in fat.	Dyed smoked cod and haddock are bright yellow.
Crustaceans Crab, lobster, shrimp, prawn, crayfish, scampi (Dublin Bay prawns)	High in protein, calcium and vitamin B_3. A good source of iron, zinc and iodine. Low in fat, except for crab.	Can cause allergies in susceptible people.
Molluscs Mussels, cockles, winkles, oysters, clams, scallops, squid, cuttlefish, octopus, snails (escargots)	High in protein, vitamin B_3 and minerals. Oysters are the richest source of zinc of all foods. Extremely low in fat.	Can cause allergies. Bivalves such as mussels are vulnerable to contamination by pollutants and sewage, so buy from a reputable source, especially oysters, which are eaten raw. The shells of fresh live bivalves should close when tapped; discard any that do not. When cooked, shells should open; discard any that do not do so.

B vitamins. However, except for poultry and game, meat is high in saturated fat (nearly half of the total fat content).

A health issue regarding meat is bovine spongiform encephalopathy (BSE), a disease of beef cattle that has been linked to the human brain disease Creutzfeldt-Jakob disease (CJD) in Great Britain. The method of transmission of the disease between cows and from cows to humans is not yet clear, although the nervous system is known to play a part. If you are concerned about eating contaminated meat, it is safest to choose organic beef.

There has been no recorded case of BSE in any British herd managed organically since before 1985.

Other health hazards from meat include food-poisoning bacteria such as salmonella and *Escherichia coli (E. coli)*. Ideally, meat should be thoroughly cooked and not pink, particularly if it is intended for children, pregnant women, invalids or the elderly. Make sure that meat does not drip on to other food when stored in the refrigerator, and thoroughly wash all utensils, surfaces and your hands after preparing it. For example, never prepare

TYPES OF MEAT AND ITS DERIVATIVES

Type		Nutritional values	Hints on using
Poultry Chicken, turkey, duck, goose, guineafowl, quail, squab		Protein, vitamins B_2 and B_3. Low in fat and saturated fat (about one third of total fat content).	Discarding skin reduces fat content enormously. Because it is susceptible to contamination with salmonella bacteria, it must always be cooked thoroughly and kept separate from all other food.
Domestic meat Beef and veal, pork, lamb		Contains protein, the B vitamins, selenium, zinc and iron. High in fat, nearly half of which is saturated.	Minced and chopped meat are more perishable than larger pieces and should ideally be eaten within a day of purchase. Chops and lamb are the most fatty types. Stewing steak, rump steak, shin, silverside and brisket are the less fatty cuts of beef. Pork can cause an allergy or intolerance.
Game Pheasant, grouse, partridge, woodpigeon, wild duck, rabbit, venison, wild boar		A good source of protein, the B vitamins, selenium, zinc and iron. High in essential fatty acids.	Wild animals and birds are lower in fat than domesticated ones (which may make them tougher). Wild boar is usually farmed and venison may be. "Hanging" (keeping game until it starts to putrefy) improves texture.
Exotic meat Ostrich, kangaroo, alligator		Lower in saturated fat than beef, lamb and pork.	Meat from ostriches and alligators comes from farmed animals.
Offal Liver, kidney, heart, tail, giblets, tongue, tripe, brains, sweetbread, foot (trotter)		Source of protein. High in vitamins A, B_2, B_3, B_{12} and folic acid, especially liver. High in fat, nearly half of which is saturated.	Highly perishable – eat within a day of purchase. Pregnant women should avoid liver because its high vitamin A content can harm the baby.
Processed meat Bacon, ham, sausage, salami, pâté, lard, gelatine		Extremely high in fat and may contain harmful additives or large quantities of salt.	To avoid contamination, keep separate from raw meat. Lower fat types available. Pregnant women should avoid liver pâté and related products.

vegetables for a salad using an unwashed cutting board and knife after you have used them for cutting meat.

To reduce the fat content, buy lean cuts of meat and trim off all visible fat. Grill or roast meat on a rack so that the fat drips through and dry fry stewing meat or mince. By not eating the skin on poultry you can markedly reduce your fat intake.

DAIRY PRODUCTS AND EGGS

Milk, yoghurt and cheese are a good source of protein (cheese has as much as meat – about 70 percent), calcium and the B vitamins. Their main value is their calcium, which is essential for healthy bones, teeth, muscles and blood (although this can be obtained from plant foods; see box, right). All dairy produce contains vitamin A, but it is also high in saturated fat. Choose semi-skimmed or skimmed milk and low-fat dairy products.

Yoghurt made with live bacteria can help stabilize the naturally-occurring bacteria in your digestive system. Some women find that it helps prevent thrush (a type of yeast infection, see pp.142–43). Dairy products can cause allergies or lactose intolerance in susceptible people and may have to be avoided by them.

Eggs are high in minerals and vitamins as well as protein, but the yolks also contain large amounts of saturated fat and cholesterol. You can avoid them in baking by using additional egg whites and eliminating the yolks. ■

CALCIUM CONTENT

The following are all good sources of calcium. The average person needs about 1000 mg a day. Pregnant and breast-feeding mothers need more.

Foods	mg per 100 g
Cheese, hard	800
Cheese, soft	400
Milk, whole	120
Milk, skimmed	130
Yoghurt, full-fat	120
Yoghurt, low-fat	180
Tofu, without calcium sulphate	200
Tofu, with calcium sulphate	680
Figs, dried	140
Broccoli, cooked	50

DAIRY PRODUCE

Type		Nutritional value	Additional information
Milk Cream Yoghurt Cheese Butter Ghee		Milk, yoghurt and cheese supply protein, calcium, vitamins B_2, B_3, B_{12} and folic acid. All dairy products contain vitamin A, but they are high in fat, two-thirds of which is saturated. Low-fat varieties are available, but these have reduced vitamin A. Cheese is high in salt and may contain additives (colourings in orange cheese and preservatives). Yoghurt may contain beneficial "live" bacteria.	A common allergen and many adults, particularly non-Caucasians, are not able to digest it because of an intolerance. Yoghurt, ghee (clarified butter) and goat's and ewe's products are less likely to cause intolerance. Do not give cow's milk to children under 12 months old. Ghee can be used for high-temperature frying. Pregnant women should avoid blue-veined, soft, goat's and ewe's cheeses (pasteurized and unpasteurized) and any other unpasteurized dairy produce because of the risk of listeria and other infections. Milk derivatives that are used as additives are labelled as casein, caseinate, lactalbumin, lactose and whey.

TYPES OF EGGS

Type	Nutritional value	Additional information
Chicken Duck Goose Quail	Contain protein, iron and other minerals, vitamins A, B_2, B_3, B_{12}, folic acid and vitamin D. Yolks are high in fat, half of which is the saturated type.	Because of possible salmonella contamination, children, pregnant women, invalids and the elderly should eat only well-cooked eggs. Adding vinegar to the raw yolk kills bacteria. Duck and goose eggs are usually baked. Eggs can cause allergies. Egg derivatives used as additives are lecithin (egg or soya) and ovalbumin.

FAT CONTENT OF MEATS, DAIRY PRODUCTS AND EGGS

The fat in meat is affected by the cooking method used. The figures given are for total fat. Not all fats are bad, but some meats, such as beef and lamb, contain high amounts of saturated fat. The figures are given for 100 g of the food – work out the size of your typical portion and adjust the figure accordingly.

Foods	g per 100 g
Oily fish	
Salmon, steamed	10.4
Sardines, tinned	13.6
Tuna, tinned, drained	21.0
White fish	
Cod, grilled	1.5
Cod, fried in batter	10.6
Plaice, steamed	1.7
Plaice, fried in crumbs	13.3
Fish fingers, fried	13.0
Molluscs, raw	
Mussels	1.9
Oysters	0.9
Crustaceans, boiled	
Crab	5.2
Lobster	3.4
Prawns	1.8
Poultry	
Chicken, roast, meat only	5.4
Chicken, roast, meat and skin	14.0
Turkey, roast, meat only	1.8
Duck, meat only	9.1

Foods	g per 100 g
Domestic meat	
Beef, grilled, lean	6.0
Beef, roast, lean	9.1
Beef, stewed	7.4
Lamb, grilled chop, meat and fat	22.5
Lamb, grilled chop, meat only	6.9
Lamb, roast, lean	8.1
Pork, grilled chop, meat and fat	18.5
Pork, grilled chop, meat only	6.7
Pork, roast, lean	6.9
Mince, stewed with onion	14.5
Processed meat	
Bacon, grilled	33.8
Sausage, pork, grilled	24.4
Frankfurter	25.6
Salami	45.5
Ham	5.5
Corned beef	11.7
Beefburger, fried	17.8
Pork pie	27.3

Foods	g per 100 g
Processed meat continued	
Meat and vegetable pie	21.5
Liver pâté	26.7
Dairy produce	
Milk, skimmed	0.1
Milk, whole	3.8
Yoghurt, low-fat	1.0
Yoghurt, full-fat	10.0
Cream, single	21.2
Cream, double	48.2
Cheese, soft, Camembert-type	23.0
Cheese, hard, Cheddar-type	34.0
Cheese, Stilton	40.0
Cheese, cottage	0.5
Cheese, cream	47.0
Butter	82.0
Eggs	
Yolk, raw	30.5
White, raw	trace
Boiled	11.7
Fried	20.0
Scrambled	22.9

Chapter 4

ESSENTIAL FIRST AID

THE TERM "FIRST AID" MEANS EXACTLY THAT: THE primary assistance given to an injured person, often before the arrival of an ambulance or professional medical help. The intentions of a person giving first aid are to preserve life and prevent the condition or injury from becoming worse. This chapter tells you about the basics so that you will be able to give that first aid if help is not available.

Emergencies and accidents are unexpected and sudden, and coping with them is not easy if you are the person providing help. When giving first aid, it is important to remain as calm as possible: don't rush into taking an action, which could cause more harm than good. Ideally, try to be prepared by taking a course.

A first aid course will train you to provide a correct and prompt response. A professional organization such as the Red Cross or St John ambulance or St Andrew's ambulance (in Scotland) can provide expert instruction. Telephone numbers for these organizations can be found in your local phone directory. ■

SEE ALSO

Resuscitation for adults
296–297

Resuscitation for children
298–299

Recovery position
300–301

Choking

You must act promptly to help someone who is choking, which occurs when there is a blockage of the windpipe. In adults, the blockage is usually caused by food "going down the wrong way"; in children, by swallowing an object — children under three years old are most at risk.

SIGNS

In an adult or older child:

■ Difficulty in speaking and breathing.

■ Hands may rise to the throat.

■ The face may turn blue, and the veins in the face and neck may stand out.

CAUTION

When trying to remove an obstruction inside a person's throat, make sure that you do not push it farther down.

FOR AN UNCONSCIOUS ADULT

I Because muscles relax during loss of consciousness, the blockage may be freed; try to remove it with a hooked finger. Open the airway and check for breathing and circulation. If necessary, start CPR (pp.296–97). If you're unable to ventilate the person, the obstruction may still be there. Go to the next step.

FOR A CONSCIOUS ADULT

I Encourage the person to cough, which may dislodge the object. If the person fails to cough up the blockage, proceed to the next step.

2 Ask the person to bend forward at the waist at about a 45° angle. Supporting the person at the waist, give her five sharp slaps with the flat of your hand between the shoulder blades. If this fails, go on to the next step.

3 Stand behind the person and put your arms around her trunk. Make a fist with a hand and place it with the thumb-side against the abdomen, just below the ribcage. Grasp the fist with your other hand and pull sharply inward and upward. Try up to five thrusts. Repeat steps 2 and 3 until the obstruction clears.

2 Turn the person on her side, supporting her head and placing it angled toward the floor. Give five sharp blows with the flat of your hand between the shoulder blades. Check in the person's mouth and remove any obstruction, using a hooked finger. If the airway is still blocked, go to the next step.

3 Turn the person on to her back. Place the heel of one hand below the ribcage and the other hand on top. With straight arms, press sharply inward and upward five times. If she stops breathing, call for an ambulance, then resuscitate (pp.296–97). If the chest doesn't rise, repeat steps 2 and 3. Place a breathing person in the recovery position (p.300).

SIGNS

In a baby or young child:
- Difficulty in breathing.
- Odd noises or no sound.
- Red face and neck.

CAUTION

If a baby loses consciousness, begin the breathing part of resuscitation (pp.298–99). If the chest does not rise, try the two steps for removing a blockage; repeat this sequence until help arrives.

CHECK SYSTEM

After each step:
- Check for an obstruction in the mouth.
- Put a breathing unconscious child in the recovery position (p.300).
- If still not breathing, give the child five artificial breaths.
- If the chest does not rise, go to the next step.

FOR A BABY UNDER ONE YEAR OLD

1 Hold the baby face-down over your forearm. The chest should be supported with your arm and the chin with your hand. Slap firmly between the shoulder blades five times. Turn the baby over and open his airway to check his mouth (p.299) – if the object was not dislodged, go on to the next step.

2 Support the baby over your knee with the head lower than the chest. Press firmly on his chest a finger's width below the nipple line with two fingers. Repeat five times, then check the baby's mouth. If the object still has not been dislodged, repeat steps 1 and 2 three times. If you still have no success, call 999, then continue the steps.

FOR A CHILD ONE TO SEVEN YEARS OLD

1 Bend the child with his head lower than his chest. Give five slaps between the shoulders with one hand. Check his mouth for the object. If not dislodged, stand or kneel behind him. Make a fist and put it against the lower breastbone. Grasp the fist with your other hand. Press into chest with a sharp inward thrust five times, once every three seconds.

2 Try five more back slaps. If choking continues, grasp your fist with your hand and place on the child's abdomen under the ribcage and above his navel. Press with a sharp upward thrust up to five times. If choking continues, dial 999. Continue the sequence until help arrives. If he starts breathing, put him in the recovery position (p.300).

3 If the child loses consciousness, lay him on his side and give five back slaps. Turn him face upward and check his mouth for object. If not breathing, give five breaths of artificial respiration (pp.298–99). Use the heel of one hand on his lower breastbone to give five sharp inward thrusts a third of the depth of his chest, once every three seconds.

4 If the obstruction hasn't been cleared, put the heel of your hand halfway between his navel and breastbone. Give up to five firm upward thrusts. Repeat the cycle of slaps and chest and abdominal thrusts described in steps 3 and 4 until medical help arrives. Put the child into the recovery position (p.300) if he starts breathing.

SEE ALSO

Asthma   28–31
Heart disease   35–39
Recovery position
                 300–301

THE ABC'S OF RESUSCITATION

- A is for open AIRWAY – keep the head tilted back.

- B is for BREATHING – look for the chest rising.

- C is for CIRCULATION – feel for a pulse.

SEEKING HELP

- If you are not alone, send someone to call an ambulance.

- If you are alone, follow the CPR procedures for a minute then call an ambulance before continuing.

- Resuscitating someone can be exhausting, so share the delivery of CPR with other people if possible.

Resuscitation for adults

The aim of resuscitation is to help a person whose breathing or heart has stopped, maybe both. If the brain does not have a constant supply of oxygen it will begin to fail after only three or four minutes. By providing artificial respiration you can breathe for a person and, combined with cardiopulmonary resuscitation (CPR), circulate oxygen.

CHECKING FOR AN OPEN AIRWAY

1 To find out whether the injured person is conscious, check for a response. Ask a question in a loud voice. If there is no response try shaking him gently by the shoulders. If there is still no response go on to the next step.

2 Open the airway by placing two fingers under the point of the person's chin and lifting the jaw. Place your other hand on his forehead and tilt the head back. If you suspect head or neck injuries, cautiously tilt the head back just enough to open the airway.

3 To check breathing, kneel beside the person and put your face next to his mouth. Look along the line of the chest for any movement. Listen for any sounds of breath. Feel for breath on your cheek. Check for up to 10 seconds. If he is not breathing go on to the next step.

4 With the person flat on his back., look for an obstruction in the mouth. Make a hook of your index finger and use this to scoop it out. Make sure you don't push an object farther down the throat. If not obstructed, go to Giving Artificial Respiration.

GIVING ARTIFICIAL RESPIRATION

1 Pinch the person's nose tightly with your index finger and thumb so that no air can escape. Take a deep full breath and place your lips around his mouth, making a seal.

2 Blow firmly and slowly into his mouth until you see his chest rise – about two seconds. Remove your lips and let his chest fall for four seconds. Repeat, then look for signs of breathing.

GIVING CPR

1 With your middle and index fingers, check the carotid pulse – located at the hollow between the windpipe and the large neck muscle – for 10 seconds. Meanwhile, look for signs of breathing or returning skin colour. If there is no pulse or sign of circulation, begin chest compressions.

2 Kneel beside the person. Using your hand farthest from his head, place your middle finger on the breastbone at the point where it meets the ribs and put your index finger above it. Place the heel of your other hand on the breastbone and slide it down until it reaches your index finger. This is where you apply pressure.

3 Place the heel of your hand on top of the hand just positioned and interlock your fingers. Leaning well over the person with your arms straight, press down and depress the breastbone 4–5 cm (1½–2 in). Release the pressure without removing your hands.

4 Compress the chest 15 times over nine seconds. Then give two breaths of artificial respiration (see above). Continue the cycle of alternating 15 chest compressions with 2 breaths of artificial respiration until help arrives.

SEQUENCE CHECKLIST

■ If a person is unconscious, open the airway and check breathing.

■ If not breathing, give two breaths of artificial respiration; check the pulse.

■ If the pulse is present, continue artificial respiration. Check the pulse every 10 breaths.

■ If the chest does not rise after two breaths, check that you have correctly followed the steps for Checking for an Open Airway and Giving Artificial Respiration. Try three more breaths, then recheck you have followed the correct procedures.

■ If there is no pulse or sign of recovery, such as return of skin colour or breathing, begin CPR, combined with artificial respiration.

■ Place the person in the recovery position (p.300) if breathing returns.

Resuscitation for children

The main cause of a child's heart stopping is respiratory failure. The resuscitation procedures depend on the child's age and size. For a child eight years of age or older, use the adult resuscitation procedures. Follow the steps here for a child one to seven years old or a baby under one year.

ABC CHECK

■ Check A for AIRWAY – is it clear? If not, open the airway.

■ Check B for BREATHING – if the child is not breathing, breathe for her.

■ Check C for CIRCULATION – Is the heart beating? If not, compress the chest.

CAUTION

Do not stick your fingers blindly down a throat to remove an obstruction – you could push the object farther down. To remove the object, use a hooked index finger to scoop it out.

SEEKING HELP

■ Send someone to call an ambulance.

■ If you are alone, follow the steps for resuscitation for one minute, then call an ambulance before continuing.

■ Resuscitating someone can be exhausting, so share doing the steps with others if you can.

FOR A ONE TO SEVEN YEAR OLD

1 Seek a response by talking to the child and gently shaking her. If she doesn't respond, open the airway by placing two fingers under her chin and a hand on her forehead and gently tilting her head back. Remove any obstruction from her mouth (pp.294–95).

2 Look for a rising chest and feel for breath on your cheek. If breathing, put her in the recovery position (p.300). If not, pinch her nose tightly; place your mouth around hers, making a tight seal. Breathe deeply until the chest rises. Give five breaths.

3 Use two fingers to feel for the carotid pulse – found in the hollow between the windpipe and large muscle on either side of the neck – for 10 seconds. If you cannot find a pulse and there are no other signs of recovery, such as returning skin colour, start chest compressions.

4 Place the heel of one hand two fingers' width above the end of the breastbone. Press down firmly to a third of the depth of the chest. Do this five times over three seconds. Give one breath of artificial respiration. Follow this sequence for a minute, call an ambulance, then continue the sequence until help arrives.

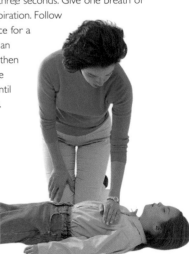

FOR A BABY UNDER 12 MONTHS

1 To find out if the baby is conscious, talk to her and shake her shoulders extremely gently. If the baby does not respond, start the resuscitation procedure.

2 Place an index finger on the chin and the other hand on the baby's forehead. Tilt the head back to open the airway. Look inside the mouth to see if anything is blocking the airway. Use a hooked index finger to remove it.

CAUTION

Do not breathe too hard when giving a baby artificial respiration: the air can go into the stomach, forcing its contents into the lungs.

3 Look for a rising chest and listen for breathing. Place your cheek by the baby's mouth to feel for breath. If the baby is not breathing after five seconds, start artificial respiration.

4 Make a tight seal by completely covering the baby's mouth and nose with your mouth. Breathe deeply enough to make the chest rise. Give five breaths, taking your mouth away after each breath.

SEQUENCE CHECKLIST

- If a child is unconscious, open the airway and check for breathing.

- If there are no signs of breathing, give artificial respiration.

- If there is a pulse, continue artificial respiration. Check the pulse every 10 breaths.

- If the chest does not rise after two breaths, check how you opened the airway and gave artificial respiration. If three more breaths fail, check for an obstruction (pp.294–95).

- If there is no pulse or sign of recovery, begin CPR (see last step), with artificial respiration.

- If child's breathing returns, put in the recovery position (pp.300–01).

5 Check the pulse, using two fingers on the brachial pulse on the inside of the arm midway between the elbow and the shoulder. If there is no pulse, go to the next step.

6 Using two fingers a finger's width below the nipple line, press the chest down 2 cm (¾ in), five times in three seconds. Give one breath. Repeat for a minute. Dial for help; continue the sequence until help arrives.

SEE ALSO
Heart disease   35–39
Resuscitation for adults
296–297
Resuscitation for children
298–299

CAUTION

If you suspect spinal or neck injuries, support the head in the neutral position: the head, neck and spine must be aligned (p.303).

Recovery position

An unconscious person who is breathing should be placed in the recovery position. The technique shown below is based on finding the person lying on her back. Not all the steps will be necessary if you discover the person lying on her side or front.

FOR AN UNCONSCIOUS PERSON

1 Kneel beside the person. Open her airway by putting two fingers under the point of her chin and one hand on her forehead and tilting the head well back.

2 Straighten the person's limbs. Gently lift the leg that is nearest you to put her hand, with the palm turned upward, under her thigh. Straighten her arm before lowering and repositioning the leg.

3 Put the arm that is farthest from you across her chest. Place the back of the hand against her cheek – the one nearest to you – and hold it there. With your other hand holding her far leg just above the knee, pull on the leg to roll her toward you. Roll her on to her side, and let her come to rest on your knees so she does not flop over.

4 Lower her gently on to her front, with her cheek resting on her hand. Move the leg closest to you so that it is bent at the knee at a right angle to her body. Check that her head is tilted back and the airway open. Make sure that the arm farthest from you is free, with the palm facing upward.

FOR A BABY UNDER 12 MONTHS OLD

Cradle the baby in your arms with the head tilted downward. This prevents the baby from choking on his tongue or from inhaling vomit. For a child older than 12 months, follow the adult procedure.

WHILE WAITING FOR HELP

■ If you suspect that a person has lost consciousness, you should confirm this by questioning her and shaking her by the shoulders.

■ While waiting for help, monitor the person's breathing by looking for a moving chest and feeling for breath against your cheek every 10 minutes. If breathing has stopped, you should begin resuscitation (pp.296–99).

■ Also check the person's pulse every 10 minutes. If you cannot find one, begin resuscitation (pp.296–99).

HEART ATTACK VICTIM

If the patient is conscious, make him comfortable by easing any strain on the heart. A half-sitting position is best, with the person's head and shoulders given plenty of support. He may be more comfortable with bent knees. Loosen any tight clothing and give reassurance. Dial for an ambulance. Keep an eye on the breathing and pulse rate and keep a record of these. If the person has a history of a heart problem, such as angina, and has medicine for it, help the person take it. If the pain continues and he is fully awake, give one tablet of aspirin to chew.

STROKE VICTIM

If the person is conscious, gently lay her down with her head and shoulders raised and supported. Use clothing if a pillow or blanket is not available. Turn her head to one side, and if there is any dribbling, place a cloth on her shoulder. If the casualty is unconscious, loosen her clothing and monitor her breathing and pulse.

Resuscitation: drowning

If you see someone drowning, your first aim is to bring her out of the water without endangering yourself. Once on dry land, treat her for drowning and hypothermia and, if necessary, call an ambulance.

CAUTION

Do not go into the water to rescue a drowning person unless it is absolutely necessary. Do not try to force water from the stomach because this can cause the contents to be inhaled. A person involved in a near drowning must receive medical attention even if she seems okay. If water has entered the lungs, the air passages can swell hours later.

1 If you are carrying the drowning person from the water, ensure that her head is lower than the rest of her body. This reduces the risk of inhaling water.

2 Lay the person down and tell someone to call for an ambulance. Open her airway by using two fingers on her chin and a hand on her forehead to tilt her head back. Check for breathing by feeling for breath on your cheek. Begin resuscitation (pp.296–99) if she isn't breathing. Because water in the lungs and being cold can cause resistance, you may need to work more slowly than normal.

REDUCING THE RISK

Drowning can result as easily from developing a cramp in a pool as from battling with currents in open water. The sea in western Europe poses an extra risk as it is cold even in summer.

Children are particularly vulnerable and can drown in the smallest amount of water. Never leave a young child alone in the bath or playing near a garden pond or where there is any collection of water such as near uncovered butts or wheelbarrows.

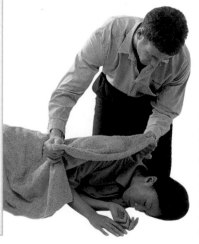

3 A drowning person may suffer from the effects of the cold. If so, treat her for hypothermia (p.308). Remove wet clothing and put dry ones on her if possible. If not, wrap her up and shield her from the wind. Put her in the recovery position (p.300). If she regains consciousness give her a hot drink. Dial for an ambulance if one has not already been called.

Head and back injuries

If you suspect a spinal injury, do not move the injured person unless she is in danger or becomes unconscious. However, if she needs resuscitating, this is more important than the risk of exacerbating an injury.

SIGNS OF BACK INJURY

- Soreness or pain in neck or back.
- A twist or curve of the spine.
- Loss of control over limbs; loss of sensation.
- Breathing difficulties.

TREATING HEAD INJURIES

All head injuries are dangerous, especially if there is concussion or unconsciousness – seek medical help.

- Signs of concussion include brief or partial loss of consciousness after a blow to the head; dizziness or nausea on recovery; and a mild headache.

- Signs of skull fracture are wounds or bruises on the head, a soft area on the scalp, a slow response or clear fluid or watery blood coming from the nose or ear.

- If a skull fracture victim is conscious, lay her down with her shoulders and head raised. Put a dressing on an ear with a discharge. Check breathing and pulse every 10 minutes.

- Put in the recovery position (p.300) if unconscious. Check breathing and pulse every 10 minutes. Call for help if unconscious over three minutes.

- Begin resuscitation if either breathing or pulse stops (pp.296–99).

SUPPORTING THE NECK

Reassure the injured person and support her head in the neutral position, with head, neck and spine aligned, and your hands over her ears. If you think there is a neck injury tell a helper to place rolled-up blankets or clothing on either side of her neck and shoulders. If there is loss of consciousness, monitor breathing and pulse. You may have to resuscitate (pp.296–99).

POSITIONING FOR CPR

Use this technique to turn an injured person on to her back for resuscitation (pp.296–99). This requires six people. Support her head with your hands over her ears. Ask five helpers to gently align the injured person's limbs until the head, trunk and toes are in a straight line. Three helpers should be on one side, two on the other. Everyone must work together, with the person holding the head directing all movements. Giving plenty of support to the spine, with the hips, thighs and calves held to steady the legs, roll the person on to her back.

For the sake of clarity, the helpers are omitted here to show how the head must be supported and aligned with the neck and back.

SEE ALSO

Resuscitation for adults
296–297

Resuscitation for children
298–299

Shock   307

Bleeding/Electric shock

If a wound is deep, first control the bleeding, then treat for shock, if necessary, and call for an ambulance. For an electric shock victim, remove the source of electricity before giving first aid treatment.

CAUTION

For bleeding

■ *Wear disposable gloves, if available, when treating a wound to prevent infection. Wash your hands in soap and water before and after treatment.*

■ *Do not use a tourniquet.*

For electric shock

■ *Do not handle electric appliances with wet hands or when standing on a damp floor – water conducts electricity.*

■ *Do not touch a person in contact with an electrical current – he may still be "live" and electrocute you.*

■ *Do not use any object that conducts electricity, particularly metal, to push away the source.*

TREATING A DEEP CUT

1 Remove or cut away any clothing from the wound, then cover it with a sterile dressing. Apply direct pressure over the wound with your fingers or the palm of your hand for 10 minutes. If an object such as a shard of glass is embedded in the wound, do not remove it. Put pressure on each side of the wound, then pad the dressing around it before bandaging.

Do not remove the original dressing.

2 Lay the person down and raise the injury above the level of the heart. Apply another sterile dressing on top of the first one if blood seeps through. Bandage it in place firmly but not too tightly or you will stop circulation. Call for an ambulance and, if necessary, treat the person for shock (p.307).

HELPING AN ELECTRIC SHOCK VICTIM

If you cannot find the mains, stand on a dry insulating material such as a telephone directory or newspapers. Using a wooden broom handle, chair or stool, push the source of electricity away from the victim or push his limbs away from the source.

ELECTRIC SHOCK

The person may be stunned, burnt or in spasm. Switch off the current at the mains or meter point. If you cannot find the mains, move the source of the electricity away from the person (see left). As a last resort, grasp any loose dry clothing to pull him away from the electricity – but do not touch him.

If unconscious, put him in the recovery position (p.300) and call an ambulance. Monitor his condition; give resuscitation (pp.296–99) if necessary. Cool any burns (see facing page).

SEE ALSO
Resuscitation for adults
296–297
Resuscitation for children
298–299
Shock 307

Burns

The priorities for treating burns are to rapidly cool the affected area and to check the person's breathing. Most people who have suffered a severe burn are affected by shock. All severe burns require medical treatment.

CAUTION

■ *Make sure you do not touch the injured area.*
■ *Do not burst any blisters.*
■ *Do not use any lotions or ointment or apply adhesive tape to the area.*
■ *Do not enter a burning building or a smoke- or fume-filled room.*
■ *Do not attempt to fight any but the smallest fire, but make sure the fire brigade has been called.*

SMOTHERING FLAMES

If the person's clothes are on fire:

■ **Stop him from running and tell him to drop to the ground.**

■ **Wrap him in a heavy non-synthetic blanket or jacket to smother the fire.**

■ **Roll him on the ground to put out the flames.**

■ **Treat any burns.**

I For a severe burn, lay the person down but keep the injury off the ground. Cool the burn by pouring plenty of cold water on it for 10 minutes. You can also use harmless cold liquids such as milk or soft drinks. Watch for signs of breathing difficulties and resuscitate (pp.296–99) if necessary. Put him in the recovery position if he loses consciousness (p.300).

2 Call an ambulance. Remove any tight clothing, watches, bracelets or rings from around the burn before the area starts to swell. Do not remove clothes that have stuck to the skin. Cut the unstuck clothes away but do not pull on them – this can cause further injury.

3 A burn has a high risk of becoming infected. Cover it with a sterile dressing if one is available. If not, use a clean cloth made from a nonfluffy material, such as a piece of bedsheet, or plastic cling film.

4 Alternatively, you can use a clean plastic bag to protect a hand, foot or lower arm or leg. No matter which dressing is used, secure it in place with a bandage or adhesive tape over the dressing – not the skin. Treat the person for shock (p.307).

SEE ALSO
Resuscitation for adults
296–297
Resuscitation for children
298–299
Recovery position 300

Poisoning

Any substance that has a harmful effect on the human body, injuring health or destroying life, can be considered a poison. You should never induce vomiting if corrosive materials were involved.

COMMON POISONS		
Cause	**Effect**	**Action**
Aspirin	Upper abdominal pain, nausea, vomiting, ringing in ears, confusion and delirium.	Resuscitate (pp.296–99). Dial for an ambulance. Look for drug containers, a suicide note or anything that may give a clue to what the person has taken. Send these with the person to the hospital.
Paracetamol	Eventually, upper abdominal pain and nausea. Can be fatal.	
Tranquillizers (Barbiturate and benzodiazepine)	Sleepiness or unconsciousness, shallow breathing and weak or abnormal pulse.	See above
Stimulants and hallucinogens (Amphetamines, Ecstasy and LSD)	Excitable frenzied, wild behaviour, tremors of the hand, sweating and hallucinations.	See above
Narcotics (Morphine, heroin)	Slow shallow breathing, pinpoint pupils in the eyes, sluggishness and confusion.	See above
Solvents (Glue, lighter fuel)	Nausea and vomiting; headache, convulsions and hallucinations.	If breathing, put the person in the recovery position (p.300). If not, resuscitate (pp.296–99) and call for help.
Carbon monoxide (Fumes from a car. solid fuel or gas fires)	Giddiness, headache, tightness of the chest, vomiting, collapse and unconsciousness.	Help the person into fresh air. Call for an ambulance.
Household corrosives (Bleach, other household cleaning fluids)	Burning pain in the mouth, throat and chest. Inflamed skin and bloodstained vomit.	Give three to four cups of water or milk by mouth at once.
Berries and fungi (Berry, toadstool, mushroom)	Pain and vomiting. Staining of the mouth or clothing may indicate the berries eaten.	Take the person to the hospital with the berries (or any stained clothes) or mushrooms.
Alcohol (Any type)	Flushed skin and weak pulse; a large amount can cause a coma, especially in young children.	Keep the patient in the recovery position (p.300); seek medical advice.

Shock

In medical terms, "shock" is the state that results when there is relative or absolute loss of circulating blood volume. It can be life threatening. Shock can develop in a number of situations, including bleeding, burns, blood poisoning, prolonged vomiting or diarrhoea and through pain and fear. It is essential to treat a person for shock in any of these instances.

SEE ALSO

Resuscitation for adults
296–297

Resuscitation for children
298–299

Recovery position 300

Bleeding/Electric shock/
Burns 304–305

CAUTION

■ *Do not give the person anything to eat or drink or allow her to move or smoke.*

■ *Do not leave the person alone except to call for an ambulance.*

■ *Do not try to warm her too quickly, for example, with a hot water bottle – this can divert blood from vital organs to the skin.*

■ *Do not confuse circulatory shock with the psychological state resulting from deep emotional trauma.*

SIGNS

■ **Pale, grey face.**

■ **Cold and clammy skin.**

■ **Fast and weak pulse.**

■ **Rapid shallow breathing.**

■ **Restlessness, yawning and sighing.**

■ **Thirst.**

■ **Untreated, unconsciousness and eventually death.**

1 Lay the victim down, and raise and support her legs at least 30 cm (12 in) from the ground. This helps the blood to flow to the upper body. If you are outside, place a blanket or coat under the victim to protect her from the cold ground. Treat any cause of shock such as bleeding or a burn.

2 Loosen any clothing that restricts the neck, chest or waist, including scarves, ties and belts. Keep her warm by wrapping her in a coat or blanket. Dial for an ambulance. Monitor and record, if possible, breathing, pulse and her level of response every 10 minutes. Be prepared to resuscitate (pp.296–99) if necessary.

SEE ALSO
Resuscitation for adults
296–297
Resuscitation for children
298–299
Resuscitation: drowning
302

Hypothermia

Elderly people, the homeless and infants are vulnerable to hypothermia, which can develop over several days in poorly heated homes. It can also be caused in the healthy by exposure to cold weather. Keep a survival bag or blanket in the car, and take it along when walking or camping.

CAUTION

■ *Do not allow an elderly or fragile person to have a bath to warm up.*
■ *Do not give the affected person alcohol.*
■ *Replace any wet clothing with dry clothes as quickly as possible.*
■ *Do not put heat sources such as hot water bottles or fires near the person.*

TREATING HYPOTHERMIA OUTDOORS
1 Put the person in any extra clothing or blankets but do not give him yours. Quickly take him to a sheltered spot.

SIGNS

■ Shivering and cold, pale skin.

■ Apathy, disorientation or irrational behaviour.

■ Lethargy.

■ Slow and shallow breathing.

Infants
■ Skin looks healthy but feels cold.

■ Limp and unusually quiet.

■ Refusal to feed.

RECOGNIZING AND TREATING FROSTBITE

The symptoms are pins and needles, then numbness and hardening of the skin and colour changes from white to mottled and blue to black. The skin is hot, painful and blistered on recovery.

■ Carefully remove any constrictions such as gloves, jewellery and boots.

■ Have the person warm his hands by placing them in his armpits. Or use your hands to warm the affected area. Do not rub it – this may harm the skin.

■ Move the person into a warm area. Place the affected part in a warm bath. Dry it and apply a dry gauze bandage.

■ Raise the limb to reduce swelling. Give an adult paracetamol and take to a hospital if necessary.

2 Place him in a foil or plastic survival bag or blanket. Or put him in a dry sleeping bag and cover him with blankets or newspapers. Use a layer of dry leaves underneath him to keep him off the ground. Send someone for help; do not leave the casualty alone. Give him a warm drink, if available.

TREATING HYPOTHERMIA INDOORS
If the victim is young and fit, he can have a bath in water of 40°C (104°F) before going to bed with a warm drink. If the victim is elderly or an infant, warm him gradually by covering him with a layer of blankets in a room temperature of 25°C (77°F). Include a hat for added warmth. Call the doctor.

SEE ALSO
Resuscitation for adults
296–297
Resuscitation for children
298–299
Recovery position **300**

Heat-related problems

Heat exhaustion occurs when the body loses too much salt and water due to excessive sweating from hot weather or too much exercise. Hot weather or a high fever can cause heatstroke, in which the body can no longer regulate its own temperature. To prevent dehydration, which occurs with heat exhaustion, drink plenty of nonalcoholic liquids.

CAUTION

Recreational drugs such as Ecstasy can cause heat exhaustion if the user fails to keep up her fluid intake.

SIGNS

Heat exhaustion

■ Headache, dizziness, confusion.

■ Loss of appetite and nausea.

■ Sweating, with pale clammy skin.

■ Cramps in arms, legs or abdomen.

■ Rapid, weakening pulse and breathing.

Heatstroke

■ Restlessness and confusion.

■ Hot, flushed and dry skin.

■ Headache, dizziness and discomfort.

■ Throbbing pulse.

■ Body temperature above 40°C (104°F).

HEAT EXHAUSTION

1 Give the affected person plenty of water to drink, if possible, with a weak salt solution (a teaspoon of salt to a litre/1¾ pt of water).

2 Take her to a cool, shady location, lay her down and raise her legs a minimum of 30 cm (12 in) to improve the blood flow to her brain. Even if the person recovers, ensure that she sees a doctor. If her condition deteriorates, put her in the recovery position (p.300) and dial for an ambulance.

HEATSTROKE

1 Take the person to a cool, shady location and remove her outer clothing. Dial for an ambulance. Place her in a half-sitting position, and wrap her in a cold wet sheet and keep it wet until her temperature drops to 38°C (104°F) under the tongue or 37.5°C (99.5°F) in the armpit. Or sponge her with cold water. You can also fan her with paper.

2 When her temperature has dropped to a safe level, replace the wet sheet with a dry one. Keep an eye on her until help arrives. If her temperature rises again, repeat the cooling process. If her responses deteriorate or she loses consciousness, follow the resuscitation procedures (pp.296–299).

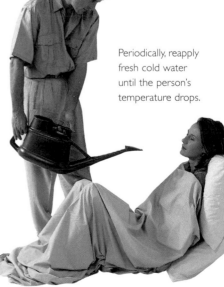

Periodically, reapply fresh cold water until the person's temperature drops.

SEE ALSO
Pregnancy   172–177
Resuscitation for adults
                    296–297
Resuscitation for children
                    298–299
Shock   307

Emergency childbirth

Labour often lasts for hours, with plenty of time to take the woman to hospital or enlist medical help. On the rare occasion when childbirth occurs unexpectedly, the mother will need reassurance. Most births are normal deliveries with mother and baby requiring little help.

THE DELIVERY AREA

Try to ensure that the area for the delivery is warm. Gather together as many of these items as are available:

■ An improvised cot, such as a box or drawer, lined with a clean, soft material such as a towel or two.

■ Disposable gloves.

■ Handkerchiefs to wear as face masks.

■ Newspapers or a plastic sheet.

■ A bowl of hot water for washing hands.

■ Clean warm towels and a blanket.

■ Plastic bags.

■ Sanitary towels.

PREPARE THE MOTHER
1 Call for help
At the first signs of labour call the midwife or doctor or dial 999 for an ambulance. Give any information you have about the mother's pregnancy history or any expected complications.

2 Find a comfortable position
Help the woman to settle into as comfortable a position as possible, often half-sitting, half-lying, with knees up. Using the heel of your hand, you can massage the woman's lower back as she lies on her side – this can help relieve the pain and have a calming influence while she waits for the delivery.

3 Cover the birth area for warmth
Lay some plastic sheeting, newspaper or towels over the bed, floor or sofa to provide warmth and to absorb any mess.

4 Prevent infection
Keep anyone with colds, sore throats or other infections away. Wear a face mask such as a clean handkerchief or folded triangular bandage. Before going anywhere near the birth canal, roll up your sleeves and wash your hands in hot soapy water, thoroughly scrubbing your fingernails. If available, wear disposable gloves. Wash your hands again after the delivery.

5 Check that an ambulance is on its way
Ring the midwife, doctor or 999 again.

Help the woman get into a comfortable position, making sure that her back and shoulders are well supported. Be meticulous in checking that everything is as clean as possible to prevent infection, and be prepared to offer practical and emotional support to mother and baby.

6 Check the mother's clothing

Help the mother to remove any clothing such as trousers and panties that could interfere with the birth. Put a blanket or sheet over her legs if she prefers to be covered.

THE DELIVERY
7 When the head shows

Ensure that the mother stops pushing and starts panting when you start to see the widest part of the baby's head. If the membrane is covering the baby's face, gently tear it away so that the baby is able to breathe.

8 Allow a natural delivery

The baby's head and shoulders will soon appear. Let the baby come out naturally, which should happen quickly. If the umbilical cord is wrapped around the baby's neck, check that it is loose, then carefully pull it over the head to prevent strangulation.

9 Put the baby on the mother's stomach

Lift the baby from the birth canal. Be careful: she will be slippery and covered in a fatty substance. Gently pass her to the mother, laying the baby on her stomach. Do not cut the umbilical cord.

10 Check that the baby is crying

The baby should begin crying once she is born. If she does not do so almost immediately, begin resuscitation (pp. 298–99).

11 Keep the baby warm

Wrap the baby in a clean cloth or blanket to protect her from hypothermia. Give her back to her mother. When laying the baby down, put her on her side with the head low so that any fluid or mucus can drain easily from the nose or mouth. Wash your arms and hands and scrub your nails.

DELIVERING THE AFTERBIRTH
12 Offer encouragement

Congratulate the mother now that her labour is almost over. Give her some encouragement while she is delivering the afterbirth.

13 Retain the afterbirth

Keep the afterbirth intact and, if possible, in a plastic bag until the midwife or doctor arrives. It will be examined to make sure that all of it has been expelled. Even a small part of the afterbirth left inside the mother can be dangerous. The midwife or doctor will also cut the umbilical cord.

14 Clean the mother

Provide warm water, clean towels and sanitary towels for the mother. Either wash her yourself or let her do it if she feels strong enough to do so.

15 Massage her abdomen

It is normal for the mother to bleed slightly. You can massage the abdomen just below the navel, which helps the womb to contract and stops the bleeding as the afterbirth peels away from the wall of the womb. If the bleeding is severe, treat the mother for shock (p.307) and alert the emergency service that she has a life-threatening condition.

WARNINGS

- *Do not let the mother have a bath if her waters have broken, because this can cause an infection.*
- *Do not pull on the baby's head or shoulders.*
- *Do not pull on or cut the umbilical cord.*
- *Do not smack the newborn baby.*

THE THREE STAGES OF LABOUR

First stage
- Contractions usually come in 10–20 minute intervals.
- The cervix begins to dilate.
- A bloodstained discharge appears if the mucus plug in the cervix is dislodged.
- The protective waters (the amniotic fluid) break.

Second stage
- There is an involuntary urge to push and stronger, more frequent contractions.
- The vagina is stretched by the descending baby and there is a stinging or burning sensation.
- The head emerges and the baby is rapidly pushed out.

Third stage
- Mild contractions expel the placenta and control bleeding from the uterus.
- The afterbirth (placenta and umbilical cord) is expelled.
- Some bleeding occurs.
- Bleeding should stop; if not, emergency treatment is needed.

CAUTION

■ *Do not move the person until the injured part is secured and supported, unless her life is in danger.*
■ *Do not let the person eat or drink anything.*
■ *Do not try to place a dislocated bone back into its socket.*

SIGNS

Fractures
■ Pain increased by movement.

■ Distortion, swelling, bruising.

■ Coarse grating of the bone heard or felt – do not try to produce this sound deliberately.

■ Tenderness over a bone if touched.

Dislocations
■ Sickening pain.

■ Pain increased by movement.

■ Person often holds arm and inclines head to injured side.

Fractures and dislocations

Some injuries such as open fractures or a dislocated thumb are plain to see, others are less obvious. Try to note as many features of the injury as possible without moving the limb – compare its shape and appearance with the uninjured side. If you are in doubt, treat it as a fracture.

SUPPORTING AN INJURED ARM

1 Have the injured person support her arm at a right angle across her chest. Use a piece of cloth as a sling, folding it in half to form a triangle – you can improvise with a scarf. Slide the cloth between her arm and body, with the long side of the triangle next to the uninjured arm. Pull the cloth over the injured arm and take the end behind her neck.

2 Knot one end snugly to the other end at the injured side. Pin any extra material in place over the elbow. If the injury is in the upper arm, shoulder or collarbone, secure the sling with a strip of cloth tied horizontally around her arm and chest, knotted on the uninjured side.

A FRACTURED LEG

1 Call an ambulance and, if it is expected shortly, support the leg by placing a hand above and below the injury until help arrives.

2 If help is seriously delayed, apply gentle traction to reduce pain and bleeding by pulling steadily at the foot in the line of the bone. Pull only in a straight line, but stop if it causes intolerable pain. Bring the sound leg next to the injured one.

If you have a helper, continue traction until the leg is stabilized.

Use towels or a blanket as padding.

3 Ease two bandages or strips of cloth under her knees; slide them above and below the injury, then place two more under her knees and ankles. Put padding between her legs. Tie a bandage in a figure of eight at the feet; then tie the other ones, starting at the ankles and knees.

SEE ALSO
Using medicines safely
18–19

The medicine cupboard

First aid kits should be kept in a suitable container (preferably airtight), which is accessible to you but out of reach of children. Keep the kit in a dry atmosphere and check it at regular intervals to be sure that the items it contains are still fit for use.

WHAT TO KEEP IN YOUR FIRST AID KIT		
Item	**Quantity**	**Use**
Paracetamol	Buy packs of 12 to prevent overdoses.	Painkiller; for headaches, colds and flu.
Aspirin	Buy packs of 12 to prevent overdoses.	In emergency, for heart attack. Painkiller; never give to child under 13 years old.
Adhesive dressing (plaster)	About 20 of various sizes.	For minor wounds.
Medium sterile dressing	Six	For bleeding, burns and large wounds.
Large sterile dressing	Two	For bleeding, burns and large wounds.
Extra-large sterile dressing	Two	For bleeding, burns and large wounds.
Roller bandage	Two	To secure a dressing, support joints or restrict movement.
Triangular bandage	Two, made of cloth or strong paper.	As sling or bandage; if sterile, a dressing.
Tubular bandage	One for joints, one for fingers or toes.	Specially shaped to give support.
Sterile eye pad	Two	To protect any eye injury.
Safety pins	Six or more	For securing bandages.
Disposable gloves	Six pairs	To dress wounds or dispose of waste.
Scissors	One pair, blunt ended	To cut dressings or clothes.
Tweezers	One pair	For removing splinters.
Thermometer	One	For taking a temperature.
Wound cleansing wipes	Pack	To clean wounds or your hands.
Plastic bags	Six	To secure over burned foot or hand.

*Ensure all medicines are kept in childproof containers and away from the reach of children. Do not use any drugs past their sell-by date.

Useful Addresses

COMMON HEALTH PROBLEMS

ALZHEIMER'S DISEASE SOCIETY
10 Greencoat Place
London SW1 1PH
Helpline: 0845 300 0336

THE ARTHRITIC ASSOCIATION
Hill House
Little New Street
London W1X 8HB
Helpline: 0800 289170

NATIONAL ASTHMA CAMPAIGN
Providence House
Providence Place
London N1 0NT
Helpline: 0345 010203

BRITISH DIABETIC ASSOCIATION
10 Queen Anne Street
London W1M 0BD
Helpline: 0171 636 6112

BRITISH HEART FOUNDATION
14 Fitzhardinge Street
London W1H 4DH
Helpline: 0990 200656

BRITISH EPILEPSY ASSOCIATION
Anstey House
Hanover Square
Leeds LS3 1BE
Helpline: 0345 089599

CANCER INFORMATION SERVICE (BACUP)
3 Bath Place
Rivington Street
London EC2A 3JR
Tel: 0171 613 2121

MIGRAINE TRUST
45 Great Ormond Street
London WC1N 3HZ
Tel: 0171 831 4818

NATIONAL ASSOCIATION FOR PREMENSTRUAL SYNDROME
PO Box 72
Sevenoaks
Kent TN13 1XQ
Tel: 01732 741709

SMOKERS' QUITLINE
Victory House
170 Tottenham Court Road
London W1P 0HA
Tel: 0171 487 3000

COMPLEMENTARY THERAPIES

AROMATHERAPY ORGANIZATIONS COUNCIL
3 Latymer Close
Braybrooke
Market Harborough
Leicestershire
LE16 8LN
Tel: 01858 434242

BRITISH ACUPUNCTURE COUNCIL
Park House
206–208 Latimer Road
London W10 6RE
Tel: 0181 964 0222

BRITISH CHIROPRACTIC ASSOCIATION
Blagrave House
17 Blagrave Street
Reading
Berkshire RG1 1QB
Tel: 0118 950 5950

BRITISH HOMEOPATHIC ASSOCIATION
27a Devonshire Street
London W1N 1RJ
Tel: 0171 935 2163

BRITISH REFLEXOLOGY ASSOCIATION
Monks Orchard
Whitbourne
Worcester
WR6 5RB
Tel: 01886 821207

BRITISH WHEEL OF YOGA
Central Office
1 Hamilton Place
Boston Road
Sleaford
Lincolnshire NG34 7ES
Tel: 01529 303233

GENERAL OSTEOPATHIC COUNCIL
Room 432
Premier House
10 Graycoat Place
London SW1P 1SP
Tel: 0171 799 2442

OSTEOPATHIC INFORMATION SERVICE
Premier House
10 Graycoat Place
London SW1P 1SB
Tel: 0171 235 5231 Tel: 0171 799 2559

THE SHIATSU SOCIETY
Suite B, Barber House
Sedgate
Petersborough
Cambridgeshire PE1 5YS
Tel: 01733 758341

SOCIETY OF TEACHERS OF THE ALEXANDER TECHNIQUE
20 London House
266 Fulham Road
London SW10 9EL
Tel: 0171 351 0828

NUTRITION

BRITISH NUTRITION FOUNDATION
High Holborn House
52–54 High Holborn
London WC1V 6RQ
Tel: 0171 404 6504

BRITISH SOCIETY FOR ALLERGY, ENVIRONMENTAL AND NUTRITIONAL MEDICINE
PO Box 28
Totton
Southampton SO40 2ZA
Tel: 01703 812124

EATING DISORDERS ASSOCIATION
1st Floor
Wensum House
103 Prince of Wales Road
Norwich
Norfolk NR1 1DW
Helpline: 01603 621414

FIRST AID
Look in your *Yellow Pages* for local branches.

BRITISH RED CROSS
9 Grosvenor Crescent
London SW1X 7EJ
Tel: 0171 235 5454

ST ANDREW'S AMBULANCE ASSOCIATION
48 Milton Street
Glasgow G4 0HR
Tel: 0141 332 4031

ST JOHN AMBULANCE
1 Grosvenor Crescent
London SW1X 7EF
Tel: 0171 235 5231

Index

Acknowledgments

Illustrations
Mike Saunders

Picture credits
t = top, **b** = bottom, **c** = centre, **l** = left, **r** = right

2–3 Iain Bagwell; **10** Matthew Ward; **12** Robert Harding Picture Library; **15** The Stock Market; **18** The Image Bank; **23** Iain Bagwell; **26** Prof. P. Motta/Dept. of Anatomy/University of 'La Sapienza', Rome/Science Photo Library; **30** Iain Bagwell; **31** Clement Clarke International; **38** Doug Plummer/Science Photo Library; **44** Sheila Terry/Science Photo Library; **50–51** Andrew Sydenham; **52** Iain Bagwell; **53** Astrid & Hanns-Freider Michler/Science Photo Library; **56** Phototake/Ace Photo Library; **58l** Mike Delvin/Science Photo Library, **58r** Princess Margaret Rose Orthopaedic Hospital/Science Photo Library; **62** Migraine art by permission of the British Migraine Association and Boehringer Ingelheim UK; **69l** National Medical Slide Bank, **69r** Richard T. Nowitz/Science Photo Library; **72t** Clinique Ste Catherine/CNRI/Science Photo Library, **72b** Larry Mulvehill/Science Photo Library; **74** Alfred Pasieka/Science Photo Library; **81** J.C. Revy/Science Photo Library; **82** Paul Baldesare/ Photofusion; **85** Mike Goldwater/Tony Stone Images; **95** P. Hawtin, University of Southampton/Science Photo Library; **102** Science Photo Library; **104** Iain Bagwell; **108** Dr P. Marazzi/Science Photo Library; **111** Dr H.C. Robinson/Science Photo Library; **117** Iain Bagwell; **120** National Library of Medicine/Science Photo Library; **127t** CNRI/Science Photo Library, **127b** BSIP PIR/Science Photo Library; **128** James King-Holmes/Science Photo Library; **131–33** Iain Bagwell; **134** M. Wurtz/Biozentrum, University of Basel/Science Photo Library; **142** Eye of Science/Science Photo Library; **150** NIBSC/Science Photo Library; **154** Stevie Grand/ Science Photo Library; **157** Iain Bagwell; **178** The Image Bank; **181** Ian West/Bubbles; **182** Mark Clarke/Science Photo Library; **185** Iain Bagwell; **186** Harry Smith Collection; **190** Andrew Sydenham; **192** Michael Busselle; **193–94** Iain Bagwell; **196** Mary Evans Picture Library; **197** Helios; **198–211** Iain Bagwell; **212** Tim Malyon & Paul Biddle/Science Photo Library; **215l** Iain Bagwell, **215r** Andrew Sydenham; **216–23** Iain Bagwell; **224** Robert Harding Picture Library; **226–29** Iain Bagwell; **232** Hattie Young/Science Photo Library; **235** Andrew Sydenham; **237** John Greim/Science Photo Library; **239–40** Iain Bagwell; **242** The Stock Market; **249–55** Iain Bagwell; **257** Mike Powell/Allsport; **258** Power Stock; **260** The Stock Market; **263** The Image Bank; **264–94** Iain Bagwell; **295t** Andrew Sydenham, **295c & b** Iain Bagwell; **296–98** Iain Bagwell; **299** Andrew Sydenham; **300** Iain Bagwell; **301t** Andrew Sydenham, **301c** Iain Bagwell, **301b** Andrew Sydenham; **302–09** Iain Bagwell; **310** Laura Wickenden; **312** Iain Bagwell